THE NURSING PROCESS
A HUMANISTIC APPROACH

Elaine Lynne La Monica
Teachers College, Columbia University

▲▼ Addison-Wesley Publishing Company
Medical/Nursing Division • Menlo Park, California
Reading, Massachusetts • London • Amsterdam
Don Mills, Ontario • Sydney

Sponsoring editor: James Keating
Cover designer: Michael Rogondino
Editorial/production services by
Phoenix Publishing Services, San Francisco

Library of Congress Cataloging in Publication Data

La Monica, Elaine Lynne, 1944–
 The nursing process.

 Includes bibliographies and index.
 1. Nursing. 2. Nursing—Addresses, essays,
lectures. I. Title.
RT41.L3   610.73   79–428
ISBN 0–201–04138–3

  BCDEFGHIJ-MA-782109

Addison-Wesley Publishing Company
Medical/Nursing Division
2725 Sand Hill Road
Menlo Park, California 94025

To my mentors
    Those who guided my journey
        during different roads in my life . . .
    Those who enabled me to form
        today's path.

Kenneth Cruze, Donald K. Carew,
Ira D. Trail, Father J. Johnson,
Elizabeth P. Hagen . . .

"And there are those who give and know
    not pain in giving, nor do they seek joy,
    nor give with mindfulness of virtue;

They give as in yonder valley the myrtle
    breathes its fragrance into space.

Through the hands of such as these God
    speaks, and from behind their eyes He
    smiles upon the earth."

Kahlil Gibran
The Prophet, 1951, p. 20.

CONTENTS

v

PREFACE

The wet, cold snow squeezed under my fleece-lined boots; wind tore through the trees; yet snow flakes melting on my nose felt like a pleasant sting embraced in warmth. I was alone and the night was dark. But out of this frosty, angry night fell pure white, delicate sculptures. I could never fully describe or share what I saw and what I felt that night. For a person to know the beauty of anger and happiness, cold and hot, pain and health, crystal and wood, darkness and sunshine, one must either experience by seeing, touching, listening, smelling, or tasting, or one must fantasize on the basis of a shared experience.

That night I was relieved at 11 P.M. from my work as a nurse in the intensive care unit of a large city hospital. The expressions of anguish and peacefulness in a dying patient, the joy and sorrow of a new mother, the pain and serenity of a human being disfigured... a paradox, I thought, a complete utter paradox. What if it were I? I would be angry with the disfigurement, I would hate, I would toss with the pain, and I would cry seeking an answer to "Why me? I have not finished yet."

Later I sat in my diningroom table meditating: If they can know and understand, why is it so difficult for me to know and understand? I should be helping them. I should bring them relief, hope, and comfort. I should understand. They knew and I did not.

The parted curtains allowed the whiteness of the snow to shine in like a warm, protective beacon. I opened my window and felt the bite of the air; I put a handful of snow to my lips and felt the numbness slowly replaced by a glowing, spreading warmth. Reflecting on myself, my form took a new shape and my mind a new form: I am a person with experience first, a teacher second. I know in each of these facets the only absolute is me as an individual.

My communion with nursing seemed a separate turmoil, but it was actually one with my experience of the night, since I believe that the strongest contribution I can offer is to be present and share me—my thoughts, my experiences, and my feelings. I also believe that, as a teacher, I should share myself and enable others to develop inner experiences and awarenesses that will be uniquely their own.*

This book grows from my experience in trying to develop effective ways to teach both prospective and practicing nurses the importance and meaning of the nursing process in the implementation of professional nursing care. Regrettably, my

*This was a personal experience of the author, previously published by Susan M. Brainerd and Elaine L. La Monica, in "A Creative Approach to Individualized Nursing Care," *Nursing Forum* 14:188–193, 1975.

experience with students and colleagues makes it all too clear that cognitive knowledge frequently does not get carried into practice behavior. Information confined to printed words and case studies essentially restricts students to "head trips" and fails to build the necessary bridge between formalized learning, attitudinal development, and resultant professional practice.

In my search for ways to provide learners with an opportunity to observe, experience, and carry out actual behavior, I have used humanistic approaches in learning with human relations techniques. The humanistic teaching process involves cognitive and affective components of learning including formalized classrooms, personalizing of vicarious experience, and actual professional practice. Learners are able thereby to study and consider theory, to employ individual resources in the educative process, and, ultimately, to enter into practice with learned, new behaviors that are truly integrated components of the learners' beliefs.

This process corresponds with our current trend in nursing to administer individualized care. Since the student is the focus in academic settings, it follows that the learning process must be individualized. Theory must be presented in a way that provides students with the opportunity to bring these ideas into step with their own personal learning processes, to adapt these ideas into their own individual frameworks and definitions of nursing, and then, to practice accordingly. The result is *knowing* the nursing process as opposed to *knowing about* it. Several years of experimenting with this teaching approach has convinced me that it is far superior to any other method with which I am familiar. The results have been learners with increased empathy for clients and colleagues; heightened sensitivity to the needs of others, as well as ways in which to meet them; and most importantly, increasing behavioral consistency between classroom and service environments.

The book follows a course that covers the entire nursing process by examining the individual components which make up the whole. The book contains humanistic, multimedia approaches to integrating theory with practice and beliefs. It is suggested that study be weighted so that greater time is devoted to the experiential elements, since enriched learning can be derived from actual and vicarious experience. Pertinent articles relating to each chapter topic are included to increase the learner's perceptions of a particular area. The reader should conceptualize the material, using knowledge from all of life's resources, and should subsequently form individual attitudinal bases for practice. The text provides the groundwork in nursing process theory. Humanistic exercises at the end of each part provide the learner with an experiential base. Careful explanations of the use of each exercise are included. The text and exercises are designed for use both in self-learning and classroom environments, for use in both individual and group learning experiences.

The primary thrust of this book is a study of the nursing process, our foundation of professional nursing practice. It is intended to be used in nursing process and practice courses at all levels of nursing education and as nursing inservice or continuing education experiences.

ACKNOWLEDGMENTS

The theory, exercises, and philosophy in this book have been derived from many personal and professional resources. Some are original, and some are from established sources to whom credit is most gratefully given; others have evolved from a constant interchange with professionals whose commitment has been to professional quality. I would like to particularly thank Eunice M. Parisi, Sister Kathleen Black, and Virginia Earles. The unending assistance from James Keating and guidance from Paula Cizmar and Rex Wolf were also appreciated deeply.

To all who have molded my beliefs, to all from whom I have received, I express my sincere gratitude.

Elaine Lynne La Monica

INTRODUCTION TO
THE NURSING PROCESS

The nursing process is the scientific method that is used to assist students and practitioners to systematically assess, plan, implement, and evaluate quality, individualized professional nursing care. It is *the* foundation for nursing practice.

By progressing through each phase of the nursing process—assessment, planning, implementation, and evaluation—the nurse ensures that the care provided to each client will be geared to individual client needs. The nursing process begins with the relatively simple methods of assessment and proceeds through analytical thinking into delivery of nursing care. The nursing process is continuously evolving.

Nursing is a human service. Yet, too often one hears of "dehumanization" in health care brought on by technologic advances in medicine as well as practitioners who function in an automatic, mechanical manner. It is hoped that dehumanization is the exception, not the rule, in health care today. And nursing, because of its unique position in the health team of being most closely and directly involved with clients, certainly has a primary goal that is vital to total client well-being: to provide humanistic care adapted to individual needs.

This book sees the humanistic approach to the nursing process as being essential to quality care—as well as the future of health care. The humanistic approach takes into consideration all that is known about an individual such as thoughts, feelings, values, experiences, likes, desires, behavior, and body. The humanistic approach involves a continual learning process in which the student is an active participant in the learning. Each facet of the learner—thoughts, feelings, body, and all others—is integrated into a learning modality that is based on content and experience. Learning then becomes an individualized experience, parallel to nursing's goal of giving individualized nursing care.

The student need not be only the student of nursing. Rather, the student is also the practicing nurse, the client, the client's entire system, and other members of the health team. The humanistic use of the nursing process yields a continuous learning experience in giving and receiving care. New data are continuously accumulated, learned, and used; new experiences are constantly occurring; and new behaviors are continuously being exchanged for old, unworkable, unhealthy ones. The client is as involved in the nursing process as the nurse. The intent of humanism, therefore, is to enable a self-aware nurse to provide care for and with an individual, whole client—that is, a client with feelings, thoughts, values, experiences, and body. (See Chapter 20 for a further discussion of humanism.)

To set the humanistic approach to the nursing process into motion, this book recommends a systems approach. The systems approach involves taking into consideration all interrelated aspects of a person, a situation, a group, or an environment. A client's system, for example, could include the client's family, employer, fellow workers, and members of the health team; each of these "components" of the client's system interact. In addition, environmental factors influence the client's system. By taking a systems approach, all persons and things affecting the client are considered.

It is important to note that each system is unique, is composed of parts which may change, and has a definite purpose. Often, by identifying the purpose of a system, it is easier to study the system and determine problems and advantages of the system.

Nursing itself is a dynamic, open system. Dynamic means it is ever-changing; open means that people and environmental factors move in and out in response to the system's purpose or goals. The client, of course, is also an open, dynamic system, as are almost all systems involved in health care-giving. For a more complete study of the systems approach, see Chapter 19.

In this book, the systems approach forms a basic organizational structure which enables the nursing student or practitioner to integrate elements of humanism with knowledge and skills. The book moves from simple to complex, beginning with simple concepts and methods and building on these to form a spiralling network of interrelated elements comprising the entire nursing process. Each chapter presents information and experiences which build upon each other. As the book progresses, the importance and inter-relatedness of each method, skill, and concept emerge with more clarity. It is the intent of this book that the nursing student and practitioner ultimately *know the nursing process, rather than know about it.*

The book is organized as follows:

- *Part I: Methods of the Nursing Process.* Methods of the nursing process are the first priority in learning nursing practice. Since the nursing process is the root of practice and is also a scientific method, the process is studied for understanding using a step by step procedure. Each step provides the foundation for the methods and concepts which follow.
- *Part II: Skills and Competencies.* Skills and competencies then become necessary to implement the nursing process in a variety of client care situations. With these skills and competencies, the nurse puts the process into action.
- *Part III: Quality Systems in the Nursing Process.* Quality systems are next presented with the rationale that once a learner knows the basics of practice, the larger system of evaluation of nursing care should be studied. Within the nursing process, many quality systems and tools of evaluation have been developed in contemporary practice. These systems provide yet another step in the move toward a total under-standing of the nursing process.

- *Part IV: Theory and Strategies for Facilitating Practice in the Clinical Environment.* Part IV presents strategies for providing actual care in different health care systems. This is valuable since there is often a discrepancy between educational ideals and actual practice. Therefore, theories of organizational behavior and change including leadership and actual models of care are provided to further strengthen the foundation established in the other chapters.
- *Part V: Nursing: A Helping Profession.* Part V takes a closer look at nursing as a helping profession in addition to providing a conceptual framework for the nursing process itself as well as the ideals of humanism. A nursing definition is provided. The goals of the nursing process are amplified using the expanse of knowledge which has accumulated throughout the first four parts of the book. These concepts of the humanistic nursing process are both the beginning and end of the nursing process. Therefore, the use of this book may wish to refer to Part V throughout the course of the book.

The purposes of the exercises following Part V are to explore the professional portion of one's life and the building of a personal philosophy of nursing. This process facilitates defining nursing within an individual and illuminates the unique experiences of each learner. The exercises commence with ice-breaking and getting-acquainted activities; these are designed to help in the formation of effective groups and may be used at the beginning of studying the nursing process.

In fulfillment of the objectives of this book, content and theory are presented first in each chapter, followed by selected readings by other authors to amplify and extend the material presented by this author. The appendix contains a key to abbreviations used in this book.

Learning exercises are provided following each part. Many can actually be done in the book and used as assignments or in discussion groups in the home, learning laboratory, or classroom. It is the purpose of these exercises to provide practice experiences that illustrate the content of the chapters, as well as to expand the nurse-reader's own range of experience. This book is seen as a learning tool that can be used in any stage of one's development.

Throughout the book, emphasis is always placed on the person as a unique individual with unique needs, desires, and feelings. It is important to remember that the nurse has needs, desires, and feelings, just as does the client. By integrating the ideals of humanism with the organization structure of system theory, the nursing process should become a workable, applicable, dynamic human process.

The ultimate goal of this book is identical to the ultimate goal of nursing: to assist the client to fullest health potential. This book provides a careful method for that assistance.

PART I

METHODS OF THE
NURSING PROCESS

Chapter 1: Data Collection
The Systems Approach
Methods of Collecting Data
Nursing Care: An Encounter

Chapter 2: Data Processing
Areas of Nursing Responsibility
Nurse's Knowledge and the Nurse
A Case Study
Method of Data Processing

Chapter 3: Nursing Diagnosis
Cognitive Dimensions of a Nursing Diagnosis
Case Example on Nursing Diagnoses and Priorities

Chapter 4: Nursing Orders
Cognitive Dimensions of Nursing Orders
Case Example on Nursing Orders

Chapter 5: Implementation
Parts of the System
Skills and Competencies Necessary in Implementation

Chapter 6: Evaluation
The Process of Evaluation
Case Examples
Continuous Evaluation, Feedback, and Data Collection

1

Data Collection

To work toward a whole process, it is necessary to proceed through specific steps. Assessment is the initial phase in the nursing process, and data collection is a primary tool in assessment. To a nurse, assessment means to evaluate critically the various conditions and situations involved in a client's system. The nurse assesses the status of the client's health, mood, family situation, responsiveness to illness or hospitalization, and any other elements necessary to assist the health team in providing treatment and care.

The assessment phase begins with the collection of data. *Data collection* is the continuous process of obtaining information needed in providing care. It is an ever-changing process with changes occurring as more data are collected and as the patient's condition alters. Data collection is done both formally and informally by such means as observation, interviewing, physical examination, research into the client's medical history, and communication, among others. Many sources are available for data collection ranging from information provided by the client personally to such things as physician's orders or results of laboratory tests.

As the member of the health team who is responsible for total care of the client, the nurse must view all data pertaining to a client's system. In addition to studying the client data which are already available, the nurse also takes action personally to obtain certain information needed to provide total client care. Among these actions is included the obtaining of a nursing history.

Sources of data collection can be grouped into primary and secondary sources. McCain (1965) cites the client as the *primary source* of data; in other words, the client provides basic, firsthand information which has not been interpreted or recounted by someone or something else. All other components of the evolving client system are *secondary sources* of data, that is, sources of data that are derived from the primary source. Secondary sources are indirect while primary sources are direct. These secondary sources may include the physician, family members, colleagues, social worker, and others. Secondary

2

sources also include written information, such as previous health records or charts, medical histories, reports of previous physical examinations, reports of x-rays and laboratory tests, and all subjective data informally and formally noted. This brief list is not all-encompassing. The nurse searches for all data available about the client from any source believed to be useful in nursing care. Of course, this should all be relative to the evolving goals of care for the client and should be reflective of priorities. Data unnecessary for planning care should never be collected. To do so is to exploit the client.

THE SYSTEMS APPROACH

Just as this book's study of the whole nursing process involves a systems approach, the study of the various steps of the process involves a systems approach as well. The systems approach requires that the client be studied concomitant with all the environmental elements (people and things) that have an effect on the client's present existence. Since the environment exerts effects and forces on an individual, all elements become both part of the problem and part of the solution. (See Chapter 19 for further study of systems theory.)

Data collection, therefore, covers the entire expanse of a client's system. Yet, it is merely the initial phase of the nursing process. This should illustrate the broad scope of the nursing process itself.

The following equation will help you visualize the initial steps of the nursing process as discussed in Part I of this book:

$$\begin{matrix} \text{Client Data} \\ \text{System Data} \end{matrix} + \begin{matrix} \text{Nursing Responsibilities} \\ \text{Nurse's Knowledge} \\ \text{The Nurse} \end{matrix} \rightarrow \begin{matrix} \text{Individualized} \\ \text{Nursing Diagnoses and} \\ \text{Nursing Orders} \end{matrix}$$

This chapter is concerned with the first elements of this equation: client data and system data. These data provide the foundation upon which the second part of the equation acts. The combination of the first two parts results in the third part of the equation: the nursing care plan consisting of individualized nursing diagnoses and nursing orders.

To study client data and system data using the systems approach, it is important to visualize the relationship of these components to the whole. See Figure 1-1. But it is equally important that a purpose is ascribed to the whole nursing process and, indeed, also to the specific components of the process. Banathy (1968) describes determining a system's purpose as a strong means of classifying the system. By determining a system's purpose, study of the system is facilitated.

Several systems are at work in the context of the nursing process. The primary system is the nursing process itself. Sub-systems include the client; the nurse; and the various components of the process, such as data collection.

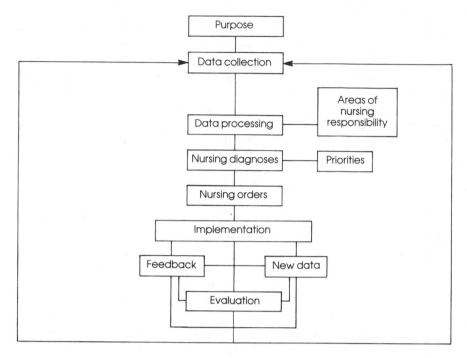

FIGURE 1-1
SCHEMATIC DIAGRAM OF THE NURSING PROCESS
ASSESSMENT FACTORS

Each system and sub-system has a definite purpose with definite goals.

The generalized, overall purpose of nursing care is to facilitate the client's growth toward a maximum health potential. The nursing process provides the systematic means to fulfilling this goal. Investigation of the purpose of the nursing process demands a response to two specific questions: (1) why does the client need care? and (2) how can and why does the nurse give care?

To respond to why the client needs care, it is necessary for the nurse to collect data. At times, the nurse collects data even before meeting the client, for example, the nurse may study a medical history provided by a physician for a patient who is scheduled to be admitted into the hospital for surgery. But despite the time or source of data collection, the overall purpose is to determine reasons for care and goals for care.

To answer the second question—how can and why does the nurse give care?—it is also necessary for the nurse to collect data. By obtaining and studying information, the nurse uses knowledge and experience to determine "how" to provide care for a particular client, as well as "why."

These questions obviously are interrelated and point to the ultimate purpose of data collection by the nurse: to provide care suited to the individual.

Before proceeding to methods of data collection, however, there is one more important point connected with the "how" and "why" of providing nursing care: the nurse's personal philosophy. This combination of the nurse's knowledge, experience, beliefs, and values is vital; Henderson (1966) eloquently calls for nurses to develop and be aware of a personal philosophy of nursing practice. And it is this author's belief that the development of a personal philosophy is an absolute for the nurse as a caring individual. Behavior is a result of our attitudes (Campbell, 1947; Hersey and Blanchard, 1977; Katz and Stotland, 1959; Lott, 1973); awareness of one's philosophy is pursued so that the basis of all actions is conscious and controllable. It is assumed that all nurses believe clients to be individuals and that individualized nursing care is the ultimate desire of practitioners. Working from this basic assumption, it follows that the human aspect of all individuals must be respected. Though the nurse and the client may be categorized as systems to provide an organized, convenient means for study and giving care, it is important to remember a basic fundamental of the nursing process: nurses and clients are people. Each is an individual person with wants, needs, and capabilities.

METHODS OF COLLECTING DATA

Even though formally discussed only in this chapter, data collection occurs throughout the nursing process since data are always changing and, therefore, always incomplete. Each passing minute for each human being results in a change in the person. Decisions, therefore, are made on limited and incomplete data. Nevertheless, each decision should be explored to the fullest degree possible as dictated by time.

All sources of data—primary and secondary—which involve the client and the client's system should be considered when making nursing decisions. The methods used to collect data with the aim of providing total care will depend on the skills necessary to carry out the task. As the practitioner gains more knowledge and more experience, more methods of data collection become available. Some methods of data collection, such as physical examination, require much technical skill and practice. Part II of this book is devoted to a discussion of major skills; in addition, the exercises following Parts I through V provide simulated learning experiences for practice.

Other methods of data collection require fewer technical skills and are an excellent means of becoming familiar with principles of obtaining information. An example of one such method is obtaining a nursing history.

When giving direct care, choose the method with which you are most comfortable. Practice those you are least familiar with outside the client/nurse environment. In this way, it becomes possible to build a reservoir of positive experiences in both the actual and the learning situations.

Methods of data collection include communication with physicians, family members, colleagues, social workers, technicians, teachers, and others. Information may also be obtained from previous health records, patient charts, medical histories, reports of physical examinations, results of x-rays and laboratory tests, admitting records, and informal observation. These methods all involve secondary sources.

Methods of collecting data from the primary source—the client—include informal conversation, formal interviews, nursing histories, and actual physical examination. Because the nursing history involves information from the primary source and because fewer technical skills are required than certain other methods of data collection (for example, the physical examination), the next section will discuss obtaining a nursing history in detail.

Nursing History

The nursing history is a foremost method of collecting data. The procedure usually involves purposeful observation and an interview or oral history; but occasionally the nursing history is written by the client first from a list of questions and is then elaborated upon by the nurse.

The nursing history is viewed by McPhetridge (1968) as a primary means of personalizing nursing care. It provides a skeleton of pertinent information from which problems can be identified initially and further pursued. This knowledge about the client is used in planning individualized nursing care as well as attempting to prevent misunderstandings or problems from arising.

The nursing history differs from the medical history. The medical history is a record of the client's previous illnesses, medical problems such as allergies, previous hospitalizations, physical traits, and familial medical patterns. By contrast, the nursing history is a record of the client's habits, emotional status, expectations, and other such factors. Though both the medical history and nursing history have the same overall purpose, that is, to provide a basis for optimum treatment and care, they differ in specifics.

Erikson (1964) describes data collection as the responsibility of the clinician for obtaining evidence relative to clinical problems, evaluation, and diagnostic inferences. McManus (1951) refers to the data collecting process as clinical thinking. The nursing history is that part of the clinical data collection process that is concerned most directly with the client as a person. Smith (1968) views the nursing history as a pathway by which the nurse can get to know a client and vice versa.

A nursing history is not an end in and of itself; rather, it is a tool to obtain what the nurse needs to provide comprehensive care. The nurse's responsibility is to assist the client *when the client is in need of help*. It follows that the nurse will not delve into areas of the client's life where intervention is not needed. Only data that are useable and that the client feels ease in providing should be obtained. Data should be collected in a way that respects the nurse's philosophy, beliefs, and expertise, as well as the environmental elements of the particular system. In other words, consider the persons, things, and situations surrounding yourself and the client.

Smith (1968) earmarked the need for a conceptual and procedural frame-of-reference in obtaining a nursing history. The following nursing history guide is a structured interview format that is intended to be a compilation of areas and questions which can be pursued by the nurse interviewer. The depth to which each area is investigated depends on the individual client and individual nurse. The following nursing history is only a guide, and is to be used according to the purposes of care with respect to the skills and techniques of the nurse. How you interview (structured or unstructured), the order of questions asked, and the depth of exploration should be flexible and should be determined by the reactions and responses of the client. Information already known should not be reintroduced; areas requiring further information can be amplified; possible problems can be noted for future study. After becoming familiar with this nursing history guide, you may wish to develop your own. Or, you may find it best to use different formats of nursing histories with different clients. The key to obtaining the nursing history is personalization.

Nursing History Guide
A. General Information
    1. Date of Interview:
    2. Date of Admission:
    3. Hours of Time Elapsed from Admission to First Interview:
    4. Patient's Name:
    5. Patient's Age:
    6. Diagnosis (Medical):
    7. Occupation:
        a.   Patient's Occupation:
        b.   Spouse's Occupation:
    8. Religion:
    9. Educational Level:
    10. Residence (City and State):
    11. Marital Status:
B. Guide Questions
    1. Family Situation

    a. With whom do you live?

    b. How many children do you have, if any?

    c. Who is caring for them while you are here?

    d. How many brothers and sisters do you have?

    e. Do your parents live nearby?

    f. Was there anything that happened to you or your family in the past year other than this illness that was upsetting to you?

2. Work Situation (including financial aspect)

    a. What type of work do you do?

    b. How long have you done this type of work?

    c. Are you on sick leave from work?

    d. Do you think your illness will interfere with your work?

    e. Do you have health insurance?

3. Patient's Activities

    a. What kind of environment and pace are you used to?

    b. What are your feelings concerning your activity schedule in the hospital?

    c. Do you have any special interests or hobbies that you would like to pursue, if feasible, while you are here?

    d. What habits have you had to change here?

4. Eating Habits

    a. Are you on a restricted diet?

    b. Are you allergic to any foods?

    c. Are there any particular foods you like or dislike?

    d. Do you eat breakfast?

    e. Do you need an early morning cup of coffee or the like?

    f. How many times do you eat each day?

    g. When do you usually eat your meals?

    h. Has being sick affected your eating habits? How?

    i. Do you foresee any difficulty with hospital food?

    j. Do you prefer plain or ice water?

    k. Are you accustomed to eating snacks? At regular times?

5. Sleeping Habits

    a. How long do you usually sleep? Between what hours?

    b. Do you sleep well at home?

    c. Do you nap? Occasionally? Regularly? Rarely?

    d. Are you an early riser?

    e. Do you need medication to sleep?

    f. Do you get up at intervals?

    g. Does light or noise disturb you?

    h. If you are awakened at night, can you go back to sleep?

    i. Do you sleep with a night light on?

    j. Do you like an extra blanket at night?

     k. Do you usually sleep with a window closed or open?

     l. Have you found that strange surroundings decrease your ability to sleep soundly?

     m. How many pillows do you use?

6. Elimination Habits
   a. What are your elimination habits at home?
   b. Do you have any difficulty with elimination?
   c. Do you take laxatives? If so, how often?
   d. Do you take any special foods to aid in elimination?

7. Allergies
   a. Do you have any allergies to drugs, food, adhesive tape, etc.?

8. Drugs or Special Diets
   a. Were you on any medications before you came to the hospital?
   b. Do you routinely take any "over-the-counter" medicines?
   c. Did you bring any of these medications with you?

9. Previous Illnesses or Hospitalizations
   a. Have you had other experiences when you or members of your family were ill?
      1) What kind of experience was it—good, bad, indifferent?
      2) What problems, if any, did you or they encounter?
   b. Have you ever been sick before?
      1) What was wrong?
      2) Were you in the hospital?
      3) How long were you sick?
      4) What do you remember most about being hospitalized?
      5) What did you like most about the hospital care, routines, etc.?
      6) What did you like least?
   c. Do you have any disability other than your present illness which may restrict your normal activity?
   d. Who cares for you when you are sick at home?
   e. What can you do when you are sick at home that makes you feel better?

10. Current Illness
    a. Why are you in the hospital?
    b. What do you think made you ill?
    c. How long have you been ill?
    d. Can you tell me what you feel concerning your illness?
    e. What kinds of things usually make you feel better when you are sick?
    f. Were there other things that happened when you first became ill?
    g. What do you feel concerning the outcome of your illness?
    h. What is causing you the most discomfort at this time?

11. Current Hospitalization

    a.   What do you think you need done for you while you are here?

    b.   What do you feel about being here in the hospital?

    c.   What do you miss most by being in this hospital?

    d.   Are there some things at home that you would like to have here with you? If so, what?

    e.   Are there things at home that might bother or worry you while you are here?

12. Personal Preferences Regarding Visitors—Family and Friends

    a.   If feasible, would you prefer to be with other patients during the day or would you rather be alone?

    b.   Would you like to have visitors?

        1) Just family?

        2) Just friends?

        3) Both family and friends?

        4) Just certain individuals? Who?

    c.   How many visitors would you like at one time and how frequently?

    d.   Is it possible for your family or friends to visit you if you so desire?

    e.   Has anyone visited with you yet or did anyone come with you when you were admitted?

    f.   (For persons with serious illness, or as hospital policy allows): would you feel better if it was possible for some of your family to stay here with you overnight?

13. Expectations of Hospital Personnel and Physician by Patient

    a.   Would you like your doctor and nurses to explain everything that is going on with you?

    b.   Would you be comfortable enough to ask them questions if they do not explain?

    c.   Would you like someone to come in frequently during the day just to talk or be with you?

    d.   Is there anything special you expect or would like me to do for you or see that it gets done, if feasible, while you are here?

    e.   What do you expect from nurses?

    f.   What do you expect from other personnel?

    g.   What has your doctor told you about your illness and what to expect while you are in the hospital?

    h.   What do you expect from your doctor?

    i.   What do you expect from the hospital?

    j.   What do you expect from hospital policy or routine?

    k.   Would you like a minister to visit with you, if possible?

    l.   How best can we help you while you are in the hospital?

C. Visual Observation on General Appearance

1. Immediate General Impression of Appearance:
2. Overall Physical Appearance:
3. Motor Activity/Posture:
4. Build and Weight:
5. Prosthesis/Limitations/Debilitations:
6. Complexion and Appearance of Skin:
   a. Color
   b. Lesions
   c. Abrasions
   d. Rash
7. Subjective Symptoms:
   a. Watery eyes
   b. Running nose
   c. Cough
8. Mouth:
   a. Oral hygiene
   b. Dentures
9. Eyes:
   a. Eye glasses
   b. Contact lenses
10. Age Group:
11. Clothing:
12. Belongings and Objects in Environment:
13. Speech:
14. Apparent Cultural, Educational, and Intellectual Levels:
15. Other Pertinent Factors:
D. Non-verbal Behavior Observations
   1. Emotional Tone, Facial Expression, Attitude:
   2. Gestures, Movements, or Activities During Interview:
   3. Main Theme of Patient's Conversation and Behavior:
   4. Topics the Patient Seemed to Avoid:
   5. Patient's Response to Interviewer:
   6. Interviewer's Response to Patient:
   7. Other Pertinent Factors:
E. Summary.

NURSING CARE: AN ENCOUNTER

Nursing care can be viewed as an encounter between persons—the nurse and the client. Carkhuff (1969) notes that the growth or deterioration of all people in a relationship depends on the interaction of all. The first person (or leader, for example) has the most critical effect on the interaction. Since the nurse is the leader in the client/nurse situation, the nurse naturally assumes added responsibility in the encounter. Moreover, since no interaction remains in neutrality, each encounter will be either harmful or helpful to all involved participants. Therefore, even though the professional is not the primary focus, the benefits and/or detriments of nursing care are experienced by all involved members of the system.

To make Carkhuff's statements meaningful in nursing, let us consider the following example. Picture yourself as a 19-year-old student who is assigned by an instructor to obtain a nursing history from Mr. Blanche. Mr. Blanche is 46 years old and has just been admitted into the hospital with a medical diagnosis of angina with a possible myocardial infarction. This is your first encounter in interviewing and the client's first admission to a hospital. You have a written history form to follow and, being an enthusiastic learner, you have studied the disease process. Entering the room, you quickly observe that Mr. Blanche is sitting in a chair watching television. His color is pink and he seems to be comfortable. You introduce yourself and tell him you would like to ask some questions to make it possible for you and your colleagues to plan nursing care reflecting his individual needs. You begin. All goes smoothly until you ask when he first noticed the pain. You ask the question and he hesitates, blushes, and hurriedly states that it was when he was having intercourse with his wife. Is this area important to pursue? Do you believe further information is necessary to help him? What questions does your training lead you to ask? Are you comfortable? Can you handle this with ease? Can you decrease the client's anxiety while interviewing? These are important questions to ask yourself. If both you and the client cannot proceed comfortably with this line of assessment, the interviewing experience will be negative. Furthermore, you will probably not be able to obtain the information needed to plan individualized care.

Pre-planning is the key in situations such as this. Since the nurse is as much a part of the data collection process (and of all nursing) as the client, it becomes crucial to look at yourself in these initial stages. A negative encounter with a client can be avoided.

Follow these steps in pre-planning your first interaction with the client. Begin by determining the purpose of nursing care. Next, specify the goals of care from the existing data and earmark those areas which need further exploration. Then, ask yourself the question: "Do I have the knowledge, experience, and ease necessary to pursue these areas with the client?" If you answer "yes," then carry on. Should your response be "no" or any combination of "yes/no," you should then get the experience needed by practicing the required skills in a safe, low-risk way. For example, you may share your feelings with your instructor. You may request that the instructor interview the client with you, giving the instructor the areas to pursue in which you are unsure or unclear. Learn by observation. Or, you may role-play the situation in a nursing laboratory or conference room with peers. The point is to learn to handle a situation positively and effectively. The myth that the best way to teach a child the effects of fire is to burn the child maintains its mythic status in nursing—and most other—situations. It is not necessary to experience pain or discomfort to learn. By placing the learning situation in the proper perspective, you assume responsibility for both yourself and the one looking to you for help. You can insure a positive first encounter.

In short, build yourself a foundation of comfort with respect to your needs, feelings, knowledge, and experience prior to encountering the client. Do whatever you must; request the help you desire; and delegate those aspects you cannot handle. As long as total care of a client is carried out by one nurse or a combination of nurses, professional responsibility is maintained. A supragoal of nursing care, as well as of learning and teaching, is that the experience be positive. Even though negative learning on the part of the nurse and/or client may occur, all attempts should be made to diminish negativity as much as possible for all concerned.

SUMMARY

Chapter 1 discusses the beginning of the nursing process—data collection. Data collection is viewed as necessary at the onset of care for the purpose of planning individualized care. Data collection is continuous throughout the nurse/patient relationship. The nursing history was earmarked as an important means of collecting information that is responsive to the goals and purposes of nursing care and is reflective of priorities. The skills used by the nurse in the process should be those with which the interviewer is most comfortable.

The following chapter discusses how to interpret the data collected. All the remaining chapters in Part I use a case study to investigate each step of the nursing process.

REFERENCES

Banathy, B. *Instructional systems.* Palo Alto, Calif.: Fearon, 1968.

Campbell, D. *The generality of social attitudes.* Doctoral dissertation, University of California, Berkeley, 1947.

Carkhuff, R. *Helping and human relations: A primer for lay and professional helpers.* Vol. I. New York: Holt, Rinehart & Winston, 1969.

Erikson, E. *Insight and responsibility.* New York: W. W. Norton Co., 1964.

Henderson, V. *The nature of nursing.* New York: The Macmillan Company, 1966.

Hersey, P., and Blanchard, K. *Management of organizational behavior.* Englewood Cliffs, N.J.: Prentice-Hall, 1977.

Katz, D., and Stotland, E. A preliminary statement to a theory of attitude structure and change. In *Psychology: A study of a science,* ed. S. Koch. Vol. 3. New York: McGraw-Hill Books, Inc., 1959.

Lott, A. Social psychology. In *Handbook of general psychology,* ed. B. Wolman. Englewood Cliffs, N.J.: Prentice-Hall, 1973.

McCain, F. Nursing by assessment—not intuition. *American Journal of Nursing* 65:82–84, 1965.

McManus, R. Assumptions of functions of nursing. In *Regional planning for nursing and nursing education.* Report of a work conference at Plymouth, N.H., June 12–23, 1950. New York: Bureau of Publications, Teachers College, Columbia University, 1951, p. 54.

McPhetridge, L. Nursing history: one means to personalize care. *American Journal of Nursing* 68:68–75, 1968.

Smith, D. A clinical nursing tool. *American Journal of Nursing* 68:2384–2388, 1968.

SELECTED READINGS

Two articles are recommended for further reading. In the first, McCain (1965) provides a rationale for assessment, underscoring that it should be a concrete and deliberative process. She introduces an assessment tool that delineates topical areas for client inquiry. In the second article, McPhetridge (1968) uses the nursing history as a means for providing individualized care and suggests a nursing history format.

Nursing by Assessment— Not Intuition

R. Faye McCain

To practice effectively, a nurse must assess. She must—consciously or unconsciously—determine the patient's nursing needs on the basis of his diagnosis, symptoms, medical orders, laboratory data, and so forth. But no precise method of such assessment has, as yet, been widely accepted. In this article, the author describes an approach to assessment which is being developed with graduate students in medical-surgical nursing.

Nursing, as it is taught and practiced today, is primarily intuitive. Unlike the professions of law, engineering, and medicine, nursing has not developed a precise method of determining when nursing intervention is needed. However, the need for a precise method has been recognized. Several years ago, Abdellah and associates described an approach to planning care, using as a guide "the twenty-one nursing problems"(1). More recently Bonney and Rothberg suggested a method of identifying the needs for nursing services of the chronically disabled person(2). But, as yet, neither of these approaches have been widely accepted by nursing educators and practitioners.

For the past three years graduate students in medical-surgical nursing at the University of Michigan have been evolving a method of systematically assessing functional abilities of patients. These assessments serve as the basis for making nursing diagnoses, for planning and evaluating the nursing therapy, and for writing the various nursing orders.

This method is far from precise and complete at this stage of its evolution. Some aspects of the method are developed to a higher degree than others; none have yet been developed in complete detail. We recognize that further experiential evidence is needed and that, ultimately, a controlled study should be done to validate the method. So far, we believe that it does have merit and does deserve further consideration by members of the nursing profession.

FUNCTIONAL ABILITIES APPROACH

The functional abilities of the patient were selected as the basis for assessment because such an approach agreed with our concept of nursing care.

Reprinted with permission from *American Journal of Nursing,* Vol. 65, No. 4. Copyright 1965 by The American Journal of Nursing Company.

This concept incorporates the belief that the primary goal of nursing care is to assist a patient to attain and maintain a state of equilibrium as he reacts to internal and external stimuli. Equilibrium, as advanced by Johnson, represents a momentary balancing of opposing forces and does not imply a state of health or well-being(3). To carry this concept further, the extent to which a patient does or does not achieve equilibrium is reflected in his physiological, psychological, and social behavior. Functional abilities, then, become another way of expressing behavior.

A patient, today, is expected to do for himself whatever he is capable of doing; in other words, he is expected to participate in his therapeutic regimen. But in order to help him be a participant, the nurse must know his functional abilities as well as his disabilities. When she plans nursing care and writes nursing orders, the nurse will capitalize on the patient's abilities but, at the same time, she will endeavor to assist him to live with his disabilities, whether they are temporary or permanent.

Before describing the proposed method of patient assessment, it is appropriate to consider some of the basic factors underlying the process. The systematic assessment of a patient's functional abilities is an orderly and precise method of collecting information about the physiological, psychological, and social behavior of a patient. The data collected from such an assessment provide a rationale for determining the patient's nursing needs and serve as a basis for planning and evaluating nursing therapy, writing nursing orders, and guiding and directing nursing activities. It is our working hypothesis that the nursing diagnosis, per se, is the identification of the patient's functional disabilities, or symptoms, as well as identification of his most important functional abilities. One can speculate, however, that with time, creativity, and sufficient precise data, symptoms that have a meaningful relationship in the nursing process can be grouped together, given a descriptive name, and be considered a nursing syndrome.

THE ASSESSMENT

Four resources are available for making an assessment: the patient, his family, health team members, and records. The primary resource, in most instances, is the patient; the other resources enlarge, clarify, and substantiate the information obtained from him. Interview and direct observation or inspection are the tools used by the nurse. Although these tools have long been recognized as essential to nursing care, in the patient assessment process they are used with direction and precision. Here again, one can speculate that with time, creativity, and sufficient precise data, specific nursing diagnostic tests could be evolved.

In assessing the patient's functional abilities, both objective and subjective data are collected and recorded. The time is long since past when the collection of only objective data should be advocated. Professional nurses can, do, and should make judgments. When professional nurses are more knowledgeable in the contributing sciences and become more competent in analytical thinking, some of these judgments probably will be independent judgments upon which nurses will make decisions without waiting for medical direction.

Patient assessment is the responsibility of the professional nurse. She initiates the assessment as soon as possible after the patient is admitted and continues to assess and evaluate, modifying the plan of care as the patient's behavior or functional abilities change.

In developing the method for systematic assessment of a patient's functional abilities, it was necessary to classify body functions. To date we have identified and used 13 functional areas: The patient's social, mental, emotional, body temperature, respiratory, circulatory, nutritional, elimination, and reproductive status; state of rest and comfort; state of skin and appendages; sensory perception; and motor ability. Although these functions are not mutually exclusive, for purposes of assessment we consider them separately. Social status may be questioned as a functional area, but after considerable thought and discussion, we decided it should be included. Our aim is to determine the patient's position in his family and community and discover, if possible, what social stimuli may be contributing to or detracting from his ability to function at an optimum level. In some instances, we decided to include a specific function under a category where the relationship cannot be validated by authorities, for example, placing the function of speech under sensory perception, and including intake and output in circulatory status.

SUGGESTIONS FOR USE OF GUIDE

Factors included in the guide we have developed are suggestive only. In a given patient, some factors will not be pertinent. The professional nurse in making the assessment, however, must consider all functional aspects and judge which ones do or do not apply.

We have included only those functional elements whose data can be collected by the professional nurse, using, primarily, the techniques of interview, direct observation, or inspection. It is well recognized, however, that more information will be needed before the nursing therapeutic regime for a specific patient can be planned and evaluated; for instance, findings from the medical history and physical examination, results of x-ray and laboratory

---

MENTAL STATUS

State of consciousness
- Alert and quick to respond to surroundings
- Drowsy and slow to respond
- Semiconscious and difficult to arouse
- Comatose and unable to arouse
- State of automatism

Orientation
- To time
- To place

• To person

Intellectual capacity
• Level of education
• Ability to recall events: recent; past

Attention span

Vocabulary level
• Use of simple, nontechnical words
• Use of complex, technical words

Ability to understand ideas
• Slow to learn meaning and make relationships
• Quick to gain meaning and make relationships
• Insight into health problems

EMOTIONAL STATUS

Emotional reactions
• Mood
• Presence or absence of anxiety
• Defenses against anxiety; such as, aggression; depression; fantasies; identification; rationalization; regression; repression; sublimation

Body image
• Effect of illness on self-concept
• Adaptation of self-concept to reality demands

Ability to relate to others
• To family
• To other patients
• To health team members

SENSORY PERCEPTION

Hearing
• Sensitivity to sound
  • Voice tone that distinguishes sounds: low; moderate; loud
  • Distance that sounds distinguished
  • Need to see speaker to distinguish sounds
• Presence of impairment
  • Partial or complete
  • Unilateral or bilateral
  • Ability to lip read
  • Use and effectiveness of supportive aid

Vision
• Acuity
• Presence of impairment
  • Partial or complete
  • Unilateral or bilateral
  • Type: hyperopia; myopia; astigmatism; color-blindness; diplopia; photophobia; nyctalopia; other
  • Use and effectiveness of supportive aid
• Enunciation
  • Unilateral or bilateral
  • Use of prosthesis

Speech
• Has auditory expression
• Aphasia
  • Verbal defect
  • Syntactical defect
  • Nominal defect
  • Semantic defect
• Anarthria
• Mute

- Laryngectomy
  - Use and effectiveness of esophageal speech
- Unusual speech patterns: such as, lisping; repetitive; staccato; stammer; stutter

Touch
- Hyperesthesia
- Anesthesia
- Paresthesia
- Paralgesia

Smell
- Anosmia
- Hyperosmia
- Kakosmia
- Parosmia

Taste
- Distinguishes: sweet; salt; sour; bitter
- Aftertaste present

MOTOR ABILITY

Mobility
- Complete bed rest
- Bed rest with bathroom privileges
- Sit in chair
- Ambulatory
  - Without assistance
  - With supportive aids: person; crutches; walker
  - Use of wheel chair
  - Use of stretcher
- Posture
  - In bed
  - Upright

Range of motion
- Passive
- Active

Gait

Equilibrium

Abnormal movement
- Clonic
- Tonic
- Spastic
- Flaccid
- Tic
- Ataxia

Muscle tone
- Spasm
- Contractures
- Weakness

Paralysis
- Hemiplegia
- Paraplegia
- Quadriplegia

Loss of extremity
- Location
- Extent
- Use and effectiveness of prosthetic

Many factors, of which those listed above are only a small sample, are taken into consideration when the graduate student first sees, talks with, and examines the patient.

tests, medical diagnosis, plan of medical management, medical prognosis, and data from hospitalizations will be needed. This information can be obtained from the patient's record or from his physician and should not be duplicated in the assessment done by the nurse.

The graduate student using the guide, approaches each patient much as a physician might in taking the patient's history and doing the physical examination—with a definite plan in mind of data to be collected. After the data are collected, she proceeds to analyze the data, make the nursing diagnosis, and decide upon a plan of care. This plan then is discussed with those who will be a part of the nursing team before it is implemented. Naturally, there will be instances when collecting data and carrying out care will be simultaneous, particularly when the patient is in acute need. At these times when symptoms are acute and may be changing rapidly, filling in the data collection forms comes after the emergency moment. However, nurses must, with the majority of patients, reach a point where their plans for care are not based on hunch alone.

Reactions to this method of patient assessment have been favorable, and there is general agreement on the wards that the nursing care plans based on the assessments take all of the nursing needs of the patients into consideration. Increased knowledge about patients and increased awareness of them have given graduate students greater satisfaction in carrying out their responsibilities. Further, we have noticed that whenever base line data are available, evaluation of the effectiveness of nursing therapy has improved.

In the beginning, we wondered how patients and physicians would react to this process. Our experiences so far indicate that patients are pleased that nurses take time to listen to their problems, demonstrate an interest in them, and obviously base nursing care on their expressed needs. Physicians' responses have been more general than those of patients, but they, too, have seen the value of the assessment process.

REFERENCES

1. Abdellah, Faye G., et al. *Patient-Centered Approaches to Nursing*. New York, Macmillan Co., 1960.

2. Bonney, Virginia, and Rothberg, June. *Nursing Diagnosis and Therapy—An Instrument for Evaluation and Measurement*. (League Exchange) New York, National League for Nursing, 1963.

3. Johnson, Dorothy E. The significance of nursing care. *American Journal of Nursing* 61:63-66.

Nursing History: One Means to Personalize Care

L. Mae McPhetridge

Early, full knowledge of what the patient perceives about his illness and hospitalization and what he prefers about his care enables the nurse, says this author, to personalize his nursing during his stay and to prepare more successfully for his departure from the hospital. Completing the history form which records this enabling information is claimed to take far less time than to gather the same facts over a period of several days' nursing care.

Personalized nursing care is increasingly difficult to achieve despite the fact that it remains a consistent goal of nurse practitioners and nurse educators. Growing numbers of patients, greater nurse participation in more and more complex plans of medical care, responsibility for larger numbers of auxiliary personnel are all cited as reasons for failure to give patient-centered nursing care.

Legitimate deterrents though these are, nurses must find a way to individualize nursing care. One means, a nursing history form, has been developed to help the nurse make maximum use of her limited time with the patient by obtaining systematically the information needed to plan his nursing care.

Any usable nursing history should identify the patient's perception and expectations related to his illness, hospitalization, and care. The history also should furnish clues to the patient's ability to meet his personal needs and to cope with problems he faces. From such data, the nurse can deduce the amount and kind of nursing assistance he requires.

A nursing history differs from a medical history in that it focuses on the meaning of illness and hospitalization to the patient and his family as a basis for planning nursing care. The medical history is taken to determine whether pathology is present as a basis for planning medical care.

One patient expressed this difference succinctly when he said during a nursing interview, "I'm glad to know someone's interested in me as well as my illness." Of course, physicians, too, are interested in patients' perceptions and ways of coping just as nurses are interested in patients' pathologies. But a history that is quite adequate for developing a medical regimen may be just as unsatisfactory for planning nursing care as a nursing history would be for planning medical care. Since information taken in a nursing history may be useful to the

Reprinted with permission from *American Journal of Nursing,* Vol. 68, No. 1. Copyright 1968 by The American Journal of Nursing Company.

physician, the two histories are complementary, valuable to both nurse and physician.

NURSING HISTORY FORMAT

Our nursing history format, developed as an interview guide, consists of questions directed to the patient and space for his answers. The recording; of direct quotes and key phrases captures the patient's meaning with a minimum of writing. His identifying data on the face sheet should be obtained from his record to avoid repetitious questioning. The history format is organized in four parts.

Patient perceptions and expectations about the meaning of illness and hospitalization to him and his family are elicited in the first section. Asking why the patient sought medical care, what he thinks caused him to get sick, and how his illness has affected his usual way of life all tend to reveal his understanding of his condition and how it has affected him. What hospitalization means to him is learned by asking what he expects will happen to him, what it is like to be in the hospital, and how long he expects to stay.

The patient's view of the effects of his illness and hospitalization on his family or other significant persons is obtained by asking with whom he lives, who is the most important person(s) to him, what effect his entering the hospital has had on his family or the person closest to him, and whether the significant person(s) are able to visit him. Inquiring what the patient does for recreation provides some guidance for considering this aspect of care. Asking how he expects to manage after leaving the hospital gives further indication of his understanding and feelings about his illness. This question also lays the foundation for early planning of care after discharge.

Basic needs are explored in the second section which investigates the patient's ability to care for himself and serves as a basis for determining whether nursing intervention will be necessary to insure comfort, rest, and sleep. Questions about these basic needs also embrace pain and personal hygiene; safety, including items related to locomotion, vision, and hearing; fluids and nutrition; elimination; oxygen; and sexuality.

Each need is considered from the patient's standpoint, from his perception of problems he is encountering at present, whether he has experienced similar problems in the past and how he coped with them, and with what success. What nursing assistance does he expect with each need at this time? The help he wants and that which the nurse thinks he should have may differ widely. This incongruity must be reconciled or it may give rise to conflict that will hinder the nurse's therapeutic effectiveness. Data concerning anticipated problems and how he expects to manage suggest the nursing assistance needed to provide continuity of care.

Additional information is secured in the third section, labeled "Other," which asks questions that do not fit logically into the first two sections. Does the patient have a history of allergy? This is important information with the widespread use of pharmaceuticals. A question asking how far the patient went in school is placed in this section rather than earlier in the interview so that he will not think the nurse measures his worth in terms of his education.

This question aids in assessing the patient's intellectual capacity, a prerequisite for successful communication and future planning. A final, open-ended question lets the patient tell anything else he thinks would help the nurse with his care. For instance, knowing whether he is being assisted by other health or social agencies is useful for continuity of care.

Nurse's impressions and suggestions, the last section, is completed after the interview. From the data, the nurse summarizes the significant findings and from this summary develops a plan for this person's nursing care. All sections except the last may be completed during the interview or the nurse may jot down a word or two as a reminder and fill in more detail out of the patient's presence.

The form is not intended to limit nurse-patient communication. Using the form only as a guide, the interviewer is free to rephrase questions and explore more deeply any areas of concern that need probing. The questions about patient's perception simply suggest material that may be significant to his nursing care and may require further discussion, depending on his response or lack of response to a given question.

After initial testing by the author with eight patients, the form was tested by junior and senior baccalaureate students during an entire school year. Students' and patients' overall reactions were positive. Questions were generally understood by patients and elicited in minimum time the information necessary to plan individualized care. Interview time ranged from 20 to 60 minutes with an average of 25 minutes. Like any nursing activity, the time varied according to the patient's response and the nurse's skill.

NURSING IMPLICATIONS

Asked why he was in the hospital and what he thought caused him to get sick, one patient with cancer of the neck responded, "I have cancer of the neck." Here, the nurse immediately learned that the patient knew his diagnosis. Accordingly she could approach him appropriately concerning his illness and thus avoid a nonverbal guessing game that is potentially destructive to a therapeutic relationship. Another person, with diagnosed lung cancer, answered these questions by saying he had had pneumonia and his lung had "closed up" so that it was hard for him to breathe. This response guided the nurse in further communication, particularly in choosing words to help the patient talk about concerns relating to his illness. A third patient, who had had a node resection for cancer of the groin, attributed this "lump" to heavy lifting. Obviously, this patient's understanding and acceptance of follow-up care was quite different from that of the man who said he had a cancer on his neck. Hence the nurse's approach must differ.

Statements about effects of illness on patients' usual ways of life demonstrated the great variation in meaning that illness holds for different persons. To one man, it meant economic disaster. To another, illness meant dependence on other people to an extent he found repugnant. To still another patient, the most significant effect had been his sexual impotence for several months. If the nurse is to assist these patients in coping with these problems, it is apparent

(Text continues on page 29)

UNIVERSITY OF KENTUCKY
COLLEGE OF NURSING
Nursing History

Date _____   Medical Diagnosis: _____
Name _____   _____
Hospital Number _____   _____
Address (city or county) _____
Age _____ Sex: M_____ F_____   Information obtained from Patient: _____
Occupation _____   Other: _____
Religion _____   Relationship: _____
Race/National Origin _____   History needs to be rechecked at later
                                      date _____

I. **Patient Perceptions and Expectations Related to Illness/Hospitalization**
   1. Why did you come to the hospital? (or go to the doctor?) _____
      _____
   2. What do you think caused you to get sick? _____
      _____
   3. Has being sick made any difference in your usual way of life? If so, how? _____
      _____
   4. What do you expect is going to happen to you in the hospital? _____
      _____
      _____
   5. What is it like for you being in the hospital? _____
      _____
   6. How long do you expect to be in the hospital? _____
   7. With whom do you live? _____
   8. Who is the most important person(s) to you? _____
   9. What effect has your coming to the hospital had on your family? (or closest
      person?) _____
      _____
   10. Are any of your family (or close persons) able to visit you in the hospital? _____
       _____
   11. What do you enjoy doing for recreation? (to pass the time) _____
       _____
       _____
   12. How do you expect to get along after you leave the hospital? _____
       _____

II. **Specific Basic Needs**
    1. Comfort, Rest, Sleep
       a. Pain/Discomfort
          1) Have you had any pain or discomfort since admission?   Yes_____
                                                                          No_____
             If yes, describe _____
             _____
          2) Did you have any pain or discomfort before coming to the hospital?
                                                                          Yes_____
                                                                          No_____
             If yes, describe _____
             _____
             How long? _____
             What did you do to relieve the pain/discomfort? _____
             Was the pain/discomfort relieved by treatment?   Completely_____
                                                                   Partially_____
                                                                   Not at all_____
          3) If you have pain/discomfort while in the hospital what would you like the
             nurse to do to relieve it? _____
             _____

b. Rest/Sleep
  1) Are you having any trouble getting enough rest or sleep since you came to the hospital?   Yes_____
      No_____

If yes, describe _____

  2) Do you usually have trouble going to sleep?   Yes_____
      No_____
     Do you usually have trouble staying asleep?   Yes_____
      No_____

If yes, describe _____

What have you done in the past to help you get enough rest or sleep?

Was it effective?   Always_____
     Usually_____
     Sometimes_____
     Never_____

  3) What would you like the nurse to do to help you get the rest and sleep you need while in the hospital? _____

c. Personal Hygiene
  1) Do you need help with your bath while in the hospital?   Yes_____
      No_____

If yes, describe _____

  2) Do you need help with brushing your teeth?   Yes_____
      No_____

If yes, describe _____

  3) Is your skin usually   Dry_____
     Oily_____
     Normal_____
  4) What, if anything, do you use on your skin?   Face_____
     Body_____
  5) How often do you prefer to bathe?_____   Morning_____
     Afternoon_____
     Evening_____
     No preference_____
  6) Do you prefer a   Tub bath_____
     Shower_____

This question is not pertinent_____

2. Safety
a. Locomotion
  1) Do you have any difficulty in walking about?   Yes_____
      No_____

If yes, describe _____

  2) Did you have any difficulty in walking before you came to the hospital?   Yes_____
      No_____

If yes, describe _____

How did you manage? _____

  3) Has anyone said anything to you about staying in bed (or getting out of bed) since you came to the hospital?   Yes_____
      No_____

If yes, what? _____

What do you think about staying in bed? (or getting out of bed?)_____

(Nursing History Form continues)

    4) Do you expect to have any difficulty getting about after you leave the
hospital?   Yes_____
                                                   No_____
                                       Don't know_____
    If yes, how do you expect to manage? _____

b. Vision
    1) Do you have any difficulty in seeing?   Yes_____
                                                   No_____
    If yes, describe _____

    2) Do you wear glasses?   Yes_____
                                                 No_____
    If #1 is yes, in what way does your limited sight handicap you? _____

    How do you manage? _____

c. Hearing
    1) Do you have any difficulty in hearing?   Yes_____
                                                 No_____
    If yes, describe _____

    2) If yes, do you wear a hearing aid?   Yes_____
                                                 No_____
    3) If #1 is yes, in what way does your limited hearing handicap you? _____

    How do you manage? _____

3.   Fluids
    1) Has the amount of fluid you usually drink been changed since you got
sick?   Increased_____
                                               Decreased_____
                                             Unchanged_____
    2) What fluids do you like to drink?
        Water_____   Coffee _____
        Milk _____   Tea _____
        Fruit juice _____   Soft drinks _____
    3) What fluids do you dislike? _____

4.   Nutrition
a. Teeth/Mouth
    1) What is the condition of your teeth?   Good_____
                                               Cavities_____
                                             Other_____
    2) Do you wear dentures?   Upper_____
                                               Lower_____
                                             Partial_____
    3) Is eating limited by the condition of your teeth?   Yes_____
                                               No_____
    If yes, describe _____

    4) Do you have any soreness in your mouth?   Yes_____
                                               No_____
    If yes, does it interfere with your eating?   Yes_____
                                               No_____

b. Do you consider yourself to be
                            Overweight_____   How much_____
                            Underweight_____   How much_____
                            About right_____
c. Appetite/Food Preference
    1) Has being sick made any difference in your eating?   Yes_____
                                               No_____
    If yes, describe _____

2) What foods do you eat mostly? _____

_____

3) Are there any foods you do not eat?   Yes_____
                                                No_____

   If yes, which food do you not eat and why? _____

_____

d. Diet
   1) Are you on a special diet?   Yes_____
                                                 No_____

   If yes, what kind? _____
   2) Were you ever on a special diet before you came to the hospital?
                                                 Yes_____
                                                 No_____

   If yes, what kind? _____
   Did you have any problems with your diet?   Yes_____
                                                 No_____

   If yes, describe _____

_____

   3) Have you had any problems with your food since you came to the
      hospital?   Yes_____
                                                 No_____

   If yes, describe_____

_____

   If yes, what do you think would correct the problem? _____

_____

   4) Do you expect to be discharged on a special diet?   Yes_____
                                                          No_____
                                                  Don't know_____

   If yes, how do you expect to manage? _____

_____

5. Elimination
   a. Bowels
      1) Has being sick changed the way your bowels function in any way?
                                                 Yes_____
                                                 No_____

      If yes, describe _____

_____

      2) Do you usually have   Constipation_____
                                          Diarrhea_____
                                          Neither_____

      3) How often do you usually have a bowel movement? _____
      4) What time of day do you normally have a bowel movement?_____
      5) Do you take a laxative Regularly_____ or an enema? Regularly_____
                                 Frequently_____   Frequently_____
                                 Occasionally_____   Occasionally_____
                                 Never_____   Never_____

      If yes, what kind? _____
      6) Do you do anything else to help you have a bowel movement?
                                                 Yes_____
                                                 No_____

      If yes, describe _____

_____

      7) Do you expect to have any problem with your bowels after you leave the
         hospital?   Yes_____
                                                 No_____

      If yes, how do you expect to manage? _____

_____

   b. Bladder
      1) Have you had any difficulty in passing your urine (water) since you came
         to the hospital?   Yes_____
                                                 No_____

      If yes, describe _____

_____

(Nursing History Form continues)

2) Did you have any difficulty with your urine before you came to the
hospital?   Yes_____
                                                                    No_____
                                                        Don't remember_____

If yes, describe _____

_____

How did you manage? _____

3) If #1 is yes, what do you think would help you pass your urine (water) while
in the hospital? _____

4) Do you expect to have a problem with your urine after you leave the
hospital?   Yes_____
                                                                    No_____

If yes, how do you expect to manage? _____

6.   Oxygen
     1) Has being sick caused any change in your breathing?   Yes_____
                                                                    No_____

     If yes, describe _____

     2) Did you have any difficulty with your breathing before you came to the
     hospital?   Yes_____
                                                                    No_____

     If yes, describe _____

     If yes, how did you manage? _____

     3) If #1 is yes, what do you think would make it easier for you to breathe
     while you are in the hospital? _____

     4) Do you expect to have any difficulty with your breathing after you leave
     the hospital?   Yes_____
                                                                    No_____
                                                           Don't know_____

     If yes, how do you expect to manage? _____
7.   Sexuality (Ask according to marital status and appropriateness to the patient.)
     1) (If Married) Has being sick made any difference in your being a
              husband_____   wife _____   Yes_____
              father_____   mother _____   No_____
     If yes, describe _____

     (If single and appropriate) Has being sick made any difference in your
     relationship with other people, particularly the opposite sex? Yes_____
                                                                    No_____

     If yes, describe _____

     2) (If appropriate) Has being sick caused any change in your sexual func-
     tioning (sex life)?   Yes_____
                                                                    No_____

     If yes, describe _____

     3) Do you expect your sexual functioning (sex life) to be changed in any
     way after you leave the hospital?   Yes_____
                                                                    No_____
                                                           Don't know_____

     If yes, describe _____

     4) Do you expect your ability to function as a husband, wife, father, mother,
     or in a social relationship to be changed in any way after you leave the
     hospital?   Yes_____
                                                                    No_____
                                                           Dont know_____

     If yes, describe _____

III. Other

1. Do you have any known allergies?   Yes_____
                                                                       No_____

   If yes, what kind? _____

   How have you managed? _____

   To what extent does the allergy handicap you? _____
   _____

2. How far did you go in school? _____
   Can you read and write? (Ask only if indicated)   Yes_____
                                                                       No_____
3. Is there anything else you wish to tell me that would help us with your nursing
   care? _____
   _____
   _____
   _____

IV. Nurse's Impressions and Suggestions

1. In your judgment which word(s) best describe this patient?

Alert_____	Homesick _____
Angry_____	Hyperactive_____
Answers questions readily _____	Hypoactive _____
Answers questions reluctantly____	Lethargic _____
Anxious____	Nonquestioning _____
Confident _____	Nontalkative _____
Confused _____	Passive _____
Cooperative _____	Questioning_____
Critical _____	Quick to comprehend _____
Demanding_____	Secure _____
Depressed _____	Seeks support_____
Disoriented _____	Slow to comprehend _____
Distrustful____	Talkative _____
Embarrassed _____	Trustful _____
Euphoric _____	Unable to comprehend _____
Fearful _____	Withdrawn____

2. Summary of findings that are significant for nursing care. _____/_____
   _____
   _____
   _____
   _____

that she must offer very different kinds of help. For the first patient, the proper assistance might be referral to social service. For the second, the nurse might plan with the patient so that he could make as many decisions as possible and thereby strengthen his feelings of independence. Perhaps the help needed by the third patient is merely to know that those caring for him appreciate his feelings.

Patients' reactions to hospitalization were equally varied. One man expressed immense relief at being in the hospital and receiving medical care from highly qualified staff. But being in the hospital meant overwhelming loneliness to one woman because of separation from her family, who were unable to visit. The man apparently did not need nursing assistance related specifically to his hospitalization, but the woman required considerable help from the nursing staff to deal with her loneliness and thus conserve the psychic energy she sorely needed to combat her illness.

Assuming that people cope better with the known than the unknown, their needs for nursing assistance will vary in proportion to their understanding and expectations during hospitalization. One patient, for instance, arrived with detailed knowledge of her proposed care, which included a proctoscopic examination and bowel x-ray. Another person had no idea what was to be done during his hospital stay or, for that matter, how long he was to stay. Some patients replied, "I don't know," to all questions related to perception of illness and expectations.

While such responses give no immediate clue to nursing needs, they do suggest questions worth further exploration. Was any information given to the patient? If so, did he comprehend it? Was he too anxious to hear? Does his pattern of response represent denial of illness? If such an explanation can be verified with the patient, the nurse can begin appropriate action. For example, assistance for a patient who does not know what to expect because he does not understand the terminology used in explanation would be very different from that for a patient whose responses stem from denial.

Asking the patient how he expects to get along after leaving the hospital also helped determine nursing needs. Some patients had specific, firm arrangements for their continued care. Others had not looked that far ahead. By asking the question early, nurses could begin discharge planning much sooner.

This question also gave a clue as to whether the patient's understanding of his illness was realistic. One woman, for example, who had a hysterectomy for a benign condition and presumably would be considered cured upon discharge, said she expected to go to bed indefinitely after leaving the hospital and be unable to do anything for herself. To help this patient plan realistically, the nurse must know not only what the patient thinks but why. If her response is based on fear of cancer, one kind of nursing action is indicated. If her answer reflects an exaggerated dependency need, an entirely different nursing measure is required.

The section dealing with the patient's basic needs yielded much useful information for planning nursing care. For example, if the patient had pain, a major nursing aim would be to relieve it. To do so, the nurse needs more information. Besides her own observations, she must consider the patient's description of his pain, whether he has had it previously, what he did to relieve it, and whether he succeeded. One patient said he gained partial relief by walking about, while another man's pain was lessened by remaining very quiet. In addition to administering their prescribed medications, some patients wanted the nurse to talk with them or help them find comfortable positions. A 28-year-old man with peptic ulcer responded that he had little faith in medications and what he wanted most was that the nurse allow him to tell her how much it hurt.

The vast majority of patients interviewed had distinct preferences about the frequency and time for bathing as well as the type of bath. There were no consistent patterns. Some patients preferred a daily bath; a few wanted to bathe only once a week. The desired time ranged from 5:00 A.M. to bedtime. Preferences for tub bath or shower were divided about equally. Giving patients a choice about personal hygiene seems to be one way to minimize the loss of identity and control associated with hospitalization. Although offering patients this choice may raise staffing problems, the overall time for bathing is not increased by changing the hour.

The physiologic and psychologic significance of food for the ill person is undisputed. Yet the best food does not nourish the patient who fails to eat because he dislikes it or because he cannot chew it. Information about food likes and dislikes, and about conditions which affect his eating, makes it possible to foster good nutrition and patient satisfaction. Two questions were particularly illuminating. One asked whether the patient considered himself underweight, overweight, or about right. The fact that nurse perceptions of a patient's weight and his perceptions of his weight do not always agree cannot be discounted if she must help in weight control.

Inquiring what foods were eaten primarily revealed some glaring deficiencies. For example, a 19-year-old girl with chronic ulcerative colitis "mostly ate macaroni, french fries, dill pickles, and vanilla ice cream." The patient's knowledge of his hospital diet, his past experiences with a special diet, along with what he expects when he goes home, all provide clues to his teaching needs.

Inquiry into elimination habits showed that what patients considered normal and the means used to facilitate bowel evacuation were highly individual. One patient dosed herself with "salts" at bedtime if she did not have two bowel movements each day. The influence of habit on elimination was demonstrated by the maternity patient who regularly had a cigarette and Coke immediately after breakfast. This practice could be followed in the hospital only if the nurse knew of it and took deliberate steps to enable the patient to do so. A 68-year-old woman, confined to bed with a fractured hip, reported that she normally had one bowel movement a week and only with the help of an enema. Because the nurse knew the effects of prolonged inactivity and knew the patient's elimination pattern soon after admission, she could institute measures to prevent a fecal impaction. Interviews documented widespread use of laxatives—a fact with clear teaching implications.

Questions pertaining to sexuality explored the effects of illness on the sexual role, as well as specific sexual functioning. While some patients did not choose to discuss this subject, others welcomed the opportunity to express concern about their inability to lead normal sex lives.

Some patients answered the nurse's questions pertaining to allergy by giving a history of allergy although they had not mentioned this to the physician. In response to the last, open-ended question, most patients did not wish to tell the nurse anything more. However, a few gave further information. One man wanted the nurse to know he "got mean" when he had pain, "cussed and everything," but that he really did not mean what he said. It appeared important to him for the nurse to understand his behavior.

CONCLUSIONS

Our testing indicates that the nursing history form is not only valuable for identifying individual patient needs, but for establishing early nurse-patient rapport. In general, patients responded cooperatively to the interview and many of them voiced appreciation for the nurse's interest in them as persons.

During follow-up visits, patients consistently picked up the discussion of their concerns where the previous conversation had ended. One patient with diarrhea for which no organic cause could be found spoke freely about recent crises in her life but denied vehemently that these could be related to her symptoms. On each successive visit she immediately began to talk about what had happened to her. After several visits with the nurse, she concluded there probably was a relationship between her recent experiences and symptoms, and added, "I've gone through enough in the past few months to give anyone diarrhea." Thus it appears that the nursing history interview, besides yielding vital information, also broadens the nurse's therapeutic effectiveness.

Must one use a nursing history form to identify needs? Obviously, no, but the form facilitates gathering data early in hospitalization. Only 30 minutes spent with the patient soon after admission yields quantities of information valuable throughout his stay. One nurse commented, after taking her first history, that she probably would have obtained almost all the information had she cared for the patient for several days. Since the length of the interview may raise a question about using this form in busy patient services, it is worth noting that while interview time can be measured readily, it is much harder to measure the time spent resolving problems which could have been prevented had information been available earlier. Priority use of the nurse's time is something that must be faced realistically. The nurse's comments about obtaining information in 30 minutes by interview which ordinarily would have taken several days of caring for the patient underscores the time value of a systematic approach to the nursing history.

So far, we have used the nursing history form only to collect data about individual nursing needs. However, the form lends itself equally well to collecting epidemiologic data relevant to the needs of a patient population. Nurses are frequently astute in their observations about individual patients, but the development of a nursing science has been impeded by the lack of data about groups of patients and their statistical analysis for characteristics common to a patient population. Plans are under way to use the nursing history form to collect epidemiologic data which will contribute to nursing knowledge.

2

Data Processing

The guiding goal in nursing is to give holistic care that encourages the client to meet a maximum health potential (Bower, 1972). As was discussed in Chapter 1, when a client needs assistance, the nurse's responsibility is to provide help while maintaining the individuality of the client and the client's system. To accomplish this, the nurse collects data with the intent of discovering what is necessary for the nursing care consumer to fulfill and further individual potential. Simply, the nurse is a helper.

Data processing is the step following data collection in the nursing process; it is a tool used to assist decision-making by both nurse and client. Data processing is an important part of the assessment phase and is necessary to integrate knowledge about clients and their systems with the responsibilities and knowledge of professional nursing as well as nursing personnel. Data processing is the act of interpreting collected data; it is the procedure of analyzing and examining information in relation to other information in the client's system. The purpose of data processing is to insure that the functioning of nursing care is in response to the individual needs and wants of the client.

Similar to data collection, data processing is a continuously occurring event. Each piece of information that an individual receives or blocks from consciousness becomes a part of past learning, experiences, values, beliefs, and goals. Behavior results from attitudes, motives, and goals. For the nurse to become more aware of the reasons for client behavior and the client's condition, and for the nurse to integrate the different perceptions of others concerning the client, data processing is an important tool. In addition, it is a valuable aid in communicating requirements of client care to other members of the health team.

Let us look again at the equation presented in Chapter 1:

$$\begin{array}{c} \text{Client Data} \\ \text{System Data} \end{array} + \begin{array}{c} \text{Nursing Responsibilities} \\ \text{Nurse's Knowledge} \\ \text{The Nurse} \end{array} \longrightarrow \begin{array}{c} \text{Individualized} \\ \text{Nursing Diagnoses and} \\ \text{Nursing Orders} \end{array}$$

The first segment of the equation involved the collection of client and system data. The second segment of the equation involves data processing. It is comprised of the elements—nursing responsibilities, the nurse's knowledge, and the nurse—which act upon the collected information, interpreting it and translating it into a useful care plan comprised of individualized nursing diagnoses and nursing orders. Data collection and data processing are tools of the assessment phase of the nursing process.

The following is a discussion of data processing, the second segment of the nursing process equation.

AREAS OF NURSING RESPONSIBILITY

According to theories of professionalism (see Chapter 18), there are three essential components of the nursing profession: areas of responsibility; autonomy; and authority. The first component, areas of responsibility, makes up the basis of nursing actions and is important in processing information. Many of these responsibilities have been assigned to nurses ever since Florence Nightingale (1967) established the framework of nursing practice in 1859. The following areas of responsibility, many of which were first written about by Nightingale, are to be considered in data processing because they reflect nursing goals to be included in the total care plan. The areas of responsibility are:

1. comfort
2. nutrition
3. exercise
4. personal hygiene
5. sleep, rest patterns
6. diversional activities
7. socializing and privacy
8. elimination
9. safety
10. environmental considerations
11. teaching
12. spiritual comfort and/or assistance
13. prevention of complications
14. assurance of physiologic status—health maintenance
15. emotional support, counseling

The areas of responsibility are usually presented as part of a beginning level nursing course. Subsequent courses and experiences of the practitioner amplify the understanding of these responsibilities. Different client-care situations supply the nurse with more information about these responsibilities. The nurse grows in the understanding of responsibilities through experience.

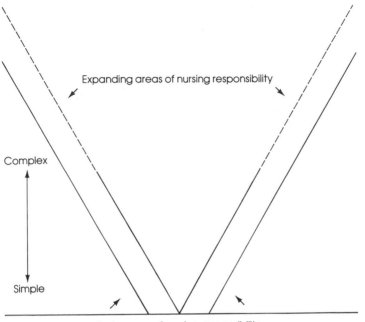

Expanding areas of nursing responsibility

Complex

Simple

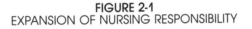

Basic areas of nursing responsibility

FIGURE 2-1
EXPANSION OF NURSING RESPONSIBILITY

This learning process is similar to Hall's (1964) model of nursing practice which portrays nursing functions as moving from simple to complex. Growth through experience requires that the funnel of knowledge always expands, even though the basic concepts are grounded. See Figure 2-1.

NURSE'S KNOWLEDGE AND THE NURSE

To process data while considering the areas of nursing responsibility, a solid body of knowledge is required. Knowing the theory framing each responsibility is important in data processing. For example, in dealing with the area of nutrition it becomes necessary to study physiology of the gastrointestinal (GI) system; physiologic responses of the GI tract to stress; normal diets; and diets that are specific for certain physiologic/psychologic alterations. The area of nutrition is related closely to elimination—overlap exists in many areas. It is important to develop knowledge of the areas of overlap to assist in processing and planning care.

Nursing knowledge and the individual nurse are closely interrelated. Nursing knowledge revolves around the areas of responsibility and combines, through the values, beliefs, and experiences of the individual nurse, to produce nursing diagnoses and orders. Lewis (1968) stresses that nursing care should be designed to provide interventions that meet the clients' needs in an individual manner. According to Sundeen, Stuart, Rankin, and Cohen (1976), the nurse is a member of a client-oriented profession; the nurse seeks to identify the unexpressed and expressed needs of the client, find meaning in the client's coping responses, and maximize the client's strengths.

Data processing provides the bridge between: (1) the nurse's knowledge and experience concerning what the client needs, including the medical diagnosis and orders, and (2) the needs as expressed by the client. The manner in which the client is most apt to receive care depends on the individual nurse. In data processing, the nurse asks: "What is it necessary for me to know about the client so that I may make a nursing diagnosis relative to my areas of responsibility?" The nurse's response to this question reflects the nurse's body of knowledge and experience, the nurse's perception of responsibilities, and the nurse's reaction to the client.

A CASE STUDY

The following case study is presented to facilitate learning how to process collected data. This case study will also follow the other steps of the nursing process throughout Part I of this book to illustrate the process in action. The skills and competencies necessary to carry out each step will be mentioned as they occur and then will be more fully discussed in Part II.

> Mr. Munson, the client, is a married, 52-year-old, white male who entered the hospital through the emergency room on June 30. Diagnosis: possible myocardial infarction. The professional nurse's first contact with him was the morning following admission in the coronary care unit on July 1. On July 7 he was transferred to an acute care unit, and then to an ambulatory care unit on July 15. July 23 marked his discharge home.*

Data collection started with the nurse's first contact and continued throughout admission. Primary nursing care was the organizational model used in the facility. The nurse taking care of Mr. Munson was a baccalaureate-prepared practitioner who had been a coronary care specialist for six years. The first step in the nursing process was to explore the purpose of nursing care:

> Though it was not definite that Mr. Munson had a myocardial infarction, he nevertheless seemed susceptible, based on symptoms.

*The case material used in this section was modified from that presented by Eugene Kresco, University of Massachusetts, 1975.

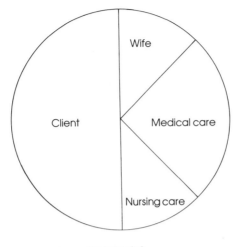

FIGURE 2-2
A CLIENT'S SYSTEM WHILE IN CORONARY CARE

Data were collected and analyzed to discover facts and habits about him and to decipher bits of information that might lead to the clarification of behaviors associated with the disease process. At the same time, strict monitoring of the client was indicated to prevent further heart damage or progression of symptoms.

It should become obvious that if nursing care was concerned just with physiologic factors and prevention of complications, expansive data collection and processing would not be necessary. These factors, however, are only one segment of comprehensive nursing care. Furthermore, physiologic nursing care generally is standardized. It would be difficult to individualize taking an electrocardiogram (ECG) and monitoring the electrical impulses of the heart in a coronary care unit.

In processing data, remember that systems change. Figure 2-2 shows the components of Mr. Munson's system in the coronary care unit. This system changes in response to his recovery and movement to different environments. Examples are shown in Figures 2-3 and 2-4.

It should be pointed out that medical care decreases as physical illness abates. Nursing care decreases as the client's home environmental factors come into play and the client requires less professional help. During the ambulatory phase, the client's work position and responsibilities also must be considered. Just as the system changes, so does the purpose. This point is cogently expressed by Hornstein (1976), a social psychologist, who says:

> Purposive behavior varies with circumstance; it is not a consistent, robotlike reaction that is unmindful of changing conditions. Warn-

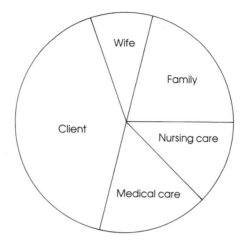

FIGURE 2-3
A CLIENT'S SYSTEM WHILE IN AN ACUTE CARE SETTING

ings are purposive if they are made *only* when another animal is endangered and they stop when the other is safe. In short, the act's beginning and end must be determined by the other's condition of distress. (p. 72)*

METHOD OF DATA PROCESSING

Once data are collected, write or list the information in any usable framework for yourself and others who may need access to it. One method is to divide the data into five columns: psychologic factors, physiologic factors, sociologic factors, and the medical regimen, and lab reports. Referring back to the case presented, the following data will be used to clarify the technique. Data processing will be done on those data collected during the beginning of the client's hospitalization.

Data Base
Physiologic Data:

1. Male, 52 years old
2. Admitted with chest pain; non-recurrent
3. Admitted through emergency room

*Reprinted with permission from Hornstein, H. *Cruelty and Kindness.* Copyright 1976, Prentice-Hall, Inc., Englewood Cliffs, New Jersey.

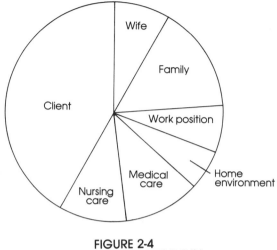

FIGURE 2-4
A CLIENT'S SYSTEM WHILE IN
AN AMBULATORY CARE SETTING

4. Low, substernal pain without radiation on admission
5. Pain was described as "dull"
6. History of intermittent dyspnea with stress
7. No respiratory distress noted
8. Normal color; circulation appears normal
9. Warm, dry skin
10. No nauses or dizziness verbalized
11. Controlled, mild diabetes for five years
12. Takes Dymelor at home, 500 mg qd
13. History of smoking 2–3 packs of cigarettes per day for 23 years
14. Quit smoking three months prior to admission
15. States he follows a haphazard diet at home
16. Seems muscular and robust, but states he tires easily
17. Height: 6'0"; Weight: 200 lb
18. Underwent a cholecystectomy 12 years prior to admission
19. Oldest brother has diabetes
20. States his appetite is usually always good, even with the diabetic diet
21. Prefers to eat at 9–2–7; hospital serves 8–12–5

Psychologic Data:

22. He is on the cardiac monitor
23. CCU standing orders places all patients on "danger list"
24. Vital signs are all within normal limits; no PVCs noted

25. Desires definite diagnosis; MI currently not confirmed
26. Wife appears to be extremely concerned, nervous, and protective
27. Left school after completing eighth grade due to father's death
28. At 15 years of age, sought employment in order to support family
29. Has worked full-time since he was fifteen
30. Father died suddenly; cause is unknown to client
31. Mother died at a young age following what the client calls a "thyroid problem"
32. Appears anxious concerning hospitalization
33. Sleeps well at home on one pillow with the exception of the last month prior to hospitalization, when he noted mild chest pain during the night
34. Verbalizes his desire to be at home with his family since they are separated only rarely
35. Seems to be outgoing, pleasant, and has a good sense of humor
36. Seems to be sensitive to the feelings of others, especially his family
37. Appears to be extremely independent and questioning
38. Maintains neat appearance
39. Demonstrates good hygiene; insists on caring for self
40. Questions why he is in the coronary unit
41. Seems to have limited understanding about diabetes or possibly does not want to be concerned with it since he states he has no problems
42. Dislikes the food served and the times it is served; occasionally refuses to eat
43. Does not seem to like being in a private room; wanders out to visit other patients often; occasionally sits at nurse's station
44. States that he dislikes being inactive

Sociologic Data:

45. One previous hospitalization for gall bladder surgery
46. Unaware of purpose of coronary care unit or why he is in it
47. Married for 30 years; wife works as dietary aid in hospital
48. Three children: two sons and one daughter
49. Elder son and daughter are married; one son in college
50. Avid sportsman: likes sailing, water skiing, scuba diving, and tennis
51. Captain of bowling league which meets two times per week
52. Plays golf frequently
53. Takes flying lessons; expects to be licensed in about one year
54. Is involved with karate as an instructor; holds a black belt
55. Drinks alcohol rarely and only socially
56. Works as a foreman at Smith & Wesson in quality control
57. Feels that his job is secure
58. Visiting hours are restricted to ten minutes every hour

Medical Regimen:

59. Defibrillate for ventricular fibrillation, PRN
60. Xylocaine 50 mg IV, PRN, for PVC's
61. Atropine 0.5 mg IV for sinus bradycardia below 40/min PRN
62. O² PRN (via nasal cannula) at 4 liters/min
63. Record intake and output; OOB with commode privileges
64. Frequent vital signs
65. On 2000 calorie diabetic diet: 3 eggs per week, no added salt, no coffee, tea, soda; may have Sanka
66. MS 5 mg SC if O² is not effective
67. Maalox 2 tbl PC and Q 2h PRN
68. Optilets 1 QD
69. Urines for clinitest and acetone–AC and HS
70. Dalmane 30 mg PO QHS PRN
71. Valium 5 mg PO QID
72. S/A urine coverage (with regular insulin–U-100) 3/31
           4+ = 10 units
           3+ = 5 units
        2+ or 1+ = no insulin
73. Daily FBS and 3 pm blood sugar
74. ECG's QD
75. Cardiac blood profile QD

Lab Reports

76. Negative chest x-ray
77. CBC: within normal limits
78. Electrolytes: within normal limits
79. Admission urine analysis: 4+ sugar and small amount of acetone
80. FBS 286 on 7/1
81. Cholesterol 270 on 7/1
82. Cardiac profile on 7/1: within normal limits
83. FBS 220 on 7/2
84. Cardiac profile on 7/2: within normal limits
85. Blood sugar and cholesterol levels are elevated
86. ECG changes consistent with subendocardial ischemia; 6/31
87. ECG: comparison shows continued STT wave changes in inferolateral leads consistent with ischemia; 7/1
88. ECG: shows continued STT wave changes over the inferolateral leads consistent with subendocardial ischemia; 7/2

One method of integrating these client data with the areas of nursing responsibility is to number each datum and then look at each nursing respon-

DATA PROCESSING IN CASE STUDY

Areas of Nursing Responsibility	Applicable Data
Comfort	2, 4, 5, 6, 7, 16, 21, 22, 32, 33, 37, 44
Nutrition	11, 12, 15, 17, 18, 20, 21, 32, 41, 42, 55, 63, 65, 68, 69, 72, 73, 79, 80, 81, 85
Exercise	1, 2, 4, 5, 6, 7, 8, 9, 10, 11, 16, 17, 21, 23, 24, 32, 35, 36, 37, 43, 44, 50, 51, 52, 53, 54, 63, 71, 86, 87, 88
Personal hygiene	1, 22, 37, 38, 39, 63, 72, 74, 79
Sleep, rest patterns	1, 16, 32, 33, 43, 58, 64, 70, 71
Diversional activity	1, 2, 6, 7, 8, 9, 16, 22, 26, 27, 28, 29, 32, 34, 35, 36, 37, 40, 43, 44, 46 50, 51, 52, 53, 54, 63, 64, 86, 87, 88
Socializing and privacy	1, 16, 22, 32, 34, 35, 36, 43, 44, 50, 51, 52, 53, 54, 58, 71
Elimination	11, 12, 15, 20, 37, 39, 42, 63, 65, 67, 72, 79, 86, 87, 88
Safety	10, 17, 37, 39, 40, 43, 44, 46, 71
Environmental considerations	3, 21, 22, 23, 34, 35, 37, 40, 42, 43, 44, 45, 63
Teaching	1, 6, 13, 14, 15, 16, 25, 26, 27, 28, 33, 35, 36, 37, 38, 39, 40, 41, 42, 44, 46, 50, 51, 52, 53, 54, 55, 65, 69, 71, 85
Spiritual comfort and assistance	26, 34, 36, 37, 43
Prevention of complications	2, 3, 4, 5, 6, 7, 8, 9, 10, 11, 12, 14, 15, 16, 22, 25, 32, 37, 40, 42, 44, 50, 51, 52, 53, 54, 55, and all data in the medical regimen
Assurance of physiologic status— health maintenance	6, 11, 12, 14, 15, 16, 17, 20, 25, 26, 29, 32, 33, 34, 41, 44, 47, 50, 51, 52, 53, 54, 55, 56, 57, 65, 67, 68, 69, 72, 73, 74, 75, 86, 87, 88
Emotional support and counseling	2, 3, 4, 5, 6, 7, 15, 22, 23, 24, 25, 26, 27, 29, 31, 32, 34, 35, 36, 37, 40, 41, 42, 43, 44, 46, 47, 48, 49, 57, 58, 71

sibility in terms of the applicable data. Place the number associated with each piece of pertinent datum alongside each area. In this way, data are categorized and organized for easy reference. Areas of overlap can be seen. You can locate possible problem areas by referring to the number of a potentially troublesome bit of information and by determining under which area(s) of responsibility this number occurs.

This process can be equated with a computer system. The input is client/ system data, the program and memory bank correspond to areas of nursing responsibility, and the output involves the integration of data and responsibility, yielding conclusions or nursing diagnoses.

With the results of data processing, the nurse has a profile of the individual client broken down according to the areas of nursing responsibility, facilitating the development of nursing diagnoses and subsequent orders that are based on the uniqueness of the client. Chapter 3 will use these data in the next step of the nursing process. It should be noted that experience using the presented data processing technique will enable one to carry out the format with greater ease. It may become unnecessary, for example, to write out this process in the lengthy detail described. In initial steps of learning, however, the author feels that detail while learning the process is necessary so that subsequent shortcuts can provide the same comprehensive, individualized care.

SUMMARY

This chapter discussed the data processing segment of nursing. It was presented as the bridge connecting rote nursing responsibilities with individualized client consideration. A case example was used to illustrate the concept; it will be followed through this section of the book.

Chapter 3 discusses the nursing diagnoses emerging from processing. Each will be arranged into a priority format.

REFERENCES

Bower, F. *The process of planning nursing care.* St. Louis: C. V. Mosby, 1972.

Hall, L. Nursing: What is it? *The Canadian Nurse* 60:150–154, 1964.

Hornstein, H. *Cruelty and kindness.* Englewood Cliffs, N.J.: Prentice-Hall, 1976.

Lewis, L. This I believe...About the nursing process—key to care. *Nursing Outlook* 16:26–29, 1968.

Nightingale, F. *Notes on nursing: What it is and what it is not.* New York: Dover Publications, 1967.

Sundeen, S., Stuart, G., Rankin, E., and Cohen, S. *Nurse-client interaction.* St. Louis: C. V. Mosby, 1976.

SELECTED READING

The reading following this chapter (Harrison, 1966) follows a case example through the nursing process to show individualized nursing care in action. It focuses on the uniqueness of the client and ways in which the nurse respects such individuality in planning care. Data processing as developed in this chapter provides a framework for beginning practitioners to accomplish the same personalization of nursing care plans.

Deliberative Nursing Process versus Automatic Nurse Action— The Care of a Chronically Ill Man

Cherie Harrison, M.A.

A PROBLEM PATIENT

Mr. C. was first observed by the present writer sitting up in bed, leaning forward slightly, breathing forcefully and rapidly through his mouth. He was very thin, unshaven, slightly cyanotic, and he talked with difficulty. He stated that he had been nauseated earlier and that he could not shake a "sick feeling"; he had been unable to eat or to get out of bed to use the Bennett machine. He declined my offer to bring the Bennett machine to his bedside by stating that the machine would not help him feel better. He used his hand nebulizer twice during the interview. The patient's apprehension and despair were evident in his manner, and he stated, "No use fooling myself, it's the way it is."

Mr. C., a patient in a large metropolitan general hospital, was considered by the ward staff as an "uncooperative patient." Conversations with the ward personnel revealed that the two staff physicians viewed him as a "typical emphysema personality" with "neurotic dependency patterns" who was "not motivated to conscientiously cooperate with the prescribed treatment." The doctor who was directly responsible for Mr. C's medical care stated that the patient would have to be hospitalized for the rest of his life since he required "constant medical supervision." The head nurse felt that "Mr. C. just doesn't want to do anything for himself and wants to be left alone."

She had recently moved him into a room with another emphysematous patient in an attempt to gain Mr. C.'s cooperation in his medical regimen. The nurses' notes reflect Mr. C.'s behavior at this time: "——[patient] does not use Bennett machine full amount of time——. [He is] refusing aminophylline suppositories for dyspnea as he views this [medication] as causing stomach distress and substernal pain." The chart further revealed that Mr. C. required "nerve pills" (Compazine and placebos) for "tension" and Darvon capsules for chest pain several times each night. Groceries and cigarettes were found in his bedside table.

Mr. C., 56 years old, had lived and worked in a city most of his life. He had never married; he left school after the eighth grade to support his parents until their death. He had lived with his sister since 1961. Mr. C. was a member of the Episcopal Church and had been an active member of Alcoholics Anonymous since 1948 (the ward staff did not know that Mr. C. belonged to

Reprinted with permission from *Nursing Clinics of North America*, Vol. 1, No. 3, pp. 387–397.

A.A.). Until three years ago he had smoked approximately three packs of cigarettes a day. He had a steady employment record; he worked in the engineering department of a large medical center from 1937 to 1961.

The patient had been hospitalized nine times at the medical center where he worked. In 1940 he was diagnosed as suffering from chronic bronchitis. He developed asthma and was hospitalized for pneumonia in 1944. In 1957 chest x-rays revealed diffuse bullous emphysema. The increased dyspnea forced Mr. C. to retire from his work in 1961. The Personnel Clinic provided the patient with a Bennett intermittent positive pressure breathing machine and a hand-bulb nebulizer for home use. Later that same year he was digitalized with Digoxin; this medication had been continued to date. It was necessary for Mr. C. to be hospitalized twice during 1963. The last admission to the medical center was in January, 1964, for breathing difficulties and somnolence. Early in 1964, Mr. C. was transferred from the medical center to the present hospital for chronic care of pulmonary emphysema with cor pulmonale.

On admission to this hospital, Mr. C. was 5 feet 10 inches tall and weighed 103 pounds. He had lost 65 pounds over the last three years. The progress note stated that on admission Mr. C. was "very apprehensive, frightened, exhausted, depressed." In January, April, and again in August, Mr. C. required treatment in the Drinker respirator in the intensive care unit for impending CO_2 narcosis. In September, 1964, Mr. C. was transferred to a convalescent ward, where this investigation took place.

PATHOPHYSIOLOGY OF EMPHYSEMA

Emphysema is a disease known to result in the impairment of pulmonary ventilation and in resulting disturbance of gas exchange.[5] Its development in most instances is characterized by a repetitive history of bronchial and pneumonic infections. These inflammatory processes result in the gradual and irreversible destruction of the small bronchioles, pulmonary blood vessels, and alveoli, and in a consequent loss of lung elasticity. The loss of lung elasticity significantly interferes with the mechanics of breathing.

In Mr. C.'s case alveolar ventilation, the amount of gas exhaled from the surface of the lung that takes part in gas exchange, was decreased greatly. Because of a loss in elasticity, there is an ever increasing accumulation of residual air in the lungs. The intrapleural pressure becomes less negative and during expiration the patient must expend great effort to force the air from his chest. The diaphragm, most important in maintaining normal negative intrapleural pressure, is pushed downward and works inefficiently. The rib cage becomes fixed in the inspirational pattern and expiration is chronically embarrassed.[5,9]

Elwood[4] states that there are three distinguishing features of this disability: marked arterial hypoxia, hypercapnea, and chronic cor pulmonale with recurring episodes of right heart failure. Mr. C. suffered from all three complications. Hypoxia, the depressed intake of oxygen into the alveoli, was evidenced by the decreased O_2 saturation level in arterial blood of 80 to 84% (normal 97%). Hypercapnea, the excess amount of carbon dioxide in body fluids, was seen in the elevated pCO_2 of the arterial blood of 54 to 58 mm. Hg (normal 40). The hypercapnea results in respiratory difficulties in the tissue cells and causes varying degrees of respiratory acidosis. Mr. C.'s compensated respiratory acidosis was reflected by the blood pH of 7.35 to 7.45 (normal 7.4).

In chronic cor pulmonale the heart is subjected to a greater effort by the necessity to pump blood through a restricted vascular pulmonary bed. This increase of work by the heart causes right ventricular heart failure with hypertrophy of the ventricle and hypertension in the pulmonary artery.[4,5,9] Mr. C.'s electrocardiograms had indicated sinus arrhythmia but not right ventricular hypertrophy.

The chronic hypoxia causes polycythemia to develop because in the presence of an arterial O_2 saturation of less than 80%, more red blood cells are produced. This compensating mechanism has physiological limitations and the resulting polycythemia becomes a disease secondary to pulmonary emphysema. This condition increases the viscosity of the blood, not only adding to the burden of the right ventricle but decreasing the renal blood flow rate.[5,9] Phlebotomies were performed on Mr. C at the beginning of the study to decrease the blood viscosity; his hematocrit stayed within normal range following the phlebotomies.

The hypoxia, the hypercapnea, and the kidney compensating mechanism present a paradox in treatment. Treatment of the hypoxia with conventional oxygen therapy increases the severity of the hypercapnea by removing the lack of O_2 as the stimulus to the respiratory center, and increasing CO_2 retention. The rising pCO_2 level is accompanied by a proportionate rise in sodium bicarbonate, i.e., the kidney compensating mechanism. However, the compensating sodium ion reabsorption by the kidney tubules, with subsequent fluid retention, adds a burden to the heart in patients with cor pulmonale.[2,4] Diuretics were given daily to the patient to regulate this compensatory kidney mechanism by medical means to prevent acid-base imbalance, pulmonary edema, and heart failure.

When the compensating kidney mechanism fails, CO_2 narcosis threatens. This is a common cause of death in these patients and it is important that it be recognized at the onset. The patient begins to get drowsy and shows some mental vagueness; he has a slight cyanosis at rest. As the CO_2 retention increases he becomes sleepier, more confused, and more deeply cyanotic. One sign may be twitching of the fingers at rest which disappears on movement. Intermittent positive pressure breathing must be carefully supervised when early signs of impending CO_2 narcosis are present.[4]

I became aware that Mr. C. did not use the I.P.P.B. machine correctly. When Mr. C. demonstrated how he used the machine, it was obvious that he did not expire the compressed room air properly. He stated, "after six or seven minutes I become sleepy and sometimes fall asleep." Upon further investigation the surprisingly limited knowledge and understanding he had of his disease, except in the area of prognosis, became apparent.

Mr. C.'s complications (chronic cor pulmonale with mild episodes of right heart failure, chronic compensated respiratory acidosis, chronic arterial hypoxia, and hypercapnea) have required close medical supervision and intervention. Four primary medical objectives were identified: (1) To facilitate more effective breathing by decreasing the bronchiolar obstruction using bronchodilators, expectorants, and the Bennett intermittent positive pressure breathing machine in order to decrease arterial hypoxia and hypercapnea. (2) To maintain electrolyte and fluid balance by medication and diet in order to prevent CO_2 narcosis. (3) To decrease the burden of the right ventricle by medication, phlebotomies, and the previous two objectives. (4) To keep the patient hospitalized for the rest of his life in order to provide close medical supervision and "symptomatic relief."

THE DELIBERATIVE NURSING PROCESS

It is my firm belief that a patient must work through his problems in his own way. The patient should be supported by an environment that allows him to do this: an environment that provides the skills, the knowledge, and the assistance the patient requires in solving his individual problems. The problems of the patient and the challenges involved were the central reason for further investigation of Mr. C. and his needs. The problem-solving process was used in an effort to help Mr. C. cope more effectively with the difficulties which beset him and to assist him in strengthening his resources and his problem-solving capacities.

Basic to this problem-solving process was the establishment of a working relationship between Mr. C. and myself. This was effectively accomplished by using Orlando's[8] deliberative nursing process. Orlando presented a conceptual framework from which a nursing care model might evolve. The basic concept underlying her theoretical model involves the "nursing situation" which is comprised of three elements: the patient's behavior, the responses of the nurse, and the nursing action. The interaction of these three elements, when in action and moving through time and space, is the "nursing process." The nursing process is based on the nurse's knowledge (principles that underlie health, environment, and people). This knowledge allows the nurse to attach specific meanings to her observations of the patient's behavior and to plan for the nursing action needed. Orlando believes that nursing action offers whatever the patient may require in order for his needs to be met.

Specific steps in this deliberative nursing process are: (1) The nurse observes the patient's behavior and explores with him its meaning. She pursues the subject until she knows the meaning of the patient's behavior and the specific activity that is required to meet his need(s). (2) The nursing action is carried out in such a way that the patient is helped to inform the nurse as to how the action affects him (an element of basic trust is involved). (3) The nurse follows through on her action to see if the need was relieved. The meaning of the behavior and the nurse action is reevaluated until the need is met and the nurse's purpose in having helped the patient is achieved. (4) The nurse is available to respond to the patient's need and she conveys this to him. (5) The nurse knows how the nursing process affects the patient.

If the nursing process is carried out without exploration for the patient's need or consideration of how the process affects the patient, it constitutes what Orlando calls an "automatic process of activity." Automatic nurse action is usually ineffective in meeting the patient's need except in an emergency situation. This type of "situational" need may be defined as a requirement of the patient which (if and when supplied) diminishes his immediate distress or improves his immediate sense of well-being.

Employing the deliberative process the nurse proceeds to fulfill her independent role as a professional, as described by McManus.[7] Via the problem-solving approach she identifies the nursing problem of the patient and makes a nursing diagnosis. She further determines the objectives of nursing for the patient and his capacity for self-direction, and decides on a course of action. An individual program of nursing care is thus developed, incorporating psychological support and guidance as needed.

The nurse then sees to it that the nursing care program is carried out, either by herself when the patient's need dictates this, or by other members of the health team. She gives continuous direction and supervision of those who assist her, and evaluates and modifies the plan of nursing care as needed. She coordinates the nursing care program with the services of the medical and allied professional practitioners.

ILLUSTRATION OF THE PROBLEM-SOLVING APPROACH USING THE DELIBERATIVE NURSING PROCESS AS A GUIDE TO ACTION

Nursing objectives for Mr. C. were formulated at the beginning of the investigation; deliberate activity toward these objectives was initiated during weekly contacts with him for nine weeks. An evaluation of the nursing process used in meeting Mr. C.'s needs was continually validated by the patient's reactions and behavior.

Nursing Diagnosis

Mr. C.'s behavior suggested that he was depressed, anxious, unaccepting of assistance offered, and that he was not employing any spiritual, social, or intellectual resources. He had little knowledge or understanding of his disease entity except in the area of prognosis. His functional level was inconsistent with his physiological capabilities.

Nursing Objectives

Three primary objectives were identified: (1) To apply the deliberative nursing process with Mr. C. in order to assist him in changing this negative behavior to more positive interdependent behavior; to validate with Mr. C. his needs and his response to the nursing action, and to assist him in maintaining his capabilities, inner strengths, and interest in living. (2) To provide the acceptance, reality-support, and assistance required to help Mr. C. work through his problems with alveolar hypoventilation, thereby enhancing his participation in maintaining the maximum ventilation possible. (3) To support and assist the patient with the designated medical care, teaching the patient the scientific facts about his disability (within the limits of his understanding) and the reasons for the medical measures used.

Examples of Nursing Therapy

1. Problem Identified   The ward staff felt Mr. C. was "uncooperative." His need was to promote the development of productive interpersonal relationships.[1]

Approach used. The concept of Orlando's deliberative nursing process was used to ascertain and validate with Mr. C. his needs and problems.

Reason for approach. "Ineffective patient behavior is used to mean any behavior which prevents the nurse from carrying out her concern for the patient's care or from maintaining a satisfactory relationship to the patient. . . . The nurse must view it as a possible signal of distress or a manifestation of an unmet need."[8] Hildegard Peplau states, "The purpose of nursing has never been merely to help cure. Rather, it has been to offer a warmly human relationship through which people could develop and use their assets and external resources toward the solution of their health problems. The mission of nursing must continue to be creative interpersonal relationships through which patients will achieve self-actualization."[11]

Seven psychosocial needs that are directly related to therapeutic relationships with patients were identified by Biestek[3]:

NEED	PRINCIPLE
•To be dealt with as an individual rather than a case, type, or category	•Treatment as an individual
•To express feelings, both negative and positive	•Purposeful expression of feelings
•To be accepted as a person of worth, regardless of dependency, weakness, faults, or failures	•Acceptance as he is, not as you would want him to be
•Understanding of and response to feelings expressed	•Controlled emotional involvement of the nurse, relating to the patient's needs only
•To be neither judged nor condemned for the difficulty in which he finds himself	•Nonjudgmental attitude
•To make his own choice concerning his life	•Patient self-determination; the environment provides the reality
•To keep confidential information about himself as secret as possible	•Confidentiality

Evaluation of approach. The patient responded to the deliberative nursing process and began to participate actively in his medical regimen. With the aid of the Bennett machine, he was able to get out of bed more often and do things for himself. He began to feel better, to be concerned about other patients near him, and to take an interest in his personal appearance. "I've felt well enough to go in and see Mr. W. next door; he is getting breathing exercises with me and does them better."

2. Problems Identified   Three related problems were: alveolar hypoventilation, moderate to severe dyspnea, and drowsiness when using the Bennett machine. His need was "to facilitate the maintenance of a supply of oxygen to all body cells."[1]

Approach used. I explored with Mr. C. why the I.P.P.B. machine and hand nebulizer were not helping him breathe better and why he was refusing the aminophylline suppositories.

Reason for approach. I could not understand why the Bennett machine was not assisting him in improving his ventilation. Slow, forced expiration should have improved his vital capacity and lowered the residual capacity, which should have improved the ventilation to the lung tissue. Aminophylline suppositories act chiefly on the smooth muscle of the bronchi, decreasing the hypertonicity.

Evaluation of approach. The patient was not expiring properly when using the Bennett machine and was exhibiting symptoms of CO_2 narcosis. Explanation of the physiological reasons for this and instructions on how to expire more adequately helped Mr. C. breathe out slowly and forcibly. He practiced forced expiration with and without using the Bennett machine. I taught Mr. C. to exhale forcibly before using the hand nebulizer so that the medication would be inhaled deeply into the bronchial tree.

The patient improved his technique in using the Bennett and began to use it at the prescribed times. Drowsiness did not recur and some relief of dyspnea was maintained, especially at rest. Mr. C. asked the doctor if breathing exercises might help him and these were ordered. He conscientiously tried to learn the breathing exercises, taught to him by a physical therapist, but was limited in abdominal inspirational breathing and tried too hard to establish the abdominal breathing rhythm.

It was suggested to the patient that he use the breathing exercises and the hand nebulizer for relief of his dyspnea so that he would not become entirely dependent on the Bennett machine. Mr. C. refused aminophylline suppositories because he felt they caused his "stomach distress"; but after an explanation of the bronchial action of the medication, he started using them to assist in breathing.

3. Problem Identified   Mr. C.'s fatigue threshold was low; therefore, he had a decreased capacity for activities. His need was "to promote optimal activity; exercise, rest and sleep."[1]

Approach used. The doctor ordered assistance in dressing activities and instructions in cane walking. These activities were begun cautiously, with progressive increase in activity level as pulmonary ventilation improved.

Reason for approach. Mr. C.'s hematocrit was within normal limits and the potential for thrombus formation did not seem to be a factor. Caution against overstepping his fatigue threshold was stressed because activity may cause an increase in metabolic lactates and increased acidosis. Hypercapnea greatly affects metabolic activity and oxidating processes within the cells, thereby causing a low fatigue threshold and a limit on the patient's activity.

Activities therefore were limited to what Mr. C. felt he was capable of doing. We worked together on increasing his activities progressively, stopping when he became tired or more dyspneic.

Evaluation of approach. At times Mr. C. walked in his room holding onto a wheel chair. He was able to dress himself but he tired easily and became dyspneic when he used his arms above shoulder height. He continued to become fatigued while attempting to eat or ambulate, but felt that he had improved since starting the breathing exercises and since using the Bennett machine. During our last visit, he stated that he could sit up longer each day and that he was sleeping better without any need for his "nerve pills."

4. Problem Identified Mr. C. appeared distressed, apprehensive, and complained of "nervous tension," "jitters," and chest pain (burning pain under the sternal notch). His need was for information and support to enable him to identify and accept his illness emotionally.

Approach used. The deliberative nursing process: The questions that he asked were answered and he was supported during the times he explored his illness emotionally. He was not reprimanded when he did not follow the medical regimen, e.g., when he was observed smoking.

Reason for approach. "Conquest of anxiety implies the acceptance of reality, the acceptance of divinity in ourselves. . . .Knowledge alone is not enough, for with knowledge alone we cannot vanquish anxiety. . . .We must strengthen our confidence in life."[10] Improving the nurse-patient relationship and the patient's ventilation should reduce his restlessness and apprehension. Mr. C. suffered burning chest pain each night for months. The pain was sometimes relieved by Darvon, a synthetic non-narcotic analgesic. The patient requested "nerve pills" several times each night, and placebo capsules were given to replace the Compazine that had been given for months previous to this study.

Evaluation of approach. Mr. C. stopped asking for "nerve pills" after the deliberative process was begun. He began to decrease his requests for medication whereas previously he had required several p.r.n. medications, especially during the night. He spoke at length about himself and his family and of the three years after his discharge from the service. He could not "settle down" and he drank too much. Mr. C. cried during this part of the interview. He related how active he had been in A.A. "It became my life, and I miss working with those guys." He said that the doctor had caught him smoking the other day; "I was so sure I could give it up when they told me to, especially after being able to give up drinking. . . .Maybe tomorrow I can resist smoking that cig when I wake up." During our last interview Mr. C. stated that he had not smoked a cigarette in five days. "Mr. Y. and Mrs. W. [patients] have the same problem and I am trying to help them."

Near the end of the interview Mr. C. thanked the writer for coming to see him every week: "You know, I would rather know what's wrong than to have someone shoot the bull with me."

Outcome

Although all of the nursing care objectives were not achieved, Mr. C.'s behavior did change from negative dependence to a more positive interdependent approach to therapy and activities of living in general. Of course this behavior change, whether real or apparent, will be fully evidenced only by time, for as Orlando[8] warns: "The improvement is always relative to what the nurse and patient start with, to the length of their contact and to what they are able to accomplish."

CONCLUSIONS

Patients and nurses do not always communicate with one another. Sometimes the patient may not be able to communicate effectively and his nonverbal behavior may be the only clue to his plea for help. The behavior becomes meaningful to the nurse if she is aware of the interactions between herself and the patient. We need to look at our communications, verbal and nonverbal, and ascertain how effective they are.

Automatic nurse action tends to stereotype a patient or place him in a fixed category. All emphysematous patients are not alike, any more than any of us are alike; stereotyping is a poor foundation for an effective nurse-patient relationship.

The deliberative nursing process stems from a theoretical model that seems to lend itself to a consistent, meaningful, and productive relationship with the individual patient. When the patient and his family are active participants in the planned program of care the basic purpose of nursing is more likely to be achieved and the planned care is successful: the nurse helps the patient meet his need(s). Inherent in the deliberative nursing process is the problem-solving approach which guides the nursing process.

A vital component of the problem-solving approach is the nurse's *acceptance of the patient as he is* when he enters the hospital. Many times we expect the patient to behave at or progress to a level which he never has achieved and is incapable of achieving. The nurse should consider the patient's resources (his personality, his family, and his community) and then keep in mind that he achieves his self-actualization level from these resources; they are the foundation upon which realistic individual planning for patient care can be achieved. The deliberative nursing process provides for effective nursing care because the nursing care goals are in harmony with the patient's goals, his capabilities, and his resources.

REFERENCES

1. Abdellah, F. G., et al. *Patient-Centered Approaches to Nursing.* New York, The Macmillan Co., 1960, p. 16.

2. *Basic Respiratory Physiology Taken From Standard Texts.* Bird Institute Lecture Series, Publication No. 9262. Palm Springs, California.

3. Biestek, F. P. *The Casework Relationship.* Chicago, Loyola University Press, 1957.

4. Elwood, E. *The Battle of Breathlessness. Nursing Care of the Disoriented Patient.* Monograph No. 13. New York, American Nurses' Association, 1962, pp. 5–15.

5. Guyton, A. C. *Textbook of Medical Physiology.* 3rd Ed. Philadelphia, W. B. Saunders Co., 1966.

6. Haas, A., and Luczak, A. *The Application of Physical Medicine and Rehabilitation to Emphysema Patients.* Monograph No. 21. New York, Institute of Physical Medicine and Rehabilitation, 1963.

7. McManus, R. L. Nurses want a chance to be professional. *Modern Hospital,* 64:89, October, 1958.

8. Orlando, I. J. *The Dynamic Nurse-Patient Relationship.* New York, G. P. Putnam's Sons, 1961.

9. Sodeman, W. A. *Pathologic Physiology.* Philadelphia, W. B. Saunders Co., 1956.

10. Steiner, H., and Gebser, J. *Anxiety: A Condition of Modern Man.* New York, Dell Publishing Co., Inc., 1962, pp. 11, 105.

11. Peplau, H. E. Automation: Will It Change Nurses, Nursing, or Both? *Technical Innovations in Health Care: Nursing Implications.* Monograph No. 5. New York, American Nurses' Association, 1962, p. 37.

3

Nursing Diagnosis

After the assessment phase of the nursing process comes the planning phase. In Chapter 3, the initial steps of the planning phase are discussed. After collecting data and processing this information according to the areas of responsibility of nurses, it becomes necessary to make a decision—a *nursing diagnosis*—on the areas of care in which the client needs assistance from the nurse. The nursing diagnosis is the first part of the nursing care plan; orders are the other part. After making a diagnosis, these areas must be ranked in priority according to the health status of the client within a given time, space, and recovery framework.

Bower (1972) states that as a client, one is free to make decisions about oneself and to be involved in one's own care. This coincides with the writings of May (1960), an existential psychologist who emphasizes the dimensions of will, decision, and choice in one's life. Therefore, the nurse must recognize the client as an important contributor to decision-making.

Chapter 3 will discuss the cognitive dimensions of establishing a nursing diagnosis and the importance of responding to priorities. The case presented in Chapter 2 will then be used to demonstrate the establishing of diagnoses and setting of priorities.

Referring back to the equation

$$\begin{array}{c} \text{Client Data} \\ \text{System Data} \end{array} + \begin{array}{c} \text{Nursing Responsibilities} \\ \text{Nurse's Knowledge} \\ \text{The Nurse} \end{array} \rightarrow \begin{array}{c} \text{Individualized} \\ \text{Nursing Diagnoses and} \\ \text{Nursing Orders} \end{array}$$

it can be seen readily that the nursing care plan consisting of nursing diagnoses and orders results from a combination of various types of input: client data, system data, responsibilities, knowledge, and, of course, the nurse. This third segment of the equation represents the planning phase of the nursing process. It is the decision segment and is highly dependent on the first two parts. For strong, individualized nursing decisions to be made, sufficient data and knowledge are necessary.

COGNITIVE DIMENSIONS OF
A NURSING DIAGNOSIS

Rothberg (1967, p. 1040) defines the nursing diagnosis as "an evaluation by nurses of those factors affecting the patient which will influence his recovery." She includes intrinsic factors, such as physical and emotional states, and external conditions, such as work, family, and environmental situations. Durand and Prince (1966, p. 52) amplified their earlier discussion of a nursing diagnosis by noting it is "a statement of a conclusion resulting from a recognition of a pattern derived from a nursing investigation of the patient." They included two aspects: the process of diagnosis and the decision.

The nursing diagnosis is viewed as a conclusive statement concerning an individual's nursing needs, based on scientific determination (Komorita, 1963). It is based on every known and surmised factor within an individual that can have an effect on his dignity, rights, well-being, recovery, and pursuit of a meaningful life style. It provides the basis for nursing orders (Yura and Walsh, 1973). Webster (1971) defines diagnosis as an investigation of the facts to determine the nature and cause of a condition, situation, or problem and the resultant decision of such examination.

Clear, simple, and specific statements should characterize nursing diagnoses. They should articulate succinctly an identified problem in the client's sytem. Furthermore, they should address problems and needs of the client and all significant variables in the identified system. Problems include those considered to be potential as well as actual (Mayers, 1972). Diagnoses are dynamic since they change in response to data. Because the area for which nursing is responsible spans a broader field than medicine's, nursing diagnoses have the effect of being greater in number with evident progression.

Because nursing terms are not standardized, it is necessary to discuss the diversity in nursing language as it relates to the diagnostic function in nursing. The literature uses synonymous terms for nursing diagnosis with many authors referring to "patient problems," "nursing problems," "patient needs," "nursing goals," and other terms (Andruskiw and Battick, 1964; Blair, 1971; Woods, 1966). There is also a controversy in the use of the term "nursing orders" versus "approaches." Obviously the term "diagnosis" carries an emotional connotation if one assumes that only physicians can diagnose. Even though what is the proper word should not be a paramount issue as long as intent is clear, "diagnosis" does convey the idea of accountability for a nurse's decision. As far back as 1961, Abdellah emphasized establishing a nursing diagnosis as an independent function of the nurse.

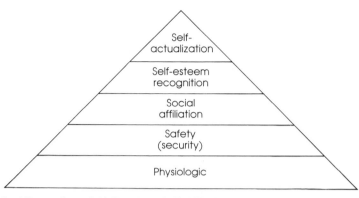

SOURCE: Paul Hersey, Kenneth H. Blanchard, MANAGEMENT OF ORGANIZATIONAL BEHAVIOR: Utiliz-ing Human Resources, 3rd edition, © 1977, p. 33. Reprinted by permission of Prentice-Hall, Inc., Englewood Cliffs, New Jersey.

FIGURE 3-1
MASLOW'S HIERARCHY OF NEEDS

There has also been energy devoted by our colleagues to develop a systematic description of nursing diagnosis which represents the entire domain of nursing (Bircher, 1975; Gebbie and Lavin, 1974). Even though these identifications can be perceived as lending unity and clarification to nurses and their responsibilities, recipes do little for individualized nursing care. There may be merit, however, in using classifications as the basis for promoting the need for individualized nursing diagnoses for each individual client.

The cognitive aspects of establishing nursing diagnoses are important in terms of providing a rationale for diagnoses and orders. The next area will focus on recognizing and responding to diagnoses as priorities.

Conceptual Framework for Establishing Diagnostic Priorities

The conceptual framework used in helping the nurse to arrange nursing diagnoses into priorities was developed by Abraham Maslow. He discussed a hierarchy into which classifications of human needs can be ordered (Maslow, 1954), as shown in Figure 3-1. In order of priority, these needs are: physiologic, safety, social, self-esteem, self-actualization. The needs are vital parts of the client's system.

According to Maslow, the physiologic needs (shown at the bottom of the pyramid) are top priority when unsatisfied and remain as having the highest priority until satisfied. Once the physiologic needs become less important or are not threatened, safety needs take priority. This format follows through to self-actualization, which is a priority only when the other four areas in a person's need system are gratified. Hersey and Blanchard (1977)* diagram this movement as shown in Figure 3-2.

*Hersey and Blanchard write for a leadership perspective. Applications to nursing are the author's.

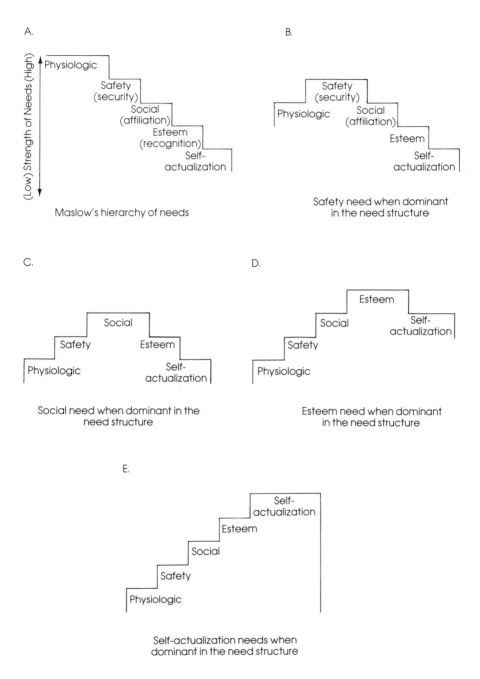

A. Maslow's hierarchy of needs

B. Safety need when dominant in the need structure

C. Social need when dominant in the need structure

D. Esteem need when dominant in the need structure

E. Self-actualization needs when dominant in the need structure

SOURCE: Paul Hersey, Kenneth H. Blanchard, MANAGEMENT OF ORGANIZATIONAL BEHAVIOR: Utilizing Human Resources, 3rd Edition, © 1977, pp. 30, 31, 32. Reprinted by permission of Prentice-Hall, Inc., Englewood Cliffs, New Jersey.

FIGURE 3-2
MOVEMENT OF PRIORITY OF NEEDS

To understand Maslow's hierarchy of needs within a nursing framework more fully, a discussion of each need will follow.

Physiologic Needs   The physiologic needs are those that are basic to life: air, water, food, clothing, and shelter. According to Chapman and Chapman's advocacy helping model (1975), needs in this area of Maslow's hierarchy fall under lifesaving (prevention of imminent death) and life-sustaining (health maintenance and prevention of complications following bodily insult) dimensions. Technologic input is high and social-emotional support and client participation is low.

Sufficient operation of the body is a foremost priority. Until threat to life is removed, these needs are paramount (Hersey and Blanchard, 1977). It follows, therefore, that when a client is in physiologic crisis and must be monitored constantly, security needs, such as socioeconomic issues, are not in priority. That is, when a client's life is in imminent danger, the client is not concerned about a possible change in work position due to the disease. When physiologic needs become satisfied, however, other levels of needs become important.

Safety (Security)   This is the second level of Maslow's hierarchy. Hersey and Blanchard (1977) define these as involved with self-preservation. Included are freedom from physical danger and deprivation of basic physiologic needs. There is an environmental awareness regarding one's own or a family's safety and preservation. Hospital costs, medical fees, and job security are all examples. Gellerman's (1968) research earmarks safety and security needs as appearing both overtly and covertly.

When basic life-threatening crises are past, safety needs emerge as priorities. In order for a client to move to higher level needs, security needs must be somewhat satisfied.

Social (Affiliation)   Included in this need structure, cogently expressed by Hersey and Blanchard (1977), are meaningful interpersonal relationships, group acceptance, and belonging. When social needs are unsatisfied, a nurse may observe boredom in clients (Mayo, 1975), apathy, desire to have friends and family visit, and other signs. There may be expression of concern for other clients in the environment and employees. This is the movement from self to others. It parallels Chapman and Chapman's (1975) third dimension of their helping model labeled "life-enhancing," that is, one's relationship with the world.

Esteem   When a client first seeks to belong, the positive values of belonging emerge as priorities and should be satisfied if a nurse desires the client to reach fullest potential. Instead of just feeling like a part of a system or group, the person who has esteem needs in focus will seek recognition and respect from others, prestige, and power. The client may want to be useful in some way, either by being personally involved in or by helping in another's case. Responsibility for helping a roommate may occur. It must be remembered that recognition involves another person. If one seeks esteem, this must be noticed and reinforced (Hersey and Blanchard, 1977). In other words, when a client tells you what she did to help herself or another, you should communicate your awareness of the achievement back to the client.

Unfortunately, needs in this area are not always acted on in a positive framework (Hersey and Blanchard, 1977). The client, for example, who has a full leg cast and impaired mobility, yet consciously disobeys his order to stay in bed or call for help when using the bathroom facilities, may be exhibiting an unfulfilled esteem need. It becomes the nurse's responsibility to satisfy this need area with measures that capitalize on the client's strengths. Once the need is satisfied by other means and in positive frameworks, maladaptive behavior will generally decrease.

Self-actualization This need structure is of the highest order, becoming prominent when all others are satisfied. It involves one's desire to reach fullest potential (Hersey and Blanchard, 1977). Moreover, this potential is with awareness of one's own strengths and weaknesses—it is reality based.

A nurse can perceive clients to be at this level if they strive to help themselves and their environment on their own—independently—yet are dependent and interdependent according to their own direction, as is necessary.

Maslow's Hierarchy of Needs in Nursing Practice

Nurses must constantly strive to satisfy the needs of clients at the level implicitly and explicitly expressed by the person. Maslow's structural framework provides a useful basis by which practitioners can determine priorities of client needs. The framework should be considered only in response to the client's nursing diagnosis.

The levels of needs Maslow delineated should not be construed in nursing as absolute. They must be interpreted in light of the client's system and the nurse's goals. In other words, one can be predominantly at a social level regarding recovery, yet may in reality be at a self-actualizing level in the work position. These levels must also be visualized as overlapping when priorities are set.

Based on the areas of nursing responsibility delineated in Chapter 2, a general framework of use may be developed. Paralleling areas of nursing responsibility with Maslow's hierarchy can be a useful base in beginning to

TABLE 3-1
MASLOW'S HIERARCHY OF NEEDS PARALLELED WITH
AREAS OF NURSING RESPONSIBILITY: GUIDELINES

Maslow	Areas of Nursing Responsibility
Physiologic	• nutrition
	• sleep, rest patterns
	• elimination
	• prevention of complications
	• assurance of physiologic status—health maintenance
Safety (security)	• comfort
	• exercise
	• personal hygiene
	• safety
	• environmental considerations
	• spiritual comfort and assistance
	• emotional support, counseling
	• teaching
Social (affiliation)	• diversional activities
	• socializing and privacy
Self-esteem	• an amplification of what has emerged before, but considering the client's need for achievement
Self-actualization	• the client can take care of self— allow it!

establish priorities of needs. See Table 3-1. The guidelines indicate where the need might emerge and also the progression through all levels of the hierarchy.

Thus far this chapter has discussed the cognitive dimensions of nursing diagnosis, in addition to Maslow's theory as the conceptual framework for determining priorities of diagnosed needs. The last portion of this chapter will use the case example begun in Chapter 2 to illustrate how to establish nursing diagnoses as well as how to rank priorities.

CASE EXAMPLE ON NURSING DIAGNOSES AND PRIORITIES

Nursing diagnoses are decisive statements concerning a client's nursing needs. Nursing diagnoses should be framed by the uniqueness of the client. Needs of the client should be arranged according to priorities. One useful means for making diagnostic statements is to follow this formula:

The client needs _____
because _____

The first part of the formula becomes the diagnosis; the latter is rationale. The rationale gives the specific reasons behind an individual client's requirements. The rationale also becomes helpful in developing nursing orders (see Chapter 4).

It is possible to have more than one diagnosis from each area of responsibility. Moreover, since there is overlap, it is important that the designer of nursing care gives comprehensive consideration to diagnosing rather than worrying about the proper place for diagnoses relative to the nurse's areas of responsibility. *The important goal is that all areas should be considered.*

The classification of nursing diagnoses by rationale and priorities is illustrated in Table 3-2 on pages 64–69, based on the case of Mr. Munson, as begun in Chapter 2. According to this method, aspects of organizing this information include: areas of nursing responsibility, a formula nursing diagnosis and rationale (the client needs _____ because _____), a nursing diagnostic statement, and a priority rating.

As can be seen in Table 3-2, diagnoses are established and then are classified according to levels on Maslow's hierarchy; next, the decision is made determining which are present or future (or both) oriented. Nursing care should be progressive, moving from what is absolutely essential to preserve life to all other areas. The actions of putting the diagnoses into operation or specifying nursing orders also reflect Maslow's need hierarchy. A diagnosis may be pertinent in a past framework, but its relevance may change with respect to the reality of here-and-now.

To follow the priority and diagnosis process step by step, let us first look at the specific needs which were delineated:

NURSING DIAGNOSTIC STATEMENT	TYPE OF NEED
• Self-maintenance of personal comfort measures	Physiologic
• Assurance of balanced diet, respectful of diabetes; investigation and treatment of anorexia	Physiologic
• Knowledge of disease process and its link with physical exercise	Safety
• Paced physical activity schedule	Safety
• Self-maintenance of hygiene needs	Physiologic
• Teaching to chart I & O, care for monitor leads and testing urine	Safety
• Adequate rest patterns; built-in periods of quiet throughout the day	Physiologic
• Diversional activities, respectful of environment and need for rest	Social
• Recognition for what he does for himself and others	Self-esteem
• Maintenance of privacy as much as possible	Safety/Self-esteem
• Expansion of social contacts	Social
• Self-maintenance of bowel and bladder elimination	Physiologic
• Prevention of elimination difficulties	Physiologic

(Table continues)

NURSING DIAGNOSTIC STATEMENT	TYPE OF NEED
•Safety of self within new environment	Safety
•Awareness and understanding of environment	Safety/Social/Self-esteem
•Acceptance and understanding of his diabetic condition	Safety
•Self-control of his own balanced diet	Safety
•Regulation of his own insulin needs	Safety
•Respectful, trusting, nurse/patient relationship	Social
•Physical signs and symptoms relating to an MI and diabetes closely monitored	Physiologic
•Understanding of his overall life style and what is important to consider	All levels
•Design for building in a leadership position at work, in exercise, and in relation to his diabetic condition so that stressors are paced evenly throughout	All levels
•Awareness of himself when stress mounts	All levels
•Control of his own body stress patterns	All levels

The next step is to separate those diagnoses that are important to consider in the present system from those that should be dealt with in the future or are of no immediate concern. Overlapping areas may occur. Keep in mind Maslow's hierarchy—physiologic and safety needs predominate, if pertinent at the present time.

PRESENT-ORIENTED DIAGNOSES	FUTURE-ORIENTED DIAGNOSES
•Physical signs and symptoms relating to an MI and diabetes closely monitored	• Knowledge of disease process and its link with physical exercise
•Safety of self within new environment	• Paced physical activity schedule
•Prevention of elimination difficulties	• Diversional activities, respectful of environment and need for rest
•Adequate rest patterns; built-in periods of quiet throughout the day	• Expansion of social contacts
•Assurance of balanced diet, respectful of diabetes; investigation and treatment of anorexia	• Acceptance and understanding of his diabetic condition
•Respectful, trusting nurse/patient relationship	• Self-control of his own balanced diet
•Awareness and understanding of environment	• Regulation of his own insulin needs
•Maintenance of privacy as much as possible	• Understanding of his overall life style and what is important to consider
•Self-maintenance of hygiene needs	• Design for building in a leadership position at work, in exercise, and in relation to his diabetic condition so that stressors are paced evenly throughout
•Self-maintenance of personal comfort measures	• Awareness of himself when stress mounts
	• Control of his own body stress patterns

- Teaching to chart I & O, care for monitor leads and testing urine
- Self-maintenance of bowel and bladder elimination
- Recognition for what he does for himself and others

The next step of the procedure is to number the present concerns, moving from those needs that are absolutely essential to meet immediately to those that can be put off for a while. There will be variance between practitioners in this area, but exact sequence is not an issue.

Nursing Diagnoses Arranged According to Priorities
1. Physical signs and symptoms relating to an MI and diabetes closely monitored
2. Safety of client himself within new environment
3. Prevention of elimination difficulties
4. Adequate rest patterns; built-in periods of quiet throughout the day
5. Assurance of balanced diet, respectful of diabetes; investigation and treatment of anorexia
6. Respectful, trusting nurse/patient relationship
7. Awareness and understanding of environment
8. Maintenance of privacy as much as possible
9. Self-maintenance of hygiene needs
10. Self-maintenance of personal comfort measures
11. Teaching to chart I & O, caring for monitor leads, and testing urine
12. Self-maintenance of bowel and bladder elimination
13. Recognition of what he does for himself and others

This listing ranks the diagnoses in order of importance. You can see that there is more of a horizontal than a vertical priority between nursing diagnoses 1 and 6, as well as between 7 and 12. The client's needs should be met in this order. Future-oriented diagnoses must be kept in mind when designating orders because they probably will emerge as priorities at a future point. It must be recognized, however, that there is a limit as to what should be expected for accomplishment—it is impossible to encompass all needs, situations, and changes in one given time and space. Furthermore, it is stressful to overload a client and the nurse.

It is important to note that the diagnoses resulting from data processing are not perceived specifically as pertinent only to the client in the case example—the essence of the diagnoses may be applicable to many clients. This process, however, insures that you have knowledge of the individual client so

(Text continues on page 70)

AREAS OF NURSING RESPONSIBILITY	FORMULA NURSING DIAGNOSIS	RATIONALE	NURSING DIAGNOSTIC STATEMENT	PRIORITY OF DIAGNOSES
				P=Present F=Future P/F=Both
Comfort	The client needs: • To continue to maintain his own personal comfort measures	Because: • He is not in any present distress; chest pain has not recurred and no respiratory distress is noted. Even though he is usually fairly active, it must be noted that he tires easily and has a history of intermittent dyspnea with stress. He sleeps with one to two pillows as he is comfortable. He is independent. It seems that he can care for this aspect himself.	(Remember that this should be a statement concerning what client needs from you; it can be called a "nursing goal.") • Self-maintenance of personal comfort measures	P Physiologic need, fulfilled by himself
Nutrition	• To receive balanced nutrients respectful of a 2,000-calorie diabetic diet	• Client is not receiving proper nutrition; he does not like the food sent by the kitchen and refuses meals since they are not in line with his usual eating patterns. This is contributing to a caloric deficit and insulin regulation becomes difficult. At home he is controlled and has a good appetite. Neither is evident in the hospital. Anxiety may be a causative factor in his lack of an appetite. Teaching is needed and will be addressed in that section.	• Assurance of balanced diet, respectful of diabetes; investigation and treatment of anorexia.	P Physiologic need necessary for life

64

Exercise	•To continue his usual state of exercise (above average), but to recognize that he must always respond to his feelings of fatigue and pace himself accordingly	He is a very active individual, engaging in many physical sports. Physically he looks muscular and robust even though stating he tires easily. With the presence of a possible MI, he may have to plan a more clearly paced schedule of physical activity and exercise. It is felt that he needs to become more receptive to changes through knowledge of his physical boundaries. When he accepts this—and because of his independent traits—he probably will be able to respond wisely to the exercise needs of his own body.	•Knowledge of disease process and its link with physical exercise •Paced physical activity schedule	P/F Safety (self-preservation) need, although some aspects relate to other areas P/F Same as above
Hygiene	•To be able to maintain his own hygienic measures	•He is independent and seems totally capable of caring for himself. He can get OOB but since he is on intake and output, he must be taught to chart himself. S/A coverage must be considered and care of monitor leads taught.	•Self-maintenance of hygienic needs •Teaching him to chart I & O, care for monitor leads and test urine	P Physiologic Needs P Safety (self-preservation) need
Sleep, rest patterns	•To be assured of adequate rest around coronary care environment and procedures	•He tires easily and is anxious concerning hospitalization. At home he sleeps well with one or two pillows, whichever he desires. Monitoring of vital signs during the night is necessary. Medication for sleep is PRN and he is on Valium for muscle relaxation, QID.	•Adequate rest patterns; built-in periods of quiet throughout the day	P Physiologic need

(Table 3-2 continues)

TABLE 3-2 (continued)

AREAS OF NURSING RESPONSIBILITY	FORMULA NURSING DIAGNOSIS	RATIONALE	NURSING DIAGNOSTIC STATEMENT	PRIORITY OF DIAGNOSES P=Present F=Future P/F=Both
Diversional activity	The client needs: • To be introduced to diversional activities in his present environment reflecting his likes and his rest schedule	Because: • He is in the hospital because of a possible MI, even though no pain or respiratory difficulty is evident. Limited activity is important, with the diversion necessity. Tiring easily, he still seems to have difficulty accepting restrictions. He is anxious, wants a definite answer to his medical diagnosis, wants to go home, and enjoys visiting with other patients. His dislike of inactivity pervades all. Exercise as diversional activity was previously discussed in that area.	• Diversional activities, respectful of environment and need for rest	P Social need
Socializing and privacy	• To have his need for recognition and affiliation met and maintained	• He seems to be socially active and a leader in outside groups. Not being able to participate in a bowling competition—and since he is captain of the team—he feels guilty. He maintains his independence but likes to talk with other patients. Commode privileges should be handled with finesse.	• Recognition for what he does for himself and others • Maintenance of privacy as much as possible • Expansion of social contacts	P/F Self-esteem need; can be filled in part by present environment but will become more important later. P Safety (self-preservation) need P Social needs
Elimination	• To continue to privately maintain elimination needs	• He is independent and able to care for self. Urine must be tested for insulin coverage and even though no bowel constipation is evident, the nurse must be alert for any dysfunction due to the nature of disease process.	• Self-maintenance of bowel and bladder elimination (charting of I & O previously discussed) • Prevention of elimination difficulties	P Physiologic need P Safety need

66

Safety	•To be able to plan and secure his own safety	•He is an above average sized man who seems totally capable of ensuring his own safety. Since he is on Valium, he must be aware of its effects even though no dizziness or nausea have been noted.	•Safety of self within new environment	P Safety need
Environmental considerations	•To adjust to the environmental limitations by understanding rationale for the policies in existence. He also needs to have his social needs met (addressed previously in that area)	•Setting is a coronary care unit. He is on a monitor and has commode and OOB privileges. Visiting hours imposed by institution make client unhappy since he feels secluded from his family and close friends. He wants to be with them for a longer period of time. Also a dislike for being in a private room is obvious.	•Awareness and understanding of environment	P Safety need Social need Self-esteem need
Teaching	•To understand the nature of diabetes and his control of the process through proper diet and insulin administration. Education regarding pacing of his exercise regimen was previously discussed	•Capitalizing on the independent, responsible, leader-like person that the client portrays, he obviously has problems owning the diabetic process as part of himself. This is conclusive in his haphazard diet, high FBS and cholesterol, and statement that he has "no problems."	•Acceptance and understanding of his diabetic condition •Self-control of his own balanced diet •Regulation of his own insulin needs	P/F Safety need, but not a priority at this time. P/F Same P/F Same

[Table 3-2 continues]

TABLE 3-2 (continued)

AREAS OF NURSING RESPONSIBILITY	FORMULA NURSING DIAGNOSIS	RATIONALE	NURSING DIAGNOSTIC STATEMENT	PRIORITY OF DIAGNOSES
				P = Present F = Future P/F = Both
Spiritual	The client needs: •To be provided a respectful and trusting relationship so that needs can be verbalized with the nurse if they emerge in the client	Because: •He seems to be sensitive and be part of a close family structure. His need for spiritual support is not presently evident; however, the nurse must establish a close relationship to be available for guidance, should a need emerge in the client within this area. Having a possible MI may be very frightening.	•Respectful, trusting nurse/patient relationship	P Social need
Prevention of complications	•To be closely watched for signs and symptoms of a moderate-severe MI	•The client is in a critical period; the diagnosis of MI is not established. The nurse must be keenly alert for signs affirming the diagnosis. Also, recurrent MI symptoms can be lethal and all fine discriminations pointing to that end must be observed, noted, and acted upon with haste. Awareness of arrhythmias evidenced on the cardiac monitor are earmarked.	•Physical signs and symptoms relating to an MI and diabetes closely monitored	P Physiologic need

| Assurance of physiologic status—health maintenance | • To adapt overall life style to a pace that is keenly responsive to his bodily signs of stress | • He has diabetes and is extremely physically active. Being sensitive and bright, he constantly questions, verbally and nonverbally, and becomes anxious. As a foreman, he must look at his position responsibilities to ultimately design a pattern for his overall life style that includes all activities but evenly meshed and paced. | • Understanding of his overall life style and what is important to consider
• Design for building in a leadership position at work in relation to exercises to his diabetic condition so that stressors are paced evenly throughout
• Awareness of himself when stress mounts
• Control of his own body stress patterns | P/F
Physiologic, safety, and social needs with the aim to have the client become self-actualized in controlling all. |
| Emotional support and counseling | • To have relief from anxiety of not being sure of his diagnosis. At the same time, he should be aware of all that is happening | (Emotional support and counseling should be a thread through all the identified areas. Those aspects not covered, however, can be discussed here.)
• He is pervasively anxious and wants to control himself. He must be aware of all that is going on regarding his care. Sometimes he hesitates to question and the respectful, trusting, helping relationship diagnosed under spiritual needs carries into play here. | • Relief of anxiety that pervades areas of present situation and environment | P
Safety/social needs |

that personalized care will be ordered and implemented as it relates to the diagnoses. By following the design in this chapter, the nurse should have at her fingertips the rationale for every action and what should be done to capitalize on the client's status and potential.

SUMMARY

Chapter 3 has focused on nursing diagnoses, exploring the cognitive dimensions as well as a conceptual framework for establishing priorities. A case example constructed in Chapter 2 was used to exemplify these two processes.

The next chapter is concerned with writing nursing orders for each diagnosis. The content of Chapters 3 and 4, nursing diagnoses and orders, generally comprises the nursing care plan.

REFERENCES

Abdellah, F. Meeting patient needs—an approach to teaching. Paper presented at the biennial convention of the National League for Nursing, Cleveland, Ohio, April 10–14, 1961.

Andruskiw, O., and Battick, B. Identification of nursing problems. *Nursing Research* 13:75–78, 1964.

Bircher, A. On the development and classification of diagnoses. *Nursing Forum* 14:10–29, 1975.

Blair, K. It's the patient's problem—and decision. *Nursing Outlook* 19:587–589, 1971.

Bower, F. *The process of planning nursing care.* St. Louis: C. V. Mosby, 1972.

Chapman, J., and Chapman, H. *Behavior and health case: A humanistic helping process.* St. Louis: C. V. Mosby, 1975.

Durand, M., and Prince, R. Nursing diagnosis: Process and decision. *Nursing Forum* 5:50–64, 1966.

Gebbie, K., and Lavin, M. Classifying nursing diagnoses. *American Journal of Nursing* 74:250–253, 1974.

Gellerman, S. *Motivation and productivity.* New York: American Management Association, 1968.

Hersey, P., and Blanchard, K. *Management of organizational behavior: Utilizing human resources.* Englewood Cliffs, N.J.: Prentice-Hall, 1977.

Komorita, N. Nursing diagnosis. *American Journal of Nursing* 63:83–86, 1963.

Maslow, A. *Motivation and Personality.* New York: Harper and Row, 1954.

May, R. *Existential psychology.* New York: Random House, 1960.

Mayers, M. *A systematic approach to the nursing care plan.* New York: Appleton-Century-Crofts, 1972.

Mayo, E. *The social problems of an industrial civilization.* Boston: Howard Business School, 1945.

Rothberg, J. Why nursing diagnosis? *American Journal of Nursing* 67:1040–1042, 1967.

Webster's Third International Dictionary. Springfield, Massachusetts: G. & C. Merriam Company, 1971.

Woods, N. Measuring a patient's need and progress. *Nursing Outlook* 14:38–41, 1966.

Yura, H., and Walsh, M. *The nursing process.* New York: Appleton-Century-Crofts, 1973.

SELECTED READINGS

In the first of the two readings, Durand and Prince (1966) provide further discussion on the procedure for building a nursing diagnosis. They used an inductive approach. Rothberg (1967) gives rationale for the need for nursing diagnoses in nursing practice. This is based on the diagnosis as a requisite for goal-directed care plans.

Nursing Diagnosis:
Process and Decision

Mary Durand Thomas, R.N., M.S.N.
Rosemary Prince Coombs, R.N., M.N.

The diagnostic process is not unique to any one occupation or profession. The medical history, the physical examination, and the laboratory tests which lead to the physician's diagnosis have been compared to the work of the police detective, who asks questions, examines clues and submits material to a crime lab for the data he needs to identify a criminal accurately.[1] When a student is not achieving at the expected level, educators seek out the strengths and weaknesses of his performance so as to make an educational diagnosis.[2] A social worker gathers facts from the client and the client's family "to make as exact a definition as possible of the situation and personality of a human being in some social need."[3] In recent nursing literature, the term "nursing diagnosis" has occurred with increasing frequency.[4]

If everyone is diagnosing, how is nursing diagnosis similar to and different from the diagnoses made by other professions and occupations? There are similarities. Every diagnosis begins with the gathering of facts. The facts may be a hematocrit of 30 percent, the location of a stray bullet, the inability to add a column of figures, or the report that the father of a large family has lost his job. At some time during or at the completion of the fact-gathering, the practitioner in a given field recognizes a pattern. He then states his conclusion.

Differences in diagnoses arise from each practitioner's view of his role behaviors and responsibilities and from the knowledge necessary for the practice of each profession. The nurse's definition of nursing determines both her view of nursing responsibilities and the knowledge those responsibilities require. Our definition of nursing is consistent with Hall's conception of nursing as a professional process involving three over-lapping aspects: (1) *the nurturing aspect—a close interpersonal relationship concerned with the intimate bodily care of patients;* (2) *the medical aspect shared with the medical profession and concerned with assisting the patient through his medical, surgical, and rehabilitative care;* and (3) *the helping aspect, shared with all professional persons and involving therapeutic interpersonal skills to assist the patient in self-actualization.*[5]

With a working definition of nursing in mind, a nurse can make a nursing diagnosis which specifies an aspect of the patient's condition that requires

Reprinted with permission of Nursing Publications, Inc., 194-B Kinderkamack Road, Park Ridge, New Jersey, from *Nursing Forum* Vol. 5, No. 4, pp. 50–64.

nursing care. How does a nurse make a nursing diagnosis? What is a nursing diagnosis?

We define a nursing diagnosis as *a statement of a conclusion resulting from a recognition of a pattern derived from a nursing investigation of the patient.* We visualize this definition as implying the two aspects of diagnosis— (1) *the process of diagnosing* and (2) *the decision, or actual diagnosis.* (Figure I). We will explain this definition as we have used it to make nursing diagnoses. In practice, the process of diagnosing, including the nursing investigation and the thought process leading to the recognition of a pattern, precedes the actual diagnosis.

NURSING INVESTIGATION

The nursing investigation begins with a collection of facts. Some of these facts are gained from members of the health team through written and spoken communication.

The patient's chart is the major means of written communication. The admission, or face, sheet gives us facts regarding the patient's age, sex, marital status, occupation, religion, and place of residence. The medical history and physical examination provide us with the patient's past and present experiences of illness. In the physician's progress notes we find an overview of changes in the patient's condition since hospitalization. The physician's orders

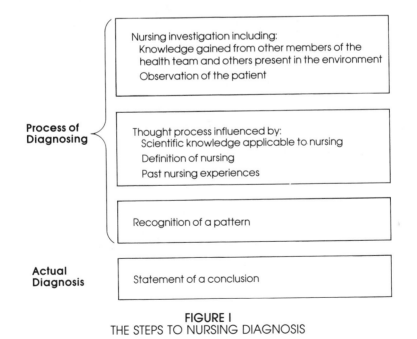

FIGURE I
THE STEPS TO NURSING DIAGNOSIS

outline the plan for diagnostic studies and therapy. Reports of diagnostic studies add to our information about the patient's present illness. The nurses' notes are reviewed for nursing observations of the patient.

Spoken communication with nurses who have cared or are caring for the patient complement the information gained from the chart. These nurses may be asked such questions as: "Tell me about Mr. G. What is he like as a person?" and "What signs and symptoms did you observe?" Other health team members, such as the medical social worker, the physical therapist, the occupational therapist, and the inhalation therapist, may be asked questions relevant to their information about the patient.

Communication with the patient's family and friends may yield information regarding the patient's prehospitalization habits. A question such as "What was he like before he became ill?" may elicit facts not obtained from the health team members.

A major source of fact collection is our own observation of the patient. Observation, as we use it, implies the use of four of the five senses. We visually observe the patient to detect overt physical and psychological signs of illness. We talk to the patient and listen to his responses, and we may listen to sounds from the heart or chest or abdomen. We may touch the patient at the site of a subjective complaint, such as pain. We may smell discharges from body orifices or from a wound.

We make statements or ask questions in order to elicit further information from the patient regarding his expectations about hospitalization, his views of his illness, and his prehospital daily activities concerning food, exercise, elimination and rest and sleep. We utilize information already obtained from other sources to guide our statements or questions and to prevent our subjecting the patient to repetitive questioning.

RECOGNITION OF A PATTERN

As we proceed in fact collection, we continually ask ourselves questions to determine the relatedness of facts and to structure our data collection. Mr. T mentions that his barium enema showed a "mass" in his abdomen. On his history it is noted that he had a cancerous lesion removed from his lip four years previously. Could he be concerned about a recurrence of cancer?

We ask ourselves how our present observations compare or contrast with those made previously by other health team members. A nurse observes that Mrs. E's newly applied cast is saturated with a blood stain measuring one inch in diameter. Fifteen minutes later we find the blood stain is two inches in diameter. Information concerning the possibility of hemorrhage may be sought by measurement of the blood pressure and heart beat, by inspection of skin color, and by consultation with the physician about his expectations regarding bleeding. Thus, one fact helps us to structure further observations.

The thought process through which the relatedness of facts is seen is influenced by our background of scientific knowledge, by past nursing experiences, and by our definition of nursing.

Scientific knowledge applicable to nursing may be drawn from such sciences as psychology, sociology, anthropology, anatomy, physiology, pathology, and bacteriology. Our education in these sciences forms our background working knowledge. Referral to new scientific findings keeps us informed about changing trends. Scientific knowledge is reinforced and expanded by our past nursing experiences with patients exhibiting similar signs and symptoms. Together, scientific knowledge and past experiences provide a mental card file of facts and principles to which we refer as we seek the significance of our obervations.

Thus, as we seek the relationship of facts, we are influenced by these considerations: a certain scientific mechanism may be present; an observation from past experience is similar to that seen in this patient; a nurse has a responsibility in this area. Gradually or suddenly our thought process draws the facts into a pattern. The end result of this process we have named the recognition of a pattern.

STATEMENT OF A CONCLUSION

The actual nursing diagnosis is the statement of a conclusion. The diagnosis may be descriptive as "Communicates exclusively through gestures" or "Limited response to auditory and tactile stimuli." The diagnosis may be etiological as "Lessened intestinal peristalsis" or "Inadequate understanding of hospital environment because he does not speak English." As more facts are obtained through nursing investigation, a descriptive diagnosis may become an etiological diagnosis. Knowledge of the etiology may suggest more pertinent nursing care.

We have made diagnoses which are primarily physiological ("Lessened intestinal peristalsis") and others which are primarily psychological ("Feelings of powerlessness"). Some nursing diagnoses—for example, "Nausea"—imply both physiological and psychological aspects. "Nausea" is also an example of the use of a major medical symptom as suitable terminology for a nursing diagnosis.

A nursing diagnosis might be anticipated in a certain medical diagnosis; for example, "Pain" may be the nursing diagnosis in a patient with a myocardial infarction. Or, a nursing diagnosis may be distinct from the medical diagnosis; it may describe a condition due to hospitalization ("Lonesomeness") or to a complication of the primary illness ("Urinary retention" in a patient with benign prostatic hypertrophy).

We have made the same nursing diagnoses in patients with different medical diagnoses, since the same physiological or psychological processes may be present even when the total patterns as viewed by the physician are different. "Inadequate oxygenation" may be a nursing diagnosis in patients whose medical diagnosis is "asthma," "postoperative pneumonectomy," or "congestive heart failure."

The nursing diagnosis may be the same as the medical diagnosis. This occurrence is most likely in emergency situations when the nurse's therapeutic actions are the same as the physician's. An initial diagnosis of "Cardiac arrest" may be both a medical and a nursing diagnosis calling for immediate respiratory and cardiac resuscitation. Following emergency treatment the medical diagnosis may become "Ventricular fibrillation" or "Myocardial infarction" and the nursing diagnosis may become "Ineffective cardiac output" or "Fear of pain."

With the exception of such an emergency, a nursing diagnosis is not a medical diagnosis. A nursing diagnosis tends to be more individualized. Where a medical diagnosis serves to summarize a group of signs and symptoms, a

(Text continues on page 81)

EXAMPLES OF NURSING DIAGNOSIS

FACTS OBTAINED DURING NURSING INVESTIGATION	MAJOR POINTS IN THE THOUGHT PROCESS LEADING TO RECOGNITION OF A PATTERN	NURSING DIAGNOSIS
Mr. A was a 55-year-old man hospitalized for a pneumonectomy complicated by a cerebral embolus, which in turn necessitated a tracheotomy and a gastrostomy.		
Vocal cords bypassed by tracheotomy		
Had difficulty covering the opening of the tracheotomy tube with his finger	Physical discomfort and physical disability when attempting spoken or written communication	
Said "It hurts there (pointing to gastrostomy) when I talk."		
Had difficulty holding tablet while writing because of paresis of left arm		Limited ability to communicate 1) by vocal sounds 2) by writing
Nodded or shook head		
Exaggerated changes in facial expression		
Rubbed his stomach	He is trying to express himself in the way in which he experiences the least frustration—usually through gestures or changes of facial expression	
Pointed to his hip		
Shook his finger		
Held out hand to shake hands		
Waved		
When he does speak, he says only one or two words		

EXAMPLES OF NURSING DIAGNOSIS

FACTS OBTAINED DURING NURSING INVESTIGATION	MAJOR POINTS IN THE THOUGHT PROCESS LEADING TO RECOGNITION OF A PATTERN	NURSING DIAGNOSIS
At times shrugs shoulders or shakes head when nurse is unable to understand him	Repeated frustrations may lead to anxiety	Anxiety as a result of frustration at inability to communicate
Requested by wave of hand that tube feeding be stopped	Signs indicative of mild stimulation of vomiting center	Nausea
Held right hand over abdomen		
Lying very still		
Two days postoperative from hiatal hernia repair	May have lessened gastric capacity from surgical trauma or lessened gastric motility	
Nurse reported episodes of hiccoughs and indigestion		
Feeding regurgitated	Excessive stimulation of oropharynx	
Coughing one ounce of mucus per hour		
Anxiety	Anxiety may stimulate the cerebral cortex to send afferent impulses to vomiting center	

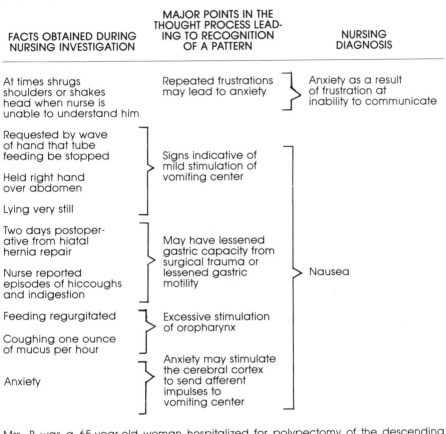

Mrs. B was a 65-year-old woman hospitalized for polypectomy of the descending colon.

Stated "My stomach hurts."	Little evidence of gastro-intestinal activity	Lessened intestinal peristalsis
Abdomen distended		
No flatus passed		
Few bowel tones		
Miller-Abbott tube in place	No peristaltic stimuli	
Receiving continuous intravenous therapy		
Medical consultation suggested intestinal obstruction		

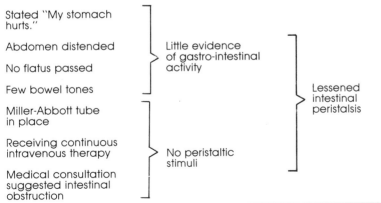

FACTS OBTAINED DURING NURSING INVESTIGATION	MAJOR POINTS IN THE THOUGHT PROCESS LEADING TO RECOGNITION OF A PATTERN	NURSING DIAGNOSIS
Face flushed, skin hot to touch Oral temperature fluctuating between 100°F and 102°F Moderate diaphoresis	Signs of fever	Pathogenic bacteria infecting incision site
Leukocyte count elevated. Presurgical: 7000/cu.mm. One week postsurgical: 12,000/cu.mm. Red, swollen, indurated area around lower half of midline incision site No evidence of healing in lower half of incisional wound Serosanguineous discharge from wound	Signs of infectious process	
Talked of coming into hospital feeling well and now being sick Said she had expected that the polyps could be removed by way of the proctoscope and "now all this"	Expectations regarding hospitalization and treatment have not been met	Feelings of powerlessness
"I'm told it will take time to get well. But I don't know what they mean by time— a day, a week, a month."		
"I don't understand why the doctor left the inhalator here. He knows. I don't know why he left it, but he knows."	Does not feel she can plan what is to come or what she can do	
"I don't know why I have to have the intravenous tubes. The doctor probably knows best."	Does not understand or feel in control of her environment	

FACTS OBTAINED DURING NURSING INVESTIGATION	MAJOR POINTS IN THE THOUGHT PROCESS LEADING TO RECOGNITION OF A PATTERN	NURSING DIAGNOSIS
"All these tubes— I just want to get rid of them so I can be on my own."		
Gross jerky movements of limbs		
Picking at bed clothes	Signs of central nervous system disturbance	
Unable to stand without assistance		R/O Electrolyte imbalance 1) hypocalcemia 2) hypopotassemia
Disoriented as to time, place and family		
Gastrointestinal decompression for one week		
Intravenous therapy with replacement of electrolytes KCl and NaCl	Loss of body electrolytes	
Five to six loose stools per 24-hour period for last three days (Presurgery pattern of one stool per day)		

Mr. C was a 44-year-old man hospitalized for thrombophlebitis of the right leg and headaches in the left frontal region.

Had cerebral vascular accident one year ago which resulted in the loss of vision in the left half of visual field		
Lost job because of impairment of vision	Has experienced losses	
His daughter was to be married in two months		Depressed; has thoughts of suicide
Reported that he had had approximately four hours of "restless" sleep per night for the last two months		

EXAMPLES OF NURSING DIAGNOSIS

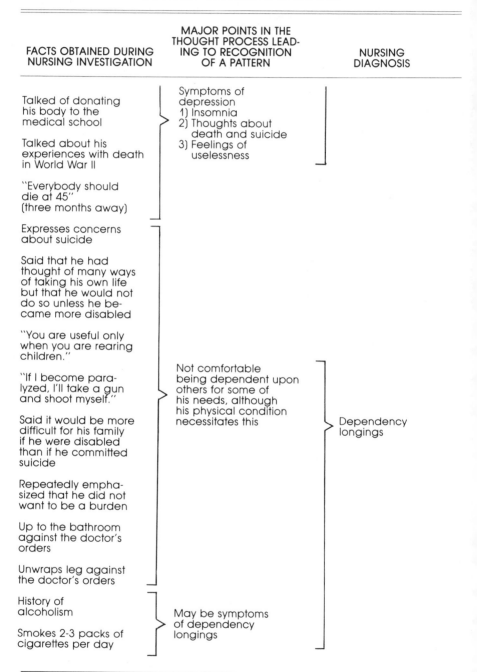

FACTS OBTAINED DURING NURSING INVESTIGATION	MAJOR POINTS IN THE THOUGHT PROCESS LEADING TO RECOGNITION OF A PATTERN	NURSING DIAGNOSIS
Talked of donating his body to the medical school Talked about his experiences with death in World War II "Everybody should die at 45" (three months away)	Symptoms of depression 1) Insomnia 2) Thoughts about death and suicide 3) Feelings of uselessness	
Expresses concerns about suicide Said that he had thought of many ways of taking his own life but that he would not do so unless he became more disabled "You are useful only when you are rearing children." "If I become para-lyzed, I'll take a gun and shoot myself." Said it would be more difficult for his family if he were disabled than if he committed suicide Repeatedly emphasized that he did not want to be a burden Up to the bathroom against the doctor's orders Unwraps leg against the doctor's orders	Not comfortable being dependent upon others for some of his needs, although his physical condition necessitates this	Dependency longings
History of alcoholism Smokes 2-3 packs of cigarettes per day	May be symptoms of dependency longings	

EXAMPLES OF NURSING DIAGNOSIS

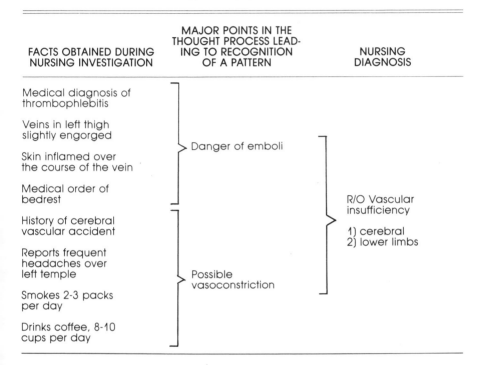

FACTS OBTAINED DURING NURSING INVESTIGATION	MAJOR POINTS IN THE THOUGHT PROCESS LEADING TO RECOGNITION OF A PATTERN	NURSING DIAGNOSIS
Medical diagnosis of thrombophlebitis		
Veins in left thigh slightly engorged		
Skin inflamed over the course of the vein	Danger of emboli	
Medical order of bedrest		R/O Vascular insufficiency
History of cerebral vascular accident		1) cerebral 2) lower limbs
Reports frequent headaches over left temple		
Smokes 2-3 packs per day	Possible vasoconstriction	
Drinks coffee, 8-10 cups per day		

nursing diagnosis may consist of one sign or symptom that focuses on the patient's particular response to his illness. A nursing diagnosis tends to reflect the progress of the patient. Whereas a medical diagnosis may remain the same until the patient has recovered or died, a nursing diagnosis indicates the significant responses the patient makes at the stages of his illness and therefore may change with daily changes in the patient. This individualization and reflection of patient progress make a nursing diagnosis useful in the round-the-clock performance of hospital nursing as well as in community nursing. Both are situations in which medical diagnosis is made, but in which there are many hours of nursing responsibilities in the absence of the medical practitioner.

The process of diagnosing begins as soon as the patient comes under nursing care, and it continues until he no longer needs nursing care. As the nurse learns more about the patient, she may revise the nursing diagnosis. The diagnosis may become more specific; "Fear and anxiety concerning the surgical procedure" may become "Fear and anxiety concerning the possibility of cancer." Or the diagnosis may become more generalized; "Cyanosis" may become "Inadequate oxygenation."

In some instances, because of interruptions or masking of physiological or psychological cues, the nurse does not have sufficient facts to recognize a clear-cut pattern. The facts merely suggest a pattern. The decision, or diagnosis, then becomes what we call a rule-out, or tentative nursing diagnosis. This diagnosis is, in fact, a hypothesis which structures and stimulates the nurse's search for more information. We seek this information, usually by returning to the patient, to determine the accuracy or inaccuracy of the tentative nursing diagnosis.

At this point we do not believe that all nursing diagnoses can or should be of a given degree of specificity or generalization. It may be possible to organize nursing diagnoses into a classification system comparable to the classifications used by medicine. Such a system will not be possible until nurses are skilled in diagnosing and agree about the meaning and implications of the nursing diagnosis.

What is the value of a nursing diagnosis? Nursing is seeking a scientific basis for practice. The process of diagnosing necessitates the use of scientific knowledge and requires the relation and application of this knowledge to nursing. The actual diagnosis establishes a point of departure, a basis for nursing care. George B. Shaw has been credited with saying "Diagnosis should mean the finding out of all there is wrong with a particular patient."[6] We believe a nursing diagnosis could mean the finding out of all that is necessary to know to begin a plan of nursing care.

REFERENCES

1. John A. Prior and Jack S. Silberstein, *Physical Diagnosis: The History and Examination of the Patient*. St. Louis: The C. V. Mosby Company. 1959. pp. 17-18.

2. Leo J. Brueckner, "Introduction" Educational Diagnosis. *Thirty-fourth Yearbook of the National Society for the Study of Education*. Guy Montrose Whipple (ed.). Bloomington, Ill. Public School Publishing Company. 1935. p. 2.

3. Mary E. Richmond, *Social Diagnosis*. New York: Russell Sage Foundation. 1917. p. 357.

4. Virginia Bonney and June Rothberg, *Nursing Diagnosis and Therapy*. New York: National League for Nursing. 1963.

5. Lydia E. Hall, "Nursing—What Is It?" Revised. Mimeographed. Loeb Center, New York, April 26, 1963, p. 1-5.

6. F. G. Crookshank, "The Importance of a Theory of Signs and a Critique of Language in the Study of Medicine" Supplement to C. K. Ogden and I. A. Richards, *The Meaning of Meaning*. 10th edition, London: Routledge and Kegan Paul, Inc. 1949. p. 343.

BIBLIOGRAPHY

Wilda Chambers, "Nursing Diagnosis," *American Journal of Nursing*, 62:102-104. November, 1962.

Nori I. Komorita, "Nursing Diagnosis," *American Journal of Nursing,* 63:83–86, December, 1963.

R. Faye McCain, "Nursing by Assessment—Not Intuition," *American Journal of Nursing,* 63:82, April, 1965.

Catherine M. Norris, "Toward a Science of Nursing—A Method for Developing Unique Content in Nursing," *Nursing Forum,* 3:22-24, Number 3, 1964.

Why Nursing Diagnosis?

June S. Rothberg

The author maintains that nursing diagnosis is essential to professional nursing. It insures focus on the individual. It reveals the many factors which influence the patient's progress. And it results in a goal directed plan of nursing care that can be evaluated.

Nursing diagnosis is a term which, in recent years, has been used with ever increasing frequency and often with little accuracy. For various reasons, the term can be an emotion-laden or frightening concept to nurses and to other health personnel. Before discussing what a nursing diagnosis is, let us review what it is not. It is not a medical diagnosis made by nurses. It is not a psychiatric diagnosis made by nurses. It is not a socioeconomic diagnosis made by nurses.

In making a nursing diagnosis, the professional nurse may utilize specific information from the diagnoses which other qualified persons have made. However, she will add to this information her own independent observations to form an evaluation which is uniquely nursing.

In 1961, Abdellah stated, "We must face up to the responsibility that making a nursing diagnosis is an independent function of the professional nurse."(1) I believe that for far too long a time we in nursing have abdicated this responsibility.

As a starting point, in broad and very general terms, a nursing diagnosis may be thought of as an evaluation by nurses of those factors affecting the patient which will influence his recovery. These factors may include intrinsic dimensions such as physical condition or emotional state, and, also, external influences such as economic problems. All nurses, I am certain, know of a patient whose physical progress was impeded because he was frantic over bills or who couldn't be discharged because he was unable to walk up three flights of stairs. Some of these factors will need to be referred to appropriate disciplines for action. Some are directly the responsibility of nursing.

It is precisely in the area of interdisciplinary functions and relations, that difficulties in patient care arise. There is considerable overlap at the boundaries of each profession's practice. Instead of leading to increased cooperation and communication for the benefit of the individual and all society, this overlap has led to the reverse. The various disciplines are warily watching their own vested interests—guarding their particular prerogatives and preserves. Lest I be misunderstood, I mean nursing, too.

In the past 15 years, there has been a tremendous increase in the number of persons working in the health arena. The 1960 census indicated that in a 10-year span, the health field has risen from seventh to third place among major United States industries in terms of numbers of persons employed(2). This was six years ago! Not only are numbers increasing but as knowledge expands and is intensified, becoming more advanced and more highly technical, new specialties are proliferating. In my own field of rehabilitation, there are physical, occupational, and recreational therapists, vocational and rehabilitation counselors, and prosthetists to mention only a few of the occupational specialists. It is now possible for a person to obtain a professional degree (a bachelor of science) in orthotics, the newest specialty field.

With the impetus given by recent health and social legislation which is directed toward the preparation of health workers to meet the needs of our continually burgeoning and aging population, there will be an ever larger number of persons working in health fields.

We may expect ever greater fragmentation of services than current and anticipated growth warrants unless each and all of us become completely aware of a single overriding fact—the common denominator in health or disease is the individual man. It is not an institution—not a doctor—not a nurse—not any other health worker. It is the human being who needs to be kept well and treated when sick. Without awareness and understanding of this central fact, health care and particularly nursing care has neither direction nor meaning.

The challenge to us today is to furnish the kind of health care people need, when and where they need it. To do this, we must bring the patient into the foreground. There is no one idea having greater importance for nursing than that of viewing the patient as a person. It is only when the patient is so viewed, as a person, that care is provided to him according to his needs in an appropriate, continuous, and dynamic pattern which is sometimes described as comprehensive care. Nursing diagnosis makes it possible to provide such care.

One hears much today about meeting total needs of patients. This is a reaction to a practice which has concentrated primarily on two areas: routine physical care concerned with fundamental physiologic processes such as nutrition and elimination, and highly technical complex aspects of nursing. We have emphasized the physical and the technical while ignoring or not understanding the perceptions, the responses, the social, and psychologic needs of people. To further complicate the picture, we have so fragmented our services that the basic physical care of patients has been relegated to increasingly less well-prepared personnel and we have taken to our professional bosom those highly complex and often painful procedures which were formerly the province of the physician.

All too frequently, we have centered on the medical diagnosis, the psychiatric or other diagnosis. We have carried out medically prescribed orders, briskly and efficiently applied some highly routine or ritualized procedures, and considered the whole process nursing, while neatly ignoring the patients' perceptions, feelings, and individual problems.

As a reminder of the hazard, encountered when we concentrate on physical diagnosis as the sole determining factor in planning nursing care, consider the following. The patient in bed 13 has a gastric neoplasm, the one in bed 32 has a viral pneumonia, and the one in bed 20 has a cerebral aneurysm. What do we know about these three persons? Only their medical diagnoses! The person in each bed could be any combination of either half of the following: a man or a woman, 35 years old or 75, ill for years with a chronic disease or sick for the first time in his life, a valued and loved family member or a socially isolated person living without family or friends, destitute or financially secure.

It is the combination of such factors plus many others which will strongly influence the particular patient's progress and recovery. These characteristics exert this influence because they are the resources—physical, emotional, social, and economic—which the person can call upon to overcome his illness. Nursing diagnosis is the process which identifies the patient's resources and deficits, thus indicating his needs for nursing assistance.

Historically, patient care has been considered the core of all nursing activity regardless of the setting in which it was performed or the type of nursing function required. Modern nursing extends over the broad spectrum of health services and encompasses promotion of health, prevention of illness, as well as care of patients and their families. In order to administer patient care, the nurse must identify the individual's needs for nursing services. Ever since nursing was first performed, the nurse, by a process either wholly or partially conscious, looked at the patient and determined on the basis of intuition, experience, rote learning, knowledge, or in some cases ignorance, which nursing acts were needed to relieve his distress.

What must the nurse know about the patient? This is the central question in determining, in a professionally responsible manner, the patient's requirements for nursing services. What must she understand of the intrinsic processes (physical, physiologic, emotional), occurring within him? What must she know of the extrinsic factors (sociologic, economic) surrounding him, and the influence these exert upon him? How well does he manage himself in relation to the stresses he faces? What probable results can she expect from her nursing? When the nurse is able to answer these questions accurately, she is ready to provide appropriate comprehensive nursing.

Answering these questions in a clearly ordered, reasoned manner, based on scientific fact, requires the establishment of a nursing diagnosis and nursing therapy. Nursing diagnosis is an evaluation within the framework of current knowledge, of the patient's condition as a person including physical, physiologic, and behavioral aspects.

Let us examine the key word of this definition: *evaluation.* An evaluation is a process, implying a continuing operation. There are many kinds of evaluations which go on all the time, continually influencing our choice of actions. Some are not conscious evaluations but are implicit or intuitive. At this moment, you are evaluating what you read. As I write, I am subconsciously evaluating your possible response to my words. But neither of us is sharply aware of this evaluation process as it goes on—it is almost automatic.

However, these kinds of evaluations—intuitive, implicit, and automatic —are not what is required in making a nursing diagnosis. It is definitive, clearly focused, and completely conscious evaluation which is necessary for our decision making about patients. In order to be of help to ourselves and especially to others, we must practice evaluation in an explicit manner as a consciously planned activity. It may be practiced informally. However, it frequently is carried out within the framework of a formal evaluation instrument.

What is it we are evaluating? We are determining the patient's condition— the relative state of health or ill health in physical, functional (or physiologic), and behavioral areas. We are looking for both strengths and weaknesses in these areas and for both overt and covert problems.

How are we evaluating? We are consciously and systematically observing physical signs and activities, physiologic indications and reports, and observing social and interpersonal behavior. The interpretation of observations is based on principles from the biologic, physical, and social sciences which have been integrated into a nursing science.

Why are we evaluating? The purpose of such assessment is to determine the patient's (or the family's) need. We are trying to appraise the situation of the patient to learn what we as professionals can do for him.

Thus, the prime element in the process of evaluation or diagnosis is identification of individual needs. The second element is clear definition of goals for the patient's care. One such goal, in the physical realm, might be to obtain the maximum possible improvement in the patient's condition. Another goal might have to be more modest such as the maintenance of his present condition without further deterioration. An even more modest but imperative goal must be the prevention of superimposed disabilities(3). A different kind of goal might be to increase the patient's verbal interaction with his roommates. Several categories of goals must be packaged together, since the patient being diagnosed is a person with a variety of responses, facets, and problems. Therefore, goals include desired physical, functional, and behavioral targets.

The nurse making a diagnosis determines which of the identified care needs are amenable to nursing. Once nursing problems have been defined clearly by the diagnosis, a course of nursing activities purposefully directed toward increasing the positive health of the patient can be initiated. The nurse selects the appropriate methods, resources, and personnel to meet the identified needs. Those needs which are beyond the scope of nursing are referred to the appropriate health workers. Thus, the unique function of the professional nurse is being performed—that of the diagnosis of the patient's need for nursing services and the decision upon a course of action to follow(4).

We have now moved into the realm of nursing therapy. Nursing therapy is defined as knowledgeable intervention in the form of nursing activities, based on the nursing diagnosis, and directed at moving the individual toward positive health(5). Nursing care plans are a step toward nursing therapy. There is absolutely no point in making a nursing diagnosis unless it leads directly to action in the form of nursing therapy. And, of course, appropriate comprehensive nursing therapy is impossible without a prior diagnosis of need. Nursing therapy is derived specifically from the diagnosis. Direction for the nursing intervention is given by the nursing diagnosis. The three elements of diagnosis—identification of individual need, establishment of goals, and selection of appropriate methods—together provide the knowledge required in order to act appropriately to move the individual toward more positive health.

New knowledge in the health sciences is expanding and pyramiding at a fantastic rate. Predictions about nursing practice of the future, made only five years ago, were considered by a majority of nurses to be science fiction, but today are reality. Nurses are working with patients treated in hyperbaric chambers, with bioelectric monitoring devices, with electronic cardiac, bladder and muscle pacemaker and implants. Microminiaturization techniques developed for outer space explorations have opened untold opportunities for the alleviation of man's physical ills.

In view of these technological changes, what happens to the fragility and importance of the individual? One way to meet the challenge is to consciously and clear-sightedly assess the patient's needs as an individual utilizing keen professional observation plus all the mechanical gadgets to obtain highly accurate information about his condition and to utilize skilled professional judgment to interpret and evaluate the information. Then, at all times remembering that all people have a diversity of needs, make a diagnosis and institute a plan of therapy to meet the individual problems of the person in our care.

REFERENCES

1. Abdellah, Faye. *Meeting Patients Needs—An Approach to Teaching.* Paper presented at biennial convention of the National League for Nursing, Cleveland, Ohio, April 10-14, 1961.

2. Manpower in health. *Progressive Health Services* 10: May 1961.

3. Rothberg, June, ed. Foreword, [to the] Symposium on chronic disease and rehabilitation. *Nursing Clinics of North America* 1:352–354, Sept. 1966.

4. Abdellah, *op. cit.*

5. Bonney, Virginia, and Rothberg, June. *Nursing Diagnosis and Therapy; an Instrument for Evaluation and Measurement.* New York, National League for Nursing, 1963.

4

Nursing Orders

Nursing orders are the second part of the nursing care plan. Chapter 4 begins with the theoretical aspects of designating and writing nursing orders. A discussion of nursing care plans and the creative process for developing and writing nursing orders frames the chapter. From this point, the case followed in Part I of the book will be carried out with *nursing orders,* that is, specific nursing actions with specific objectives, developed for the diagnoses presented at the conclusion of Chapter 3.

Let us recall the equation used to illustrate these first chapters:

$$\begin{matrix} \text{Client Data} \\ \text{System Data} \end{matrix} + \begin{matrix} \text{Nursing Responsibilities} \\ \text{Nurse's Knowledge} \\ \text{The Nurse} \end{matrix} \rightarrow \begin{matrix} \text{Individualized} \\ \text{Nursing Diagnoses and} \\ \text{Nursing Orders} \end{matrix}$$

As the equation shows, nursing orders are a part of the results of data collection and processing. With individualized nursing diagnoses, they make up the planning phase of the nursing process.

COGNITIVE DIMENSIONS OF NURSING ORDERS

Care Plan Framework

The nursing care plans observed on charts, the kardex, and clinical unit care plan books generally denote the nursing diagnoses and orders for each client. Often, the nursing history will be attached.

Care plans can be observed in a variety of forms, and nursing literature has devoted many pages to the need for a diversity of types from written formal plans to informal ones (Ciuca, 1972; Harris, 1970; Palisin, 1971; Wagner, 1969). Considering the responsibility of the nurse to perceive and plan for an array of overt and covert patient needs for a group of patients, and considering that the plans will be implemented by a variety of professional and technical care-givers, systematic and formal planning is considered to be essential. Little and Carnevali (1967) designate formal planning as absolutely necessary to incorporate all health care efforts and to maintain a goal of providing quality, comprehensive care to consumers. Furthermore, care plans knit together the aspects of care required for a client—various data, histories, diagnoses, orders—and communicate the essentials to every member of the nursing and health team. Progress can be noted and new data integrated constantly. Client transfer to other in-house units or community agency referrals can be made more efficiently when accompanied by a concise, systematic report of client needs of the past and present, as well as potential needs of the future.

Writing Nursing Orders

A nursing order should be a specific statement of what actions to take based on what objective(s) a nurse wishes to achieve with and for a client, relative to an established diagnosis. It can be equated with such terms as the *aims* of nursing care (Taba, 1962), objectives (Conley, 1973), terminal behaviors (Mager, 1962), goals (Zimmerman and Gohrke, 1970), or just explicit statements of things needing to be done; nursing orders can be identified with any one of these terms, depending on the preference of the writer.

A brief discussion of the aforementioned terms is appropriate. Use of any or all should be guided by the nursing care plan designer's understanding of the terms, as well as the implementer's understanding.

The term "goals" suggests a broader area than "aims," "objectives," or "terminal behaviors," and, therefore, does not suit this book's use of the term "nursing orders" as that which needs to be done by the nursing team.

"Objectives," "aims," and "terminal behaviors" have connotative and denotative meanings which better suit our purposes, however, and which will be used interchangeably in this book. Perhaps one of the clearest descriptions of terms is Mager's definition of a terminal behavior as "the behavior you would like your learner to be able to demonstrate at the time your influence over him ends (Mager, 1962, p. 2)." This is also an apt description of "objectives," the term primarily used to describe nursing orders in this book.

There are two aspects of Mager's statement that require amplification. First, "demonstrate" implies behavior that is visible and measurable to some degree (Mager, 1962). Logically speaking, therefore, an objective must be specific, succinct, and observable. It should not be composed of general statements, such as "the patient will experience relief of anxiety and acceptance of his illness," or "relieve anxiety of patient." Instead, specific statements such as how relief of anxiety concerning a certain factor will be accomplished or attempted should be used. Clear objectives include statements on where the client is heading (Smith, 1971), relative to the diagnosis at hand. They should not portray nursing behaviors such as "giving emotional support (Smith, 1971)," but should be action oriented, indicating desirable client behaviors as well as those to be employed by the nurse in assisting the client to reach optimal health.

Second, Mager's statement that an objective refers to behavior patterns that should be fulfilled by the time your influence ceases must be adapted to a nurse/client relationship. Specifically, the system of health care should be considered as "your influence." Short- and long-term nursing orders can then be developed and progress reports or evaluations written and communicated to the care-givers in various parts of the health system and in accordance with the client's presence within the structure. In other words, orders that may be begun in a coronary care unit and emerge as a number one priority in a rehabilitation unit should be considered even though the nurse writing the order will not move with the client.

In writing orders, it may be necessary to write a primary objective and then write sub-objectives that elucidate the process and content of the primary one more clearly. An example would be:

Primary Objective

Ms. F., the client, will be able to give her own insulin every morning in any setting.

To move from the point where a client is totally unfamiliar with diabetes, insulin, needed equipment, and giving herself an injection to fulfillment of this objective, the specific steps for accomplishment should be delineated. These specific steps are the action part of nursing orders and are useful in progressively evaluating where the client is in relation to objective fulfillment. This facilitates continuity of care.

Three basic areas must be considered when writing nursing orders for each diagnosis. According to Bloom (1954), there are three aspects of the order system: cognitive, affective, and psychomotor. Cognitive aspects refer to the theoretical (or content) domain such as knowledge of diabetes as a disease. The affective domain covers feeling and attitudinal processes: one's acceptance of an illness, relief of anxiety, and the like. Psychomotor refers to necessary skills, such as competence in giving one's own insulin using aseptic technique. All three areas must be considered in writing orders for a given diagnosis. In addition, it is obvious that the nurse's overall order system should integrate medical orders with nursing aims.

Note that all nursing orders should be stated in a behavioral format. The purpose for writing orders is to delineate the steps required to move a client's behavior toward an objective or relief of a designated problem.

Creative Order Writing   Nursing literature has commented on the paucity of nursing interventions in care plans and the magnitude of physician orders in the same (Kelly, 1966). Moreover, even with all the steps delineated in this section of the book, aimed at *individualized* nursing care, sometimes it is easy to fall into a pattern of writing nursing orders that are nonspecific to the client. These tend to be bland and impotent, and adhere to hospital policies and procedures at a much greater ratio than to specific client needs and the *best* way to fulfill these needs.

Following general procedure may become automatic. It becomes easy to do again what has been done before. This process leads to preconceived notions or *mental* sets concerning what *should* be done with the client. As these automatic mental sets are formulated and reinforced, perceptual fields may narrow. This can result in routine orders and ways of implementing them. It is necessary to foster expansion of perceptual fields through creativity in nursing orders that respond to the individuality of the client's system and the best ways to enable clients to reach their fullest potential as they use their own assets.

Eisenman (1970) conducted an investigation that unfortunately found student nurses becoming less creative during nursing education. He later (1972) researched whether or not student nurses high in creativity, as measured by perceptual preferences for complexity, would be accepting of clients labeled mentally ill or physically disabled. He contrasted this with student nurses low in creativity. Results indicated that those who had a preference for complexity displayed increased acceptance of these clients while others who preferred simplicity displayed decreased acceptance. These studies have important implications in nursing practice and education. First, creativity must be specifically developed, not dampened. Second, if a system (education or practice) dampens creativity to any degree, it becomes the responsibility of practitioners themselves to insure that overt, conscious measures are taken to compensate for the natural tendency to formulate mental sets, make care routine, or be blocked from thinking by the system's policies *before* one actually thinks of newer approaches in care and ways to implement them.

It becomes essential to look upon an individual, a disease, a strength, or a weakness and form opinions that are based upon an expansive perceptual field and creative ways of setting decisions in motion. McNeil (1973), in discussing the aesthetic educational process, states that a teacher with only one or two ways of teaching is limited in meeting the learners' differences as to the way each learns best. If one relates this to nursing practice, routine orders may not be what is best for the client.

Table 4-1 compares the nursing process with the components of the creative process.

TABLE 4-1
NURSING PROCESS AND THE CREATIVE PROCESS

NURSING PROCESS	CREATIVE PROCESS
Assessment •Collection of data from many sources •Classification, analysis, and summarization of data to determine nursing problems and/or needs Note: At this point in the nursing process it is very easy to get caught in the routine, trite methods of problem-solving and fail to study the "individual" need of the "individual" patient/client.	**Motivation** •Assumes that a person is creating because of internal and external forces **Exploration** •Observes, surveys, and explores all the possibilities that are available for use **Improvisation** •Outgrowth of what is discovered through exploration •Unplanned, impromptu manipulation of ideas, thoughts, concepts •Working with the interrelatedness and movements that are suggested in the explored possibilities
Planning •Design for action •Development of strategies or alternative approaches to meeting the needs of patients	**Experimentation** •Combining and planning structure of ideas, materials, and concepts in a certain area •Designing alternative methods and structures suitable for implementation
Implementation •"Trying on" and carrying out of the proposed plan of care	**Application** •Experimentation and application involving strategies and designs that are then "tried on"
Evaluation •Based on available feedback, use of new information to revise the care plan as necessary	**Evaluation** **Extension** •New avenues of ideas opened and experimented with; repeating the process •Extended or implied further areas of study

SOURCE: The components of the creative process as herein described were developed by Susan M. Brainerd, 1971.

The step that can be used first to foster creativity and develop orders that reflect the individuality of the client is exploration. Here, and before nursing orders are designated, brainstorming takes place. This process involves freeing the mind of rights/wrongs and can-do's/cannot-do's. It is the process of expanding possibilities. It answers the question: "If I could develop orders for this client, ideally doing anything I want, being as specific and personal to the client as possible, and reflecting what I know about the client, what would I want done and how?" Any ideas are important and no values of good or bad are operative. After the ideas are listed, choose those that can be implemented with ease. Pick out one or two that require minor alterations of agency or hospital norms. Then implement them according to the brainstormed "how." In this way creativity is fostered rather than dampened. Moreover, care is not routine and guided by sets, because one is always considering and working on something new, in relation to a unique person. It follows, of course, that new modes of client care have the ability to become part of the system, with changes occurring as necessary and documented as effective. It follows, also, that just because a procedure is standard, it is not necessarily ineffective or not suited to a particular client. The nurse must use judgment.

Thus far Chapter 4 has discussed cognitive aspects of nursing orders and components of objective writing for nursing orders. The creative process of brainstorming was introduced to facilitate individualization of nursing care plans.

Next, following the established diagnoses in Chapter 3, the same case study will be discussed in the next portion of this chapter. Nursing orders will be the focus.

CASE EXAMPLE ON NURSING ORDERS

The case example will be developed more completely by dealing with the nursing diagnoses that are essential at the present time in the client's system and in order of priority. Diagnoses of less than immediate priority will become a focus of emphasis in the rehabilitation phase of the client's progress, that is, when plans for discharge are in the picture. It is important to remember that medical orders are included in the nursing orders, since this is one aspect of nursing responsibility. To personalize nursing orders, it is often necessary to refer back to the data collection and processing stages and obtain and examine client data necessary to make the orders come alive in the client's system.

An example of nursing orders developed for the client, Mr. Munson, according to the priorities of his needs is given on pages 95–98. Nursing orders are developed for each diagnosis including objectives and specific actions related to the objectives.

SUMMARY

Chapter 4 has focused on the cognitive aspects of nursing orders. This area forms the bulk of a nursing care plan and should contain statements concerning what is needed to bring the client towards goal accomplishment and diagnosis eradication. The creative process was emphasized as a means for providing the nurse with a tool to develop nursing care that is truly indi-

(Text continues on page 98)

NURSING DIAGNOSES IN ORDER OF PRIORITIES	NURSING ORDERS

Physical signs and symptoms relating to an MI and diabetes closely monitored

Primary objective
• The client will be closely monitored to prevent complications relating to the disease states MI and diabetes.

Sub-objective
• The client will be monitored for pain and given treatment accordingly.

1. Monitor constantly—be alert for arrhythmias.
2. Monitor vital signs QIH. Be alert for changes.
3. Listen to lungs for signs of congestion, QID.
4. Be alert for nonverbal signs of chest pain or related pain. Check with client frequently.
5. Be alert for signs of dyspnea and utilize oxygen at 4 liters/min. PRN.
6. Observe skin color and body temperature frequently for flushing or pallor.
7. Monitor lab reports for signs of abnormalities; if any exist, report them to the physician stat.
8. If arrythmias occur, treat immediately as specified by standing orders and document by running a strip on the monitor. CALL FOR A PHYSICIAN STAT.
9. Keep an accurate I & O sheet in client's room.
10. Test urine for S/A AC and HS. Give insulin as indicated.
11. REPORT ALL CHANGES IN CLIENT'S CONDITION TO PROFESSIONAL NURSE IN CHARGE.

Safety of self within new environment

Primary objective
• The client will have an understanding of the reason for his hospitalization in the coronary care unit.

Sub-objectives
• The client will be aware of purposes of procedures.
• The client will have an awareness of his diabetic condition.

1. Explain coronary care unit concept to client.
2. If feasible, give him a tour of the unit or show him pictures.
3. Familiarize him with all the equipment in his room and how it works, emphasizing the purposes of each piece. Carry this out in small steps.
4. Explain rationale for all care that he will receive: monitor, medications, treatments, I & O, S/A test, diabetic diet, visiting hours, and all others.
5. Be sure he understands by encouraging him to respond to your statements.

Prevention of elimination difficulties

Primary objective
• Because of nature of disease process, elimination difficulties are possible and should be prevented.

1. Be alert for constipation—be sure to check for bowel elimination every day.
2. Observe inconspicuously for any straining during bowel elimination.
3. Record I & O.

NURSING DIAGNOSES IN ORDER OF PRIORITIES	NURSING ORDERS

Adequate rest patterns; built-in periods of quiet throughout the day

Primary objective
- Client will be assured of needed quiet and rest.

1. Administer medications on time—Valium.
2. Give sleeping medication if necessary.
3. Since he is anxious about the hospital, sit and talk with him often—comfortably.
4. Quietly monitor vital signs at night; try to discover his sleeping patterns and do not disturb him when he is in deep sleep.
5. Keep two pillows at bedside within easy reach; he can use these as necessary.
6. Try to get a feeling for his cycle during the day; what are his periods of rest and activity. Then build treatments and procedures around these times, allowing him to rest when he can.

Assurance of balanced diet respectful of diabetes; investigation and treatment of anorexia

Primary objective
- Client will be assisted in adapting to special diet.

Sub-objective
- Hospital procedures will be adapted when possible to assist client in eating.

1. Request that his meals be sent up or kept warm until he wants to eat: 9–2–7; make special arrangements with department head in the kitchen.
2. Explain diabetes and the importance of eating well-balanced meals.
3. Tell client that you will help him in any way you can so that he receives foods that are in accordance with his likes.
4. Obtain food exchange lists from dietician and plan meals with client.
5. Be aware if this plan is not working and change accordingly.

Respectful, trusting nurse/client relationship

Primary objective
- Client will be at ease with nurse.

1. Spend time sitting down and talking with client. Do not ask questions, but rather respond to his feelings, letting him know that you have heard what he says.
2. Let him know when you will be back to talk.
3. Always be alert for signs of stress, anxiety, boredom. Notice what you see by telling client that he looks _____. Listen to what he says in response to your statement.
4. ALWAYS RESPOND TO WHAT CLIENT IS SAYING: PUT YOUR AGENDA IN THE BACKGROUND.

Awareness and understanding of the environment

Primary objective
- Client will be able to socialize as much as possible.

1. Explain rationale for visiting hours.
2. If you do not think that visitors for a longer period of time will harm anyone else in the unit, allow client's visitors to remain as long as possible. Always observe client for signs of fatigue.
3. If client is OOB, perhaps you could set up chairs in the hall and have client visit with family and friends there.
4. Move client's bed nearer to another client.
5. During quiet hours, have client sit in nurse's station, monitored directly by the large receiver.

NURSING DIAGNOSES IN ORDER OF PRIORITIES	NURSING ORDERS
Maintenance of privacy as much as possible	**Primary objective** • Client's modesty and privacy will be respected. 1. Provide privacy while client is using commode. 2. Be alert for signs of embarrassment in client—blushing, nervousness, slow speech—and intervene by engaging client in conversation aside from what you are doing. Or, note what you are doing and explain your reasons fully. Do what you feel most comfortable doing, respecting client's need. 3. Be discreet in everything you do for client.
Self-maintenance of hygiene needs	**Primary objective** • Client will care for himself independently whenever possible. 1. Allow client to care for his hygiene needs to the degree desired, respecting exercise or activity level needed for recovery. 2. Have all equipment handy for client. 3. Explain why limits are placed on his activity. 4. Involve wife in his care if he and she desire.
Self-maintenance of personal comfort measures	**Primary objective** • Client will be personally comfortable. 1. Continually be alert for what makes him comfortable and his favorite manner for having things done. Amplify these. 2. Sit and talk with him concerning things at home that he might like to bring into his room; follow through by having family obtain these items. 3. Always respond to his likes and dislikes; then respect them!
Teaching to chart I & O, care for monitor leads, and testing urine	**Primary objective** • Client will be independent in treating his disease whenever possible. 1. Talk with him regarding the importance of the three treatments. 2. Find out if he is interested in caring for these aspects himself. 3. If he does, then develop a plan for teaching that moves from your demonstration, client doing and being checked and then client assuming responsibility himself. 4. Keep chart of intake measures or equivalents on bedside table. 5. Keep I & O sheet by client. 6. Keep all equipment handy.
Self-maintenance of bowel and bladder elimination	This area has been covered in a previous nursing diagnosis and in teaching. Self-maintenance means that client is aware of the importance placed on this area of care and is responsible and accountable for his own care.

NURSING DIAGNOSES IN ORDER OF PRIORITIES	NURSING ORDERS
Recognition of what he does for himself and others	**Primary objective** • Client will feel self-satisfaction by being recognized as needed by others. 1. Always notice and verbally respond that you have seen what the client has accomplished. 2. Reinforce positively all aspects of client's growth. 3. Give client small things to do for self, you, and other clients. Examples: talk or sit with another client because he seems depressed; keep track of visiting hours for himself and others. 4. Verbalize the positive aspects of the accomplishment of the client: for example, eating better, requiring no extra insulin. Use this also as a way to reinforce teaching areas.

vidualized. The case example followed throughout Part I of the book was further developed to include orders for each diagnosis in priority.

Chapter 5 will focus on implementing the nursing care plan according to the level of maturity of the client and nurse and the skills necessary to accomplish each facet of care.

REFERENCES

Bloom, B., ed. *The taxonomy of objectives.* New York: Longmans, Green, 1954.

Brainerd, S. A curriculum for an aesthetic program for teacher education. Doctoral dissertation, University of Massachusetts, School of Education, Amherst, 1971.

Ciuca, R. Over the years with the nursing care plan. *Nursing Outlook* 20:706–711, 1972.

Conley, V. *Curriculum and instruction in nursing.* Boston: Little, Brown and Company, 1973.

Eisenman, R. Creativity in student nurses: A cross-sectional and longitudinal study. *Developmental Psychology* 3:320–325, 1970.

Eisenman, R. Creativity in student nurses and their attitudes toward mental illness and physical disability. *Journal of Clinical Psychology* 28:218–219, 1972.

Harris, B. Who needs written care plans anyhow? *American Journal of Nursing* 70:2136–2138, 1970.

Kelly, N. Nursing care plans. *Nursing Outlook* 14:61–64, 1966.

Little, D., and Carnevali, D. Nursing care plans: Let's be practical about them. *Nursing Forum* 6:61–76, 1967.

McNeil, J. The creative process. Unpublished paper, Center for the Study of Aesthetics in Education, University of Massachusetts, Amherst, 1973.

Mager, R. *Preparing instructional objectives*. Palo Alto, California: Fearon Publishers, 1962.

Palisin, H. Nursing care plans are a snare and a delusion. *American Journal of Nursing* 71:63–66, 1971.

Smith, D. Writing objectives as a nursing practice skill. *American Journal of Nursing* 71:319–320, 1971.

Taba, H. *Curriculum Development: Theory and Practice*. New York: Harcourt, Brace & World, 1962.

Wagner, B. Care plans: Right, reasonable, and reachable. *American Journal of Nursing* 69:986–990, 1969.

Zimmerman, D., and Gohrke, C. The goal-directed nursing approach: It does work. *American Journal of Nursing* 70:306–310, 1970.

SELECTED READING

The reading by Smith (1971) provides additional guidelines and discussion on writing objectives. The emphasis is on stating specifically the objectives for client behaviors. Smith also talks about articulating what the nurse must do to assist the client to achieve the stated objectives.

Writing Objectives as a Nursing Practice Skill

Dorothy M. Smith

Objectives for patient care should be written as expected patient behaviors, "The patient will circle those foods that are not appropriate on his low sodium diet," and not as personnel behavior, "Encourage fluids," says this author. Such objectives can guide nurses to where they are going in patient care and let them know when and where they have arrived, she maintains.

In the preface to his book *Preparing Instructional Objectives*, Mager tells a story of a sea horse who set out to find his fortune. On the way, he met other sea creatures who promised him a speedier trip by selling him different methods of transportation and short cuts. His last short cut took him into the mouth of a shark, and he was devoured. Mager says the moral of the fable is that if you don't know where you are going, you are liable to end up somewhere else and not even know it[1].

Commonly used words to express "where are you going" are "goal," "objective," "end," "intention," "aim." In a previous article describing a tool for collecting data and planning care, I used the word "goal"[2]. Subsequent work indicates that the word "objective" seems to be easier for staff and students to use. "Setting objectives" is a familiar phrase in education and there is much literature on the value of behavioral objectives.

Since the client of nursing is the patient I believe the objectives of nursing must be stated in terms of patient behavior. Then evaluation of practice (did you get to where you were going) consists of finding out whether the objectives were attained. Objectives of this kind can be narrow, concrete, specific, and unambiguous and clearly communicate intent to all members of the staff and to the patient and his family.

Such objectives are developed from data obtained from the patient as well as from nursing knowledge. They are developed with the patient and within the context of the patient's health and pathological states of body and mind. Thus, the objectives and the methods or strategies for achieving them are generally a series of compromises between ideal and real, known and unknown, and predictable and unpredictable (relatively sure and relatively unsure). This article will not deal with these compromises but rather with the skill that is needed to express "where you are going" in terms of patient behavior.

Reprinted with permission from *American Journal of Nursing*, Vol. 71, No. 2. Copyright 1971 by The American Journal of Nursing Company.

Writing objectives as expected patient behavior and in a way that makes evaluation possible is a difficult task. There is a tendency to write too broadly, for example, "The patient will accept his illness," or, "The patient will understand his diagnostic tests."

There is also a tendency to confuse objectives with standards. Standards are predetermined criteria for nursing care all patients have a right to expect. Standards are derived at best from research, although some may develop from long-standing unvalidated experience. Objectives are more individualized. Nevertheless, in the course of time, today's objectives may become tomorrow's standards.

Often objectives, regrettably, are expressed as personnel behavior—"to give emotional support to the patient," or "to encourage fluids," or "to teach the patient how to give his own insulin." We believe that the behavior (technical, interpersonal, and cognitive) of personnel reflects educational, professional, and institutional objectives and standards and cannot be used as a direct measurement of nursing practice objectives.

The inability to reach a nursing practice objective with a patient may be traced back to human error, negligence, ignorance, an inadequate system or procedure, or to any number of factors. But evaluating any of these factors in and of themselves does not constitute measurement of nursing practice objectives for a patient.

Personnel may perform tasks superbly, but end up in the shark's interior. On the reverse side, the state of our science and art is such that we sometimes reach the objective in spite of potentially dangerous, intuitive efforts carried on in a seemingly disorganized and unsystematic fashion. We must learn to analyze why we got where we wanted to go or why we did not get there.

EXAMPLES

The following examples of objectives are stated as expected patient behavior. Since these are real objectives for real patients, we have evidence of rationale for the objectives (data and knowledge). However, here we are concerned not with the appropriateness of the objective but with the statement of the objectives: Is the intent of the journey clear, and can we tell if we got there?

- The patient will measure his own intake and output and record it as instructed.
- The patient will demonstrate three types of antepartal exercises and state the purpose of each during each clinic visit.
- The patient has moist mouth and lips as evidenced by absence of furring on the tongue and dryness and caking of the lips.
- The patient will sleep more comfortably at night as evidenced by a decrease in the number of episodes of shortness of breath from 2300 to 0700 hours.
- When requested, the patient will list in writing from memory those foods that are not appropriate on a low sodium diet.

- Each morning, the patient will circle, from a list of foods, those that are appropriate on his low calorie diet.
- The patient will discuss with his nurse the statement that he repeated several times during the initial interview, "The wife is living a lonely life while I am in the hospital."
- The patient will discuss her labor experience with the nurse at 1400 hours.

Some of our staff prefer, "The patient is able. . . ." I prefer the stark "will." Greenwood says:

The scientist's prime aim is the description of the social world; the practitioner's prime aim is the control of that world(3).

FEELINGS ABOUT CONTROL

Nursing practitioners are seeking control. We apply knowledge for control; for the best, we hope. The word "control" may frighten some readers.

Principles of control, based on scientific knowledge, must be related to the patient, to his feelings, his perception, and his condition. Control is involved, and to deny this is to deny nursing practice itself.

Objectives are discussed with the patients (and families when appropriate), as are the methods to be employed. The patient's responsibilities and the nursing responsibilities are defined. Progress notes related to specific objectives are charted. When appropriate (with new data and knowledge), objectives are discontinued, or modified, and new ones added. It is interesting to note that the following kinds of comments were made when objectives, as described in this article, were discussed with nurses:

- We have objectives. We just cannot put them into words.
- Doing things and getting the work done is so important that there is no time for anything else.
- If I were to do this (that is set objectives) my staff would feel that I was letting them down, because I was not out helping them.
- You cannot tell a patient what the objectives are. He will get too involved, and he needs all his energy to get well.
- There is only one objective—to care for the whole patient. More objectives will only fragment the patient.
- That stuff is for students—maybe—but it is not practical when you are dealing with life and death.
- It is not possible, because patients are individuals and you cannot have a system with individuals, only with things.
- It is real interesting, but we could not do anything like that in our agency because they would not let us.
- You will never measure nursing. It is too intangible and personal.

Such feelings and thoughts are not necessarily shared by all or even a majority of nurses. In answer to such comments I say both to these nurses and to myself, because we all have some of these feelings some of the time, that it is imperative that nursing find some way to show to ourselves and the public and our colleagues in the health field that our practice is socially useful, worthwhile, tangible, and measureable.

"Nurses are such wonderful people," is not enough. Education, in and of itself, is not enough. Hard work is not enough. We must begin to measure in a systematic way what we accomplish for and with patients, and we must put this into words that can be understood. Perhaps this way is not *the* way to do it. What suggestions do you have for keeping us out of the shark's stomach (and not even knowing we are there)?

REFERENCES

1. Mager, R. F. *Preparing Instructional Objectives.* Palo Alto, Calif., Fearon Publishers, 1962, p. vii.

2. Smith, Dorothy M. Clinical nursing tools. *American Journal of Nursing* 68:2384–2388, Nov. 1968.

3. Greenwood, Ernest. Practice of science and the science of practice. In *Planning for Change,* ed. by Warren E. Bennis and others. New York, Holt, Rinehart and Winston, 1961, p. 74.

5

Implementation

Implementation, the third phase of the nursing process, is the act of putting the nursing care plan (nursing interventions) into operation; it is taking action to meet objectives. Marriner (1975, p. 109) describes it as "the actual giving of nursing care." The nurse is considered the person responsible for comprehensively coordinating the care of the client.

The client is always the primary participant in the care plan and the individualization process. The nurse, because of expertise, is co-leader. The nurse is responsible for discovering the best method for involving the client in the individual care plan and for delegating responsibility to other professional and technical care-givers as necessary. This involves four steps, three of which are covered in this chapter. The nurse's role is to:

1. Designate the parts of the health care system which will implement the care plan;
2. State the skills and competencies necessary to carry out the plan;
3. Diagnose the level of maturity (relative to each task) of the client in order to discover the leadership style needed by the nurse to implement the care plan;
4. Diagnose the level of maturity (relative to each task) of the others in the health care system who may be delegated portions of the client's care. This involves leadership and delegation activities (managing of patient care) and is covered in Chapter 16 of this book.

The case developed in Part I will form the foundation for amplifying the aforementioned steps. The following sections discuss the first three steps of the nurse's role.

PARTS OF THE SYSTEM

As previously discussed in Chapter 1, the most direct means for identifying a system is to state its purpose (Banathy, 1968); system purposes evolve and change. In the implementation phase of the nursing process, the system's purpose is to deliver individualized, comprehensive nursing care with, to, and for the client (individual or family). The system includes, therefore, those persons who will deliver the care and those who receive care. Figure 5-1 shows a hypothetical example of system components which may be important based on the case study used in Part I.

Those people directly and indirectly involved in any care must be designated as part of the network. All persons must be considered, since it is the interaction of the parts, as well as the individual entities, that produces and affects outcome.

The next step is to consider the skills necessary in order to implement the nursing orders relative to each nursing diagnosis.

SKILLS AND COMPETENCIES NECESSARY IN IMPLEMENTATION

The skills and competencies necessary to actualize the nursing orders and deal with the diagnoses must be determined. Certain skills are required of each part of the system and can be derived by answering and re-answering this simple question: What particular skills and competencies are needed by this particular person to carry out this specific nursing order? Referring to Figure 5-1, it is logical to deduce that the segments of the system involve two classifi-

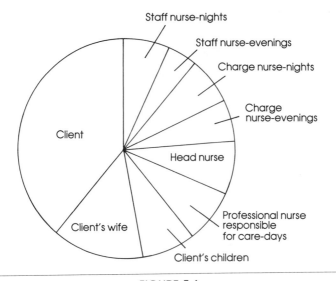

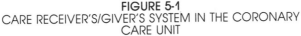

FIGURE 5-1
CARE RECEIVER'S/GIVER'S SYSTEM IN THE CORONARY
CARE UNIT

cations of persons: nursing care-givers and -receivers. An operational definition of skills and competencies for care-givers and -receivers may provide further clarity. *Skill* is "the ability that comes from knowledge, practice, aptitude and experience to accomplish a task (Webster, 1971)." *Competency* is "the quality of being adequate and qualified to carry out a responsibility (Webster, 1971)."

Referring to the nursing diagnoses and orders of the case example used in this Part, skills and competencies are listed for care-givers and care-receivers as they directly relate to fulfillment of nursing care.

(Text continues on page 110)

NURSING CARE PLAN	SKILLS AND COMPETENCIES
Nursing Diagnosis Physical signs and symptoms relating to an MI and diabetes closely monitored **Nursing Orders** 1. Monitor constantly—be alert for arrythmias. 2. Monitor vital signs Q 1 h—be alert for changes. 3. Listen to lungs for signs of congestion, QID. 4. Be alert for nonverbal signs of chest pain or related pain. Check with patient frequently. 5. Be alert for signs of dyspnea and utilize oxygen at 4 liters/min PRN. 6. Observe skin color and body temperature frequently for flushing or pallor. 7. Monitor lab reports for signs of abnormalities; if any exist, report them to the physician stat. 8. If serious arrythmias occur, treat immediately as specified by standing orders and document by running a strip on the monitor. CALL FOR A PHYSICIAN STAT. 9. Keep an accurate I & O sheet in patient's room. 10. Test urine for S/A AC and HS. Give insulin as indicated. 11. REPORT ALL CHANGES IN CLIENT'S CONDITION TO PROFESSIONAL NURSE IN CHARGE.	**Care-receivers** 1. Willingness to permit the nurse to carry out this area of care **Care-givers** 1. Knowledge and experience of the process of this illness 2. Observation 3. Listening 4. Recording I & O 5. Testing urine for S/A 6. Physical assessment 7. Interpreting ECG readings 8. Decision-making

NURSING CARE PLAN	SKILLS AND COMPETENCIES
Nursing Diagnosis Safety of self within new environment **Nursing Orders** 1. Explain coronary care unit concept to client. 2. If feasible, give him a tour of the unit or show him pictures. 3. Familiarize him with all the equipment in his room and how it works, emphasizing the purposes of each piece. Carry this out in small steps. 4. Explain rationale for all care that he will receive: monitor, medications, treatments, I & O, S/A test, diabetic diet, visiting hours, etc. 5. Be sure he understands by encouraging him to respond to your statements.	**Care-receivers** 1. Awareness of environment 2. Awareness and understanding of nursing care **Care-givers** 1. Effective interpersonal skills—empathy 2. Teaching 3. Expertise with environment

NURSING CARE PLAN

SKILLS AND COMPETENCIES

Nursing Diagnosis
Prevention of elimination difficulties

Nursing Orders
1. Be alert for constipation—be sure to check for bowel elimination every day.
2. Observe inconspicuously any straining during bowel elimination.
3. Record I & O.

Care-receivers
1. Awareness of the importance of maintaining comfortable elimination patterns

Care-givers
1. Recording I & O
2. Observation
3. Knowledge of the importance of elimination practices in relation to the disease process

NURSING CARE PLAN

SKILLS AND COMPETENCIES

Nursing Diagnosis
Adequate rest patterns; built-in periods of quiet throughout the day

Nursing Orders
1. Administer medication on time—Valium.
2. Give sleeping medication if necessary.
3. Since he is anxious about the hospital, sit and talk with him often—comfortably.
4. Quietly monitor vital signs at night; try to discover his sleeping patterns and do not disturb him when he is in deep sleep.
5. Keep two pillows at bedside within easy reach; he can use these as necessary.
6. Try to get a feeling for his cycle during the day; what his periods of rest and activity are. Then build treatments, etc., around these times, allowing him to rest when he can.

Care-receivers
1. Awareness of the need for rest and the resources available
2. Freedom to request for rest measures

Care-givers
1. Administering medications safely and with knowledge of their effects
2. Physical assessment skills
3. Observation
4. Listening
5. Effective interpersonal relationships

NURSING CARE PLAN

SKILLS AND COMPETENCIES

Nursing Diagnosis
Assurance of balanced diet, respectful of diabetes

Nursing Orders
1. Request that his meals be sent up or kept warm until he wants to eat—9-2-7; make special arrangements with department head in the kitchen.
2. Explain diabetes and the importance of eating well-balanced meals.
3. Tell client that you will help him in any way you can so that he receives foods that are in accordance with his likes.
4. Obtain food exchange lists from dietician and plan meals with client.
5. Be aware if this plan is not working and change accordingly.

Care-receivers
1. Knowledge of the importance of diet maintenance
2. Awareness of unique dietary needs

Care-givers
1. Knowledge and experience with dietary needs of diabetic clients
2. Collaboration
3. Observation
4. Listening
5. Interviewing
6. Teaching

NURSING CARE PLAN	SKILLS AND COMPETENCIES

Nursing Diagnosis
Respectful, trusting nurse/patient relationship

Nursing Orders
1. Spend time sitting down and talking with client. Do not ask questions, but rather respond to his feelings, letting him know that you have heard what he says.
2. Let him know when you will be back to talk.
3. Always be alert for signs of stress, anxiety, boredom, etc. Notice what you see by telling client that he looks _____. Listen to what he says in response to your statement.
4. ALWAYS RESPOND TO WHAT CLIENT IS SAYING: PUT YOUR AGENDA IN THE BACKGROUND.

Care-receivers
1. Trusting relationship with care-givers
2. Perception of nurse—empathy

Care-givers
1. Effective interpersonal relationships
2. Counseling
3. Empathy
4. Listening
5. Observing
6. Interviewing

NURSING CARE PLAN	SKILLS AND COMPETENCIES

Nursing Diagnosis
Awareness and understanding of the environment

Nursing Orders
In addition to orders listed under safety,
1. Explain rationale for visiting hours.
2. If you do not think that visitors for a longer period of time will harm anyone else in the unit, allow client's visitors to remain as long as possible. Always observe client for signs of fatigue.
3. If client is OOB, perhaps you could set up chairs in the hall and have client visit with family and friends there.
4. Move client's bed near to another client.
5. During quiet hours, have client sit in nurse's station, monitored directly by the large receiver.

Care-receivers
1. Awareness and understanding of environment and constraints of same

Care-givers
1. Teaching
2. Expertise with environment
3. Observation
4. Empathy

NURSING CARE PLAN	SKILLS AND COMPETENCIES

Nursing Diagnosis
Maintenance of privacy as much as possible

Nursing Orders
1. Provide privacy while client is using commode.
2. Be alert for signs of embarrassment in client—blushing, nervousness, slow speech—and intervene by engaging client in conversation aside from what you are doing. Explain your reasons fully. Do what you feel most comfortable doing, respecting the client's needs.
3. Be discreet in everything you do for client.

Care-receivers
1. Awareness that he is respected
2. Awareness of procedures that must be accomplished

Care-givers
1. Respect for client's integrity
2. Observation
3. Empathy
4. Effective interpersonal behaviors

NURSING CARE PLAN	SKILLS AND COMPETENCIES

Nursing Diagnosis
Self-maintenance of hygiene needs

Nursing Orders
1. Allow client to care for his hygiene needs to the degree required, respecting exercise or activity level needed for recovery.
2. Have all equipment handy for client.
3. Explain why limits are placed on his activity.
4. Involve wife in his care if he desires.

Care-receivers
1. Knowledge of environment
2. Respect for his physical condition
3. Awareness of what he is able to do
4. Familiarity with use of equipment

Care-givers
1. Teaching
2. Collaboration
3. Decision-making
4. Observation

NURSING CARE PLAN	SKILLS AND COMPETENCIES

Nursing Diagnosis
Self-maintenance of personal comfort measures

Nursing Orders
1. Continually be alert for what makes him comfortable and his favorite manner for having things done. Amplify these.
2. Sit and talk with him concerning things at home that he might like to bring into his room; follow through by having family obtain these items.
3. Always respond to his likes and dislikes; then respect them!

Care-receivers
1. Trusting relationship with care-givers
2. Perception of nurse—empathy
3. Knowledge of environment

Care-givers
1. Observation
2. Listening
3. Interviewing
4. Advocacy
5. Effective interpersonal communications

NURSING CARE PLAN	SKILLS AND COMPETENCIES

Nursing Diagnosis
Teaching to chart I & O, care for monitor leads, and testing urine

Nursing Orders
1. Talk with him regarding the importance of the three treatments.
2. Find out if he is interested in caring for these aspects himself.
3. If he is, then develop a plan for teaching him that moves from your demonstration, client doing and being checked and then client assuming responsibility himself.
4. Keep chart of intake measures or equivalents on bedside table.
5. Keep I & O sheet by client.
6. Keep all equipment handy.

Care-receivers
1. Recording I & O
2. Care of monitor leads
3. Testing urine for S/A
4. Familiarity with equipment
5. Knowledge of disease process

Care-givers
1. Teaching
2. Observation
3. Listening

NURSING CARE PLAN	SKILLS AND COMPETENCIES
Nursing Diagnosis Self-maintenance of bowel and bladder elimination This area has been covered in a previous nursing diagnosis and in teaching. Self-maintenance means that client is aware of the importance placed on this area of care and is responsible and accountable for his own care.	Previously covered

NURSING CARE PLAN	SKILLS AND COMPETENCIES
Nursing Diagnosis Recognition of what he does for himself and others **Nursing Orders** 1. Always notice and verbally respond that you have seen what the client has accomplished. 2. Reinforce positively all aspects of client's growth. 3. Give client small things to do for self, you, and other clients. 4. Verbalize the positive aspects of the accomplishments of the client: eating better, requiring no extra insulin. Use this also as a way to reinforce teaching areas.	**Care-receivers** 1. Awareness of his accomplishments 2. Listening 3. Awareness of environment **Care-givers** 1. Effective interpersonal skills 2. Positive reinforcement behaviors 3. Creativity 4. Teaching 5. Listening

It becomes evident that care-receivers' skills are relatively smaller in number than those of the providers when an acute phase of illness is involved. This is explained in Chapman and Chapman's (1975) advocacy helping model where the degree of client participation decreases as severity of illness increases. Therefore, as the seriousness of illness decreases, the level of client participation increases. This factor lends further evidence of the dynamic processes in nursing care and the need for a system's approach to plan individualized care.

Level of Maturity of Skills and Competencies

After delineating the skills and competencies necessary to set nursing orders in motion, it is imperative to determine whether or not care-givers and care-receivers have the necessary level of maturity relative to each task. This means, simply, is the giver or receiver capable of adequately performing the skill? Maturity refers to ability and willingness to accomplish specific tasks. Levels move from low to moderate to high. This section will focus on using a model for diagnosing the level of maturity of the client and the primary care-giver. (See Chapter 16 for a discussion of diagnosing the level of maturity of other care-givers; nursing leadership is involved.)

The situational leadership theory, developed by Hersey and Blanchard (1977), is the administration model that will be helpful in discovering how it is most appropriate to actualize the nursing care plan—how to intervene most effectively to develop those skills necessary for both the care-givers and -receivers. Hersey and Blanchard's model is designed for leadership training; the integration into nursing is done by this author. It is necessary for the nurse to view herself as the leader in her own learning, as well as a leader with the client in client recovery. It is assumed that the client needs help in some areas and the nurse is expected to have this expertise. It is necessary to discern the degree of nurse intervention in relation to each task involved in the client's care. The nurse must be alert to tasks the client can accomplish independently as well as those requiring assistance.

There is a gap between expertly planning individualized nursing care and implementing individualized interventions. Even though care can be tailor-made for the unique person in focus, the communication processes, if not synchronized with the maturity of the client in relation to the task, can have the effect of being "off-the-wall" to the client. By diagnosing the level of maturity of the client and implementing nursing orders accordingly, the hope is that the effectiveness of any nursing intervention can be maximized. This means that it must be received and accepted by the client to be useful. Furthermore, those areas in which the client can carry on independently should be allowed and encouraged with support given only when needed. This follows the definition of nursing explained in Part V.

The nurse's level of maturity in relation to a task plays just as important a role in implementing a nursing order as the client's level of maturity. The nurse must engage in a self-study of maturity in relation to a task. This self-diagnosis will raise the nurse's consciousness and will illuminate areas for further study and experience. It will also designate the type of learning essential to mature growth. The next section will discuss situational leadership theory as a means of implementing nursing orders.

Situational Leadership Theory

According to the situational leadership theory (Hersey and Blanchard, 1977), as a client's ability in a task moves from low to moderate, the nurse changes her interventions by decreasing task behaviors and increasing relationship behaviors until a moderate level of maturity is reached. At that time the nurse decreases both types of behavior to that point at which no further intervention by the nurse is necessary. This is another way of saying the nurse assists the client to fullest potential. Learning has taken place in the client; the client has reached maturity on a specific task and will carry on with no outside interventions needed. The client is both able and willing. At this point, interventions can be perceived as interferences.

Before going on it is necessary to define what is meant by task behavior and relationship behavior. First of all, *behavior* consists of actions and reactions perceived by others. This is different from *attitudes*, which are emotion-based values, beliefs, and opinions. As is noted in Part V, attitudes and behaviors function best when integrated with each other. To think that "everyone knows what I really mean" is to be deluded. People truly know what a person means only by what behaviors they observe. Therefore, a nurse's behavior should reflect the nurse's attitude. *Task behavior* is the nurse's action of designating what needs to be done or learned, how it must be done or learned, when, where, and why. It involves mostly one-way communication. *Relationship behavior* is the nurse's socioemotional support, positive reinforcement, psychological strokes, and maintenance of warm personal relationships with the receiver. It involves two-way communications patterns (Hersey and Blanchard, 1977). There are four areas of task behavior involved in implementing nursing care: (1) delineating the order or intervention; (2) diagnosing the level of maturity of the client; (3) discovering the appropriate style on which to base interventions; and (4) carrying out the order.

Figure 5-2 is a diagram of situational leadership theory. Noted in the figure are two sections: the bottom refers to the maturity of the client, while the top indicates the appropriate leadership style of the nurse. The curvilinear line running through to the uppermost segments refers to the way people grow from immaturity to maturity and the appropriate leadership style necessary in facilitating learning.

It may be helpful to imagine yourself learning a skill, for example, skiing. At the onset what is probably needed is a high degree of teacher explanation of exactly what is needed to get down the mountain alive, things such as "stand up," "bend knees," "relax," "keep the skis straight." This is task behavior. As the act of descending the hill becomes easier, relationships behavior is indicated along with task behavior. This includes positive reinforcement such as: "You are looking better—not quite as stiff"; "How does it feel to fly through the air?"; "You are getting it, but remember to keep your knees bent!" Gradually, as one moves from immaturity to maturity in skiing, neither behavior nor teaching becomes necessary. The skier engages in the sport because it is now a part of personal life. The curvilinear line represents this growth process. It moves in the fashion described because of the learning theories that support this growth process in learners. If your teacher left you completely on your own after you successfully descended the mountain once, learning would not be completely or effectively fulfilled.

It becomes evident that the level of task maturity is not simple or two-pronged (yes or no; immature or mature), but rather it is multi-faceted. Hersey and Blanchard (1977) designate four benchmarks in maturity levels:

M 1 = Low maturity	**Follower is** unwilling and unable
M 2 = Moderate maturity	willing but unable
M 3 = Moderate maturity	able but unwilling
M 4 = High maturity	able and willing

It follows that if a client needs to maintain a strict 1500 calorie diabetic diet, does not have any knowledge on the subject, and is not interested in learning, the client would be diagnosed as M 1 in relationship to the task. If the client shows interest but has no knowledge, then the client would be at the M 2 level. Further, if the client has the knowledge but pays no attention to diet, M 3 is indicated. The M 4 level reflects a person with knowledge and ability in that the diet is followed independently without any intervention.

Figure 5-3 shows how the nurse can decide on the appropriate leadership style after diagnosing the maturity level of the client.

If a client is diagnosed at the M 1 level, simply draw a straight angle (90°) from the point of the immaturity-maturity continuum up to where it intersects

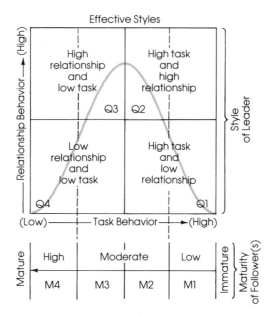

SOURCE: Paul Hersey, Kenneth H. Blanchard, Management of Organizational Behavior: Utilizing Human Resources, 3rd Edition, © 1977, p. 167. Reprinted by permission of Prentice-Hall, Inc., Englewood Cliffs, New Jersey.

FIGURE 5-2
SITUATIONAL LEADERSHIP THEORY:
Designations for styles of leadership and
maturity levels of follower(s).

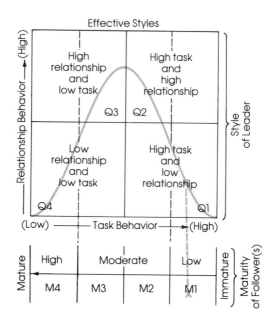

SOURCE: Paul Hersey, Kenneth H. Blanchard, _Management of Organizational Behavior: Utilizing Human Resources_, 3rd Edition, © 1977, p. 167. Reprinted by permission of Prentice-Hall, Inc., Englewood Cliffs, New Jersey.

FIGURE 5-3
SITUATIONAL LEADERSHIP THEORY:
Determining an appropriate leadership style
according to maturity level of follower(s).

the curvilinear function (Hersey and Blanchard, 1977). It is in that quadrant that the nursing intervention must be based _in relationship to the task._

As an example, let us refer to the client who is unwilling and unable to follow the diabetic diet. An S 1 quadrant—high task and low relationship—is indicated according to the situational leadership theory.* This means that the nurse must tell the client what to do (that is, the diet must be followed), how it should be followed, and the need for its accuracy. Since the purpose is to move the client to maturity on this task, as soon as the nurse observes willingness, adaptation, or receptiveness, the original diagnosis changes from M 1 to M 2 and the style of leadership from S 1 to S 2. At this point, the nurse should engage in two-way communication, providing positive support, feedback, questions, and similar input. It becomes obvious that no matter where one starts, movement should always be toward maturity because the nurse desires

*S 1, S 2, S 3, and S 4 correspond to Q 1, Q 2, Q 3, and Q 4 on Figure 5-3. S signifies the "style" of leadership represented in each quadrant (Q) of the situational leadership paradigm.

that clients eventually become able to direct and intervene totally on their own behalf.

Hersey and Blanchard (1977) delineate four verbs which help clarify the leadership styles:

Q 1 = High Task, Low Relationship   = "Telling"
Q 2 = High Task, High Relationship = "Selling"
Q 3 = High Relationship, Low Task   = "Participating"
Q 4 = Low Task, Low Relationship   = "Delegating"

Telling is reflective of one-way communication whereby the nurse must be explicit concerning what needs to be accomplished and how it must be accomplished to safeguard the health of the client. *Selling* is a leadership style whereby the nurse must still be responsible for carrying out the task, but at the same time engages in two-way communication to attempt to move the client into involvement. *Participating* is a collaborative effort between client and nurse with the nurse moving toward a supportive role, since the client is able to accomplish the task. *Delegating* involves letting the client have full control, since the client is both able and willing (Hersey and Blanchard, 1977).

This cycle may be used as a consciousness-raising exercise to determine one's own needs in relation to a specified task. To do so, simply diagnose maturity on the scale and then determine the appropriate leadership style needed. Quadrants S 1, S 2, and S 3 require that outside help is necessary; ask for it, find it, and receive it. S 4 signifies that one can carry on alone.

Referring back to the example of teaching a client about a diabetic diet, suppose in this case it is the nurse who has the desire but does not have knowledge. An M 2 level is indicated with an S 2 leadership style required. High task and relationship means the nurse must be directed to the knowledge, must be taught, and also must be involved in two-way communication processes with the teacher as well as with the client. From that point, the growth processes remain the same, moving through each quadrant as maturity increases. As another example, suppose a nurse has knowledge but is not highly motivated to work through this process with the client—this is an M 3 level. What is necessary is to seek someone who can support, listen, and help the nurse in accomplishing this task; this is high relationship, low task. To mesh attitudes with behaviors, all feelings must be worked through, recognizing that all nurses and others have both positive and negative feelings at different times, reflecting various circumstances.

Going back to the skills and competencies delineated earlier in this chapter, one must consider each as a separate entity. A diagnosis of the level of maturity of the care-giver and care-receiver must be made and followed through in implementing individualized nursing care. It should be noted that maturity levels are not consistent; any person has evidence of all facets of the continuum in his or her behavioral system. Moreover, inasmuch as maturity flows in relation to many circumstances, especially in response to environ-mental changes and illness, people can be expected to move back and forth in maturity as situations change. It is the nurse's major responsibility to respond to any changes in self as well as in clients, rediagnosing and intervening as required.

Implementation of nursing care and the appropriateness of leadership styles can be effective or ineffective; this requires evaluation and is discussed in the next chapter, which concludes the steps of the nursing process. Note that leadership in nursing is further discussed in Chapter 16 and models of nursing actions are discussed in Chapter 17.

SUMMARY

Chapter 5 focused on implementation of the nursing care plan. Designa-tion of the system involved in this implementing process and delineation of the skills and competencies of the care-givers and care-receivers was shown according to the case example used in Part I. These skills are necessary to carry out nursing diagnoses and orders. The situational leadership theory was used as the theoretical framework for determining the manner of appropriate inter-vention, with the nurse and client being considered.

REFERENCES

Banathy, B. Instructional systems. Palo Alto: Fearon, 1968.

Chapman, J., and Chapman, H. Behavior and health care: A humanistic helping process. St. Louis: C. V. Mosby, 1975.

Hersey, P., and Blanchard, K. Management of Organizational Behavior: Utilizing human resources. Englewood Cliffs, N.J.: Prentice-Hall, 1977.

Marriner, A. The nursing process: A scientific approach to nursing care. St. Louis: C. V. Mosby, 1975.

Webster's Third International Dictionary. Springfield, Mass.: G & C Merriam Com-pany, 1971.

SELECTED READING

Zimmerman's and Gohrke's (1970) article is recommended for showing another case using the steps of the nursing process in detail. The authors present a succinct and articulate care plan, making the nursing process in action easy-to-follow and necessary for individualized nursing care.

The Goal-Directed Nursing Approach

Donna Stulgis Zimmerman
Carol Gohrke

And it isn't mystical or difficult, these authors point out. They illustrate that the nursing process of assessment, goal setting, planning, action, and evaluation is orderly, usable, and useful in caring for a patient; furthermore, there is the added benefit of knowing, not guessing, the impact that nursing care has had on the patient's well-being.

The ever enlarging scope of nursing responsibilities has led us to a confrontation with routinized care.

We need to use a systematic approach to planning patient care, based on a scientific foundation, if we are to attack the multiplicity of problems which patients present. Such an approach is a process which encompasses four phases: assessment, goal setting and planning, implementation, and evaluation.

During the *first phase* all members of the nursing team, in cooperation with the professional nurse, gather information or data about the patient from all available resources. This information includes the patient's normal functioning, his present status, and tentative goals for his future level of function. The form of this assessment may involve one or more approaches. For example, the nurse may decide to assess the functioning of bodily systems; that is, she may ask herself what is the patient's ability to exchange oxygen and carbon dioxide via the respiratory system? The nurse might also employ an assessment of the patient's activities of daily living, such as his sleep pattern.

Another approach might be a "head to toe" assessment. In this approach, general observations of the patient's condition are noted, as well as more specific ones. For example, the nurse would note the general signs and symptoms of fatigue as well as the specific sign of atrophy of the lower leg musculature.

The collected information is then organized and utilized in the identification of nursing problems. We define a nursing problem as a patient's need or potential need. Concomitant with the identification of the patient's needs is the setting of realistic goals for the resolution of the problem.

Reprinted with permission from *American Journal of Nursing*, Vol. 70, No. 2. Copyright 1970 by The American Journal of Nursing Company.

The *second phase* involves utilizing the collective knowledge and experience of all members of the nursing team and gathering current scientific information related to the identified problem. To illustrate, an assessment of a bedfast patient might include the aide's observation that the patient lies on his back without alteration of position for periods of up to four hours. This observation, coupled with additional data about the patient's age, nutritional status, and skin condition, would lead the nurse to define the problem as "maintenance of skin integrity and prevention of decubitus ulcers."

Scientific information which relates to decubitus ulcer formation has indicated that continuous pressure of one hour's duration causes beginning tissue breakdown[1,2]. Having determined this and gathered other information, this leads to the *third phase:* implementing nursing actions. For the problem described above, an action derived from the literature might be to turn the patient every hour, utilizing all four of his body surfaces in succession. In this third phase, careful communication and teaching are necessary to interpret the plan of care to all nursing team members involved in the patient's care.

The *final phase* of the process involves evaluating the effectiveness of the nursing action based on specific criteria. In the case of preventing decubitus ulcers, the criteria might include absence of redness and breaks in the skin. The appearance of these signs and symptoms would indicate a need for revision of therapy. This emphasizes the ongoing nature of this process.

This method of planning nursing therapy is applicable to patients wherever they are on the health continuum and in varying environments. The application of this process is illustrated by presentation of a patient with a diagnosis of systemic lupus erythematosus. This patient with a somewhat obscure diagnosis was chosen purposely to emphasize that it is not solely the patient's medical diagnosis that dictates nursing care. Rather, nursing care is determined by the needs manifested by the particular individual.

Prior to her illness, Mrs. W., a small, thin 28-year-old wife and mother, was an active participant in such activities as bowling, skiing, and sewing. On the first encounter with Mrs. W. one saw a pale, lethargic woman with a flat facial expression. With further inspection, we found diffuse symmetrical muscle wasting, sacral, foot, and ankle edema, and moderate abdominal distention.

While Mrs. W. presented a multiplicity of needs, only two—weakness and elimination—were selected to illustrate the use of the process, as well as the interrelationship of the patient's needs and the nurse's role in reinforcing the contributions made by other members of the health team. Other problems that Mrs. W. manifested which are not dealt with in this discussion included susceptibility to thrombus formation, alteration of body image and role, beginning formation of sacral decubitus ulcers, generalized edema and fluid and electrolyte disturbances secondary to impaired renal function. Problems of short-term duration that were resolved included diarrhea secondary to antacid therapy, with its associated fluid and electrolyte imbalance.

PROBLEM: WEAKNESS

Assessment

The first encounter with Mrs. W. suggested the likelihood of weakness as a possible problem. This led to the collection of additional information beyond the initial observation of lethargy and muscle wasting, with the purpose of validating or ruling out the presence of this problem.

On further investigation, it was learned that Mrs. W. had been on bed rest and steroid therapy for two months prior to this hospitalization. Yet, when she entered the hospital, Mrs. W. was encouraged to ambulate within her ability. Specific observations revealed interference with activities requiring minimal exertion. For example, she was unable to rise unaided from a sitting to a standing position and was unable to gradually lower herself back to a sitting position. Once erect, although she was able to walk, her walking was limited to a distance of 10 feet before she had to rest. When asked about her minimal activity even in bed, Mrs. W. stated, "Even turning to my side is exhausting." She also expressed frustration at not being able to do "the everyday things in life." The findings of an electromyelogram confirmed myopathy secondary to steroid therapy and the disease process.

In assessing Mrs. W.'s strengths, we noted that she was capable of some activities of daily living and had full range of motion in all her joints. The tentative goal formulated for her was the strengthening of muscles of the abdominal girdle and the extremities to minimize her frustration and to maximize her independence.

Planning

In an effort to find a scientific basis for intervention in this problem, we investigated literature on the causes and treatment of weakness and associated fatigue.

Muscle weakness in this patient was attributed to three factors: the disease process, prolonged bed rest, and steroid therapy. Data from 15 autopsies of persons who had had lupus erythematosus revealed that 73 percent manifested muscle degeneration[3]. An earlier reference demonstrated a distinct relationship between immobilization and muscle strength, particularly in immobilized leg muscles[4]. Finally, we learned that muscle weakness from steroids is most prominent in the limbs and the abdominal musculature, to the point that activities requiring these muscles are hampered[5].

In the area of nursing intervention for weakness, exercise has been cited as being most beneficial. Therefore, we investigated the uses of isometric exercises, since these exercises require less energy expenditure and equipment and can be supervised independently by nursing personnel.

A further basis for selecting isometric exercises was the fact that the patient was currently receiving isotonic exercises five times a week from a physical therapist. One study had demonstrated that isometric contraction of the forearm flexor muscle for six seconds twice daily resulted in increased muscle strength of from 17 to 20 percent[6]. Other findings from patients on bed rest for 60 days showed that a regimen of isometric exercises was sufficient to counteract the detrimental consequences of bed rest and inactivity[7]. Although exercise is recognized as therapy for weakness, it has been noted that prolonged and strong contraction of a muscle leads to muscle fatigue.[8]

Implementation

Nursing actions were directed toward (1) providing supplementary exercise, (2) facilitating movement in bed, and (3) preventing weakness and fatigue from overexertion. Mrs. W. was given written instructions and demonstrations, and then she redemonstrated, herself, the isometric exercises for the musculature of the arms, legs, and abdomen. She was helped to do these exercises twice a day on weekdays and three times a day on weekends when physical therapy was not available. Mrs. W. expressed satisfaction in doing these exercises, saying, "This is one thing I can do on my own to help myself."

As an additional means to encourage exercise and independence with less exertion, a trapeze and footboard were applied to her bed. In an effort to avoid overexertion, a schedule of daily activities was arranged with Mrs. W., including meals, exercises, physical therapy, and rest periods (see this page).

Activity Schedule For Mrs. W.

Time	Activity
7:30	Awaken, void, wash face and hands T.P.R., weight
7:45	Rest
8:15	Breakfast
9:15	Ambulate to B.R., brush teeth
9:30	Rest
10:00	Physical Therapy
11:00	Rest
12 noon	Lunch
12:30	Rest
1:00	Bath, linen change
2:00	Rest
2:30	Isometric Exercises
2:45	Rest
3:30	Occupational Therapy
4:15	Rest
5:00	Dinner
5:30	Rest
7:00	Visiting Hours
8:30	Isometric Exercises
9:00	Prepare for sleep, wash, brush teeth, massage
9:30	In bed for night

Since physical therapy was available only in the mornings, it was agreed with Mrs. W. to schedule her bath after lunch to prevent overexertion.

Evaluation

Several measures were selected to evaluate the effectiveness of the nursing actions directed toward strengthening Mrs. W.'s musculature. These criteria included the following: (1) the distance Mrs. W. could walk, (2) the amount of assistance required by Mrs. W. to come to a standing or sitting position, (3) the consistency with which she performed the isometric exercises, (4) the frequency of use of the trapeze and footboard as a means to alter positions, and finally, (5) the incidence of frustration she expressed related to muscle weakness.

After six weeks with this plan in action, and despite further progression of her pathophysiology, Mrs. W. was able to walk unassisted for distances of up to 100 feet. Further, she was capable of standing and sitting without assistance, although this was not done with ease. She did the isometric exercises regularly, although at times she did require reminding and encouragement. She used the trapeze to assist herself in moving in bed and in coming to a sitting position. As Mrs. W.'s muscle strength increased, her comments related to frustration with the inability to perform daily tasks decreased.

While it is impossible to differentiate the contributions made by physical therapy and nursing, we believe that Mrs. W. would not have achieved this level of functioning without the supplementary nursing action.

PROBLEM: INADEQUATE ELIMINATION

Assessment

The problem of bowel elimination was manifested on admission by Mrs. W.'s complaints of constipation and inability to defecate. She reported that prior to her illness, she had had a daily bowel movement approximately 45 minutes after breakfast. She denied a history of constipation or diarrhea related to stress.

During her hospitalization, Mrs. W. was encouraged to use the toilet in the private bathroom adjoining her room. There, she was able to maintain an upright position but, because of her abdominal muscle weakness, she was unable to bear down with sufficient force to expel a stool of normal consistency.

Due to the problem of weakness, this patient spent the majority of her time in bed, and this in itself is known to decrease bowel motility. As a result of the additional problem of edema, Mrs. W.'s fluid intake was restricted to one liter a day.

Compounding the intake limitation was the fact that Mrs. W. was reluctant to take even this amount of fluid without encouragement. Her fluid intake was predominantly apple juice, ginger ale, and milk. She was receiving Colace (dioctyl sodium sulfosuccinate) 100 mg. daily which was given at 9 A.M., and milk of magnesia 30 cc. with cascara sagrada 5 cc. p.r.n. at bedtime to help alleviate her constipation.

In the assessment, Mrs. W.'s nutritional patterns were examined and a strength noted in that she consistently ate all of her general, low sodium diet. We assumed that Mrs. W. was receiving adequate bulk, since her stools were of normal size.

Planning

The long-term goal for Mrs. W.'s elimination was that she return to her normal defecation pattern of a daily bowel movement after breakfast. Collection of information related to bowel elimination again provided the guides to nursing action. It is well known that mass peristaltic movements from the upper intestines cause distention of the rectum and the urge to defecate. However, unless this urge is responded to in a few minutes it will disappear, leading to an accumulation of the wastes and constipation. Further, mass peristaltic movements usually occur after breakfast, and adequate fluid intake is essential to the prevention and treatment of constipation[9]. It is also suggested that the gastrocolic reflex may be augmented by hot coffee or warm water[10].

The act of defecation requires the assistive contraction of several abdominal muscles as well as the contraction of the muscles of the pelvic floor[11]. Leaning forward from the hips while in a sitting position also assists in raising the intra-abdominal pressure. Others have concluded that regular abdominal exercises will enhance an individual's ability to "bear down," thus assisting with defecation[10,12].

Yasuna, in studying stool softeners and laxatives, concluded that the primary action of stool softeners is that of decreasing the surface tension of the bowel. The peak action of stool softeners occurs six to eight hours after ingestion, whereas the peak action of milk of magnesia and cascara sagrada occurs approximately eight hours after ingestion. In conclusion, he suggests that if laxatives are given in combination with stool softeners, they should be administered at times that will allow their peak actions to coincide, so that the strong propulsive movements will occur in combination with the decreased surface tension[13]. The time-honored use of prunes and figs was also suggested as an adjunct[10].

Implementation

Nursing actions focused on the following four areas: (1) taking advantage of mass peristaltic movements, (2) increasing intra-abdominal pressure, (3) increasing fluid intake within the ordered limitations, and (4) utilizing the complementary actions of the laxatives and the stool softener.

Mrs. W. was already including hot coffee with her breakfast, and prune juice was substituted for the morning apple juice. Forty minutes after breakfast

Nursing Care Plan

Problem/Goal	Nursing Actions
Weakness Goal: Decrease Frustration, Maximise independence	1 Isometric exercises for arms, legs and abdomen bed 2:30 pm and 8:00pm — remind and encourage patient 2 Physical Therapy Monday thru Friday 10 am. 3 Encourage use of foot board and trapeeze 4 Avoid rushing patient with any activity 5 Observe planned rest periods — do not interrupt patient 6 Follow planned schedule of activities — do not awaken until 7:30 am.
Inadequate Bowel Elimination Goal: Return to Normal Defecation Pattern	1 Encourage fluid consumption up to 1 liter limit 7-3 700cc. 3-11 250cc. 11-7 50cc. 2 See that prune juice and hot coffee included on breakfast tray 3 Assist patient to B.R. 40 minutes past breakfast 4 Positioning on toilet: assist patient to lean forward from hips while she applies internal pressure over abdomen with hands. 5 Isometric exercise of abdomen as noted above 6 Colace 100 mgm. 10 pm; moin. 30cc. Cascara 5cc @ 9 pm. Evaluate need before giving

she was assisted to the bathroom. We discussed with her the importance of heeding the stimulus to defecate and she was encouraged to call immediately for assistance whenever she felt the urge to evacuate.

Once positioned on the toilet, she was instructed to place her hands over her abdomen and lean forward from the hips in order to increase her intra-abdominal pressure. The nursing personnel remained with her when it was necessary to help her maintain this position. Mrs. W.'s isometric abdominal exercises also helped her with this problem and, in addition, she was encouraged to move in bed using the trapeze to increase the strength of her pelvic girdle musculature.

The desirability of having the peak actions of the stool softener and laxative coincide was discussed among the nursing personnel. As a result, it was agreed that the daily order of Colace would be given at 10 P.M. rather than the routine time of 9 A.M., since the milk of magnesia and cascara were given at bedtime. This enabled the peak actions of the medications to coincide at approximately the time of the morning meal when mass peristaltic movements are most likely to occur. This time was consistent with her normal bowel pattern.

Evaluation

We used two criteria to evaluate the success of nursing interventions: (1) that Mrs. W.'s bowel evacuation pattern returned to her prehospital evacuation pattern, and (2) that her stools should be of soft, formed consistency.

For the first two weeks following the institution of these measures, little improvement of the problem was seen. However, after the third week, as Mrs. W.'s state of weakness began to show improvement with the concomitant increase in strength of the abdominal musculature, gradual improvement was observed. At this point, Mrs. W. was having daily, loose, semiformed stools, with the administration of colace, milk of magnesia, and cascara each night. At the end of six weeks, Mrs. W. was able to have formed stools with the daily intake of prune juice but without the use of laxatives or stool softeners. The frequency of the stools varied from daily to every other day.

SUMMARY

It is our belief that the effectiveness of nursing care for this patient was enhanced by the utilization of a systematic process of assessment, goal setting, planning, implementation, and evaluation. Nursing care based solely on intuition or on routine carries no assurance that the individual needs of each patient will be met. This is not to imply that the nurse does not utilize her knowledge of specific disease entities and the associated nursing care. For example, in caring for a patient with external bile drainage following a cholecystectomy and common bile duct exploration, the nurse relies on her knowledge of the purpose, function, and location of the T-tube to guide observation and nursing care. Though the diagnosis is different, this patient might also manifest problems of weakness and inadequate bowel elimination similar to those of Mrs. W. Thus, if the nurse's focus is limited solely to nursing care as it relates to the cholecystectomy, it is probable that other needs will go undetected.

It is also our belief that the implementation of such a process promotes greater satisfaction for nursing personnel on all levels. A major strength is the goal-directedness of nursing care, and the fact that the nurse can use measurable criteria to demonstrate her contribution to the patient's well-being.

REFERENCES

1. Kosiak, Michael. Etiology of decubitus ulcers. *Arch.Phys.Med.* 42:19, Jan. 1961.

2. Kottke, F. J., and Blanchard, R. S. Bedrest begets bedrest. *Nurs.Forum* 3(3):59, 1964.

3. Lowman, E. W. Muscle, nerve and synovial changes in lupus erythematosus. *Ann. Rheumat.Dis.* 10:19, Mar. 1951.

4. Deitrick, J. E., et al. Effects of immobilization upon various metabolic and physiologic functions of normal men. *Amer.J.Med.* 4:18, Jan. 1948.

5. Harrison, T. R., et al., eds. *Principles of Internal Medicine.* 5th ed. New York, McGraw-Hill Book Co., 1966, p. 1315.

6. Hislop, Helen J. Quantitative changes in human muscular strength during isometric exercise. *J.Amer.Phys.Ther.Ass.* 43:38, Jan. 1963.

7. Brannon, E. W., et al. Influence of specific exercises in the prevention of debilitating musculoskeletal disorders. *Aerospace Med.* 34:905, Oct. 1963.

8. Guyton, A. C. *Textbook of Medical Physiology.* 3d ed. Philadelphia, Pa., W. B. Saunders Co., 1966, p. 99.

9. Bockus, H. L. *Gastroenterology.* 2d ed. Philadelphia, Pa., W. B. Saunders Co., 1964, Vol. 2, pp. 627–628.

10. Palmer, E. D. *Clinical Gastroenterology.* New York, Harper and Brothers, 1957, pp. 339–340.

11. Fuerst, Elinor, and Wolff, Luverne E. *Fundamentals of Nursing.* 3d ed. Philadelphia, Pa., J. B. Lippincott Co., 1964, p. 311.

12. Harmer, Bertha. *Textbook of the Principles and Practices of Nursing.* 5th ed. revised by Virginia Henderson. New York, Macmillan Co., 1958, p. 436.

13. Yasuna, A. D., and Halpern, Alfred. Timed integration of stool hydration and peristaltic stimulation in constipation correction. *Amer.J.Gastroenter.* 28:539, Nov. 1957.

BIBLIOGRAPHY

Nite, Gladys, and Willis, F. N., Jr. *Coronary patient.* New York, Macmillan Co., 1964.

6

Evaluation

Chapter 6 begins with a discussion of the evaluation process followed by its application to the case developed for this section. Tools used in the evaluative process are then discussed.

Evaluation is theoretically the concluding step of the nursing process, nursing's scientific method. It is the act of discovering whether or not plans were fulfilled. Conley (1973) elaborates on the meaning of evaluation from an educational perspective. She states that the purpose of a nursing curriculum is to bring changes in certain directions within students; this should be a planned, rational activity. The analogy in nursing care is explicit, for the practitioner desires changes in the client(s) and self; these changes are conscious, planned, and directed. It logically follows that evaluation is the process of going back to the nursing diagnoses and determining whether the needs they signified were met and/or determining what other assistance is necessary based on the outcomes of the care plan for each client's system. It should be noted that discussion will be limited to evaluation of direct patient care and the effectiveness of nursing care plans. The broader aspect of nursing service quality assurance is covered in Chapter 14.

THE PROCESS OF EVALUATION

The simplicity of the evaluative process has a positive relationship to the clarity and comprehensiveness of the nursing diagnoses and orders. If the objectives of the nursing care plan are clear, it becomes the base for evaluation. Moreover, when care plans are not explicit, the evaluation process cannot take place, since there are no established controls of objectives. It is impossible to measure success without being aware of intent.

Broadly speaking, the goal of nursing is to assist the client to fullest health potential, thus eliminating the need for professional assistance. Again, this is based on the definition of a nursing diagnosis as an item or area in which the client requires nursing assistance. Hersey and Blanchard (1977) refer to maturity (in other words, a client's fullest potential) as that stage where neither task nor relationship behavior are required from the leader; the client can and will carry out functions and adapt independently.

All parts of the designated system involved in client care require evaluation as each fits into the nursing diagnoses and orders. Yura and Walsh (1973) underscore this point when they state that the nurse and client are the agents of the process with involvement of nursing personnel, health team members, and family. It follows that several facets of care must be evaluated:

1. Restoration of health of the client with alleviation of problems delineated in the nursing diagnoses;
2. Level of maturity of care-givers and -receivers in relation to the skills and competencies necessary to implement care; and,
3. Effectiveness of the leadership style used in implementing care (Hersey and Blanchard, 1977).

Based on outcomes of this evaluative process, the nurse becomes aware of additional data on which to plan or adapt subsequent nursing care.

The most often used method of evaluation in nursing is a behavioral method involving direct observation by the nurse planning the care. Since evaluation by one person lends less validity to the results because of the limited perceptual field of the individual, evaluation of nursing care is best when several health personnel are involved in the process. The larger the number of competent people observing the same effect, the more valid are the results. Campbell and Fiske (1959) describe this as separating method from trait variance by employing different methods for testing the same trait and obtaining construct validity for what is being tested. Their theory states that different measures of the same trait should be more highly correlated than: (1) different measures of different traits, or (2) different traits measured by the same method.

The evaluative process can be formal or informal. An example of a formal evaluation is one in which specific outcome criteria in nursing care are delineated and written down prior to implementation. These then become the bases for evaluation. Another example of formal evaluative processes is the retrospective evaluation in which the nurse makes a point by point review of the client's response to care after the nursing plan has been initiated; in retrospective evaluations, outcome criteria are not delineated before implementation. Informal processes include nonspecific professional judgment or a combination of explicit, observed phenomena such as "no arrhythmias" and "stable vital signs" plus intuitive bases for evaluation. Informal processes are used most often.

The evaluative process also can be objective, subjective, or both. *Objective* in this instance refers to evaluation that is based on specific facts, such as a record of a client's vital signs, rather than an evaluation based on intuitive concerns, feelings, or emotional responses to the client. These evaluations which involve the nurse's thoughts rather than hard facts are *subjective* evaluations. Both are valuable for different reasons. Objective methods of evaluation are most prevalent in nursing audit literature (McGuire, 1968; Phaneuf, 1966; Rubin, Rinaldi, and Dietz, 1972); however, subjective methods are most often used in actuality. This is unfortunate because while subjective evaluations are valuable in individualizing and personalizing care as well as responding to clients, objective evaluations are more reliable and valid. A combination of objective evaluation and subjective evaluation is the best method because it integrates facts with intuition; it eliminates the tendency of objective evaluation to be automatic and the tendency of subjective evaluation to be vague. In addition, it is a good way to check for error. For example, a client whose temperature registers normal yet who appears to the nurse to be chilled may need to have temperature measured again. The first reading may have been in error. Objective and subjective evaluations also provide other dimensions to the process: subjective data may include input from secondary sources which may prove valuable in determining client outcome; objective and subjective data can lead to development of research questions and nursing theory.

CASE EXAMPLES

Table 6-1 illustrates how to write objective outcome criteria based on two examples. (Note that "objective" used in this way is a descriptive word meaning "factual," whereas "an objective" used in the phrase "to develop an objective for the nursing plan" is a noun meaning "aim or goal.") The objective (factual) outcome criteria in the examples are based on the nursing diagnoses derived from the case study used throughout Part I.

In the first column are the "Nursing Diagnoses" which need to be dealt with; in the second column are the "Objective Outcome Criteria," that is, the specific signs expected to be observed before the patient can be considered at fullest health potential; in the third column labeled "Nursing Observations" are the actual signs noted by the nurse. By comparing objective outcome criteria with the nursing observations, the nurse can evaluate the client's progress toward maximum health potential.

Subjective outcome criteria may be developed and used in the same way. The nurse may write down explicit patterns of attitude and behavior to look for when evaluating the client. Thus, even though this is an intuitive, emotional judgment, it is based on specific observations to be made. For

TABLE 6-1
EVALUATION USING OBJECTIVE OUTCOME CRITERIA

NURSING DIAGNOSES	OBJECTIVE OUTCOME CRITERIA	NURSING OBSERVATIONS
Physical signs and symptoms relating to an MI and diabetes closely monitored	1. Physical signs should be monitored with normal ranges noted for five days for: a. B/P, P, R, T b. ECG pattern (no arrhythmias) c. heart and lung sounds (no congestion) d. laboratory reports e. respiratory patterns f. urine sugar and acetone g. no dyspnea h. no pain in chest 2. Client should state he feels well 3. Client's appearance should be normal: a. good color b. skin warm, dry c. alert	1. Physical signs monitored for five days show: a. B/P, P, R, T—normal b. ECG pattern—no arrhythmias c. heart and lung sounds— no congestion d. laboratory reports— normal e. respiratory patterns— normal f. urine sugar and acetone—normal g. no dyspnea h. no chest pain 2. Client states he feels well 3. Client appears normal: a. good color b. skin warm, dry c. alert
Assurance of balanced diet, respectful of diabetes	1. Client should be able to interpret diabetic diet to nurse and family 2. Client should plan balanced meals from diet sheet and eat the chosen food on time 3. Client should be able to care for himself with respect to his diabetic condition	1. Client interprets diabetic diet to nurse and family 2. Client plans balanced meals from diet sheet and eats chosen food on time 3. Client cares for himself with respect to diabetic condition; requests more information on disease; seeks more knowledge

example, the nurse may use subjective criteria to evaluate the client's visiting needs. If the client appears anxious or depressed when visitors are asked to leave by the nurse because of unit requirements, the nurse may deduce that the client needs more company or needs someone to talk to. The nurse can then make arrangements accordingly: personally talk to the client; move the client into a visiting area for a while if possible; or introduce the client to another in the same unit. The nurse uses subjective outcome criteria to determine if the client's attitude is congruent with the client's behavior.

Tools in Evaluation

There are formal tools which can be used by the nurse to assist in and amplify the evaluative process. These include progress notes, team conferences, and discharge summaries.

Progress Notes   Progress notes take many forms such as nurse's notes or notes written on the "Progress Notes" sheet by all health personnel involved in the client's care. Many health care systems require that personnel record routine care in addition to deviations from the normal health states of the client. Whatever the form, progress notes should contain statements concerning the nursing diagnosis of the client and the client's progress to date. The movement should be in relation to the goals of care explicated previously and should be changed whenever indicated.

Progress notes provide for continuity of care between health workers as the entire team works to assist the client in reaching fullest health potential.

Team Conference   At best the team conference involves all persons involved in the care of a client and family. It is a time to discuss the entire care plan, problem-solve, explain, gain competence in skills, or evaluate. With many people sharing expertise and perceptions in a given area, the results can be more reliable and creative and have a broader foundation than a single person's efforts. Team conferences also tend to solidify the system's approach by including everyone in the client's health plan system. This group approach can become the bond builder between health workers so that each can become a teacher and learner for and with one another. It strengthens *team* work and creates a support system for all people who are part of it.

Discharge Summaries   Discharge summaries can be used as referrals or summaries of the client's progress to date. They should include a synthesis of client data, nursing diagnoses and orders, evaluation of nursing care to date, and recommendations for future nursing care, if appropriate. This is important in continuing care so that the ladder effect in nursing—that is, moving from simple to complex, from low to high maturity—can be facilitated without requiring subsequent care-givers to regress to a zero base.

The summary generally and simply states the patient's progress in relation to the priority diagnoses and may give reference to those areas which are expected to emerge for priority in another time and place. Should clients be readmitted to a health facility, the discharge summary serves as a secondary source of data.

CONTINUOUS EVALUATION, FEEDBACK, AND DATA COLLECTION

The last step of the nursing process is bridged by feedback to the first step; the process begins again, and it is important that it continue dynamically. Actually, the nursing process should not be thought of as linear, but rather as circular as denoted in Figure 6-1.

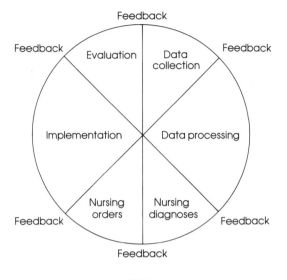

FIGURE 6-1
THE DYNAMIC NURSING PROCESS

Each facet of the nursing process pie is intersected with feedback which relates to all parts of the system. For example, the results of evaluation become new sources of data which must be processed. This data processing may change the nursing diagnosis, which must then be reflected in the nursing orders. Different orders may require changes in implementation and all must then be reevaluated, producing additional data. This cyclic process occurs continuously.

SUMMARY

Chapter 6 discussed evaluation and concluded the section on the methods involved in the nursing process. Evaluation was theoretically discussed as it applied in nursing practice, followed by examples of formal and informal evaluation processes. Team conferences, progress notes, and discharge summaries were discussed as tools in evaluation. The nursing process was then portrayed as a dynamic method of practice.

REFERENCES

Campbell, D., and Fiske, D. Convergent and discriminant validation by the Multitrait-multimethod matrix. *Psychological Bulletin* 56: 81–105, 1959.

Conley, V. *Curriculum and instruction in nursing.* Boston: Little, Brown and Company, 1973.

Hersey, P., and Blanchard, K. *Management of organizational behavior: Utilizing human resources.* Englewood Cliffs, N.J.: Prentice-Hall, 1977.

McGuire, R. Bedside nursing audit. *American Journal of Nursing* 69:2146–2148, 1968.

Phaneuf, M. The nursing audit for evaluation of patient care. *Nursing Outlook* 14:51–54, 1966.

Rubin, C., Rinaldi, L., and Dietz, R. Nursing audit—Nurses evaluating nursing. *American Journal of Nursing* 72:916–921, 1972.

Yura, H., and Walsh, M. *The nursing process: Assessing, planning, implementing, evaluating.* New York: Appleton-Century-Crofts, 1973.

SELECTED READING

The following article was written by a specialist in measurement and evaluation. The author, Elizabeth P. Hagen, has been a consultant and leader in nursing and nursing evaluation during the past several decades. She raises many questions on evaluation of nursing services that reflect expertise in an underdeveloped nursing area.

Conceptual Issues in the Appraisal of the Quality of Care

Elizabeth Hagen, Ph.D.

Concern for the quality of health care has probably existed since the first human being emerged from the primeval ooze and had his first accident. The evaluation of that initial health care has been lost in the mists of time, but you can be sure that some judgment was made about its adequacy and the way it was delivered. The concept of evaluating or judging is not new; it has always been present whenever human beings have been present.

Nor is the idea of evaluating health care services and programs new. We can go back to the writings of Graunt in 1662 and Holley in 1693 to find suggestions that vital statistics and morbidity and mortality data be used as objective indices of the state of the health of the citizens of the country. In the mid-1800s, pioneers in public health such as Chadwick (1842) and Farr (1885) pointed out the need to collect systematic data to evaluate the effectiveness of public health departments in lowering morbidity and mortality.

When the American Public Health Association was formed in 1874, it immediately appointed a committee to collect data on the condition of public hygiene in the larger towns and cities of the United States. This action initiated a series of health surveys that resulted in the development of a large number of community appraisal forms, evaluation schedules, and grading standards for use by public health agencies.

However, it was not until after World War I that the demand for critical appraisal really began to grow, and it has been growing ever since. Since World War II, citizens have become more vocal and insistent that all social systems or subsystems provide "proof" of their effectiveness to justify their continued support.

Since 1960, changes in six aspects of public service have tended to reinforce each other and produce a growing demand for evaluation of all public services including health services. These are: (1) changes in the nature of social problems, (2) changes in social values, (3) changes in the structure and function of public agencies, (4) changes in the needs and the expectations of citizens for services, (5) the continued professional growth of health practitioners and increased specialization of health practitioners, and (6) the increased costs of health care. The health field has felt the impact of all of these

Paper prepared for the conference "Assessment of Nursing Services," sponsored by the Division of Nursing, Department of Health, Education, and Welfare. Report published in May, 1975. U.S.D.H.E.W., Pub. No. (HRA) 75-40. Reprinted with permission of the author.

factors and has responded, although sometimes not rapidly enough to satisfy all of its critics.

The need for systematic assessment of the quality of health care has never been greater than it is today. At present, people are demanding more and better health services as their right. At the same time, costs for health care are increasing, and the battle between infinite demand for health services and finite funds is engaged.

The primary purpose of any evaluation is not to justify what exists; it is to provide descriptive data that will enable a person to explain the present status and to make better decisions about what to keep or what to change. Evaluation should not be viewed as a fringe activity that is undertaken to satisfy some outside agency, but it should be considered as an activity that is an integral part of the health care delivery system because the evaluation data permit us to make better decisions.

Since 1965, the literature on evaluation of health care has increased enormously. One comment that occurs frequently in the literature is that it is much easier to write or talk about evaluation than it is to do it. This is certainly true; however, in the remainder of this paper, I want to discuss some of the problems and issues that we must consider to do an adequate evaluation of health care. Most of the problems and issues relate to the "who," "what," and "how" of evaluation.

THE "WHO" OF EVALUATION

The question of "who" in evaluation studies really has three foci. One focus is *who* shall determine what shall be evaluated. A second focus is *who* is the target for evaluation or about whom shall data be collected. The third focus is *who* shall do the judging.

The issues as to who shall decide what shall be evaluated and who shall make the final judgments about the quality of health care are of critical importance. Evaluation always involves value judgments; therefore, one of the real issues is *whose* values shall be reflected or *whose* values shall predominate. The setting of goals and objectives for health care and the assignment of priorities to these goals and objectives reflect value systems.

In the evaluation of health care, physicians, in particular, have insisted upon peer review as the only valid procedure. In so doing, they have effectively indicated that their value system should have priority over all others. The question is: Should the value system of any one group determine exclusively what should or should not be evaluated? The answer is most certainly no.

The concept of quality of health care is complex; it must be examined within the framework of many value systems. The question of whose value system is appropriate to use in determining what shall be evaluated should be answered by the kind of decision that is desired.

For example, if we wish to determine whether professional nurses are practicing nursing according to accepted standards of professional nursing, then the value systems of professional nurses should be reflected in what is evaluated. On the other hand, if we want to determine whether nurses are meeting the needs and expectations of the patients or clients, then the value systems of the patients or clients provide the relevant framework for determining what should be evaluated.

The question of who is the target for evaluation or about whom shall evaluation data be collected is somewhat less value-laden than that of who determines what shall be evaluated and who makes the final judgment about quality. The target for the evaluation depends entirely upon the answer to what is to be evaluated, and this brings us to the most crucial issue or problem in the evaluation of quality of nursing care.

THE "WHAT" OF EVALUATION

Whenever the evaluations of the quality of nursing care are discussed, someone is likely to raise questions about the validity of the data or the validity of the data-gathering instruments. The questioners are really asking whether the data gathered can be used to make valid inferences about the adequacy of nursing care. In most evaluations of quality of nursing care, the validity question cannot be answered because the evaluator has not defined the term, quality of care, explicitly.

It is unfortunate that we have fallen into the trap of using the term, quality of nursing care, as a label for a somewhat heterogeneous collection of concepts or constructs. At present, the term represents nothing more than an ecological category of events that occur in the same context.

Before we can answer questions about what should be appraised in evaluating nursing care or whether a particular appraisal represents a valid measure of the quality of nursing care, we must identify more explicitly and more completely the domains or universes of variables that are encompassed by the term, quality of nursing care. This means that we must develop conceptual frameworks for studying the problem.

As pointed out earlier, what constitutes quality will vary according to the values of the individual or group of individuals making the judgment. Therefore, one requirement of a good conceptual framework is the identification of the group whose values are being reflected.

The number of groups or combination of groups from whose point of view quality of nursing care can be studied is infinite. However, we can identify four general groups whose values influence the conceptualization of quality: (1) the professional providers of health services—the nurses, physicians, and other health workers; (2) the administrators of health care delivery systems; (3) the consumers of health services; and (4) the people or agencies that provide money for the delivery of health services.

Although the values of all four groups can be reflected in the conceptualization of quality, usually the values of one particular group dominate or influence the way that quality is defined. This is the group that must be explicitly identified.

To simplify this presentation, let us assume that we are going to use the value systems of professional nurses as the primary frame of reference to develop an operational concept of quality of nursing care. The literature on the evaluation of quality of nursing care indicates that the value system of professional nurses leads to the identification of three major domains or universes of variables that are relevant: (1) the specific practices or interventions that constitute professional nursing; (2) the characteristics of the setting or the conditions under which nursing care is delivered; and (3) the effects of (1) and (2) on the consumer of nursing or on patient outcomes.

Again, we are likely to hear arguments about which universes should be studied. Some will say that the only meaningful universe to study is number (3), patient outcomes. In one sense, these people are correct. Health care systems and practices are presumed to exist because they confer benefits upon the consumer; therefore, the ultimate judgment must be made on this basis.

However, we must first be able to devise and put into operation a system or practices and make sure that both the system and practices are operating as intended before we can judge the effects of the system or practice on the consumer. One of the ultimate purposes of all evaluation is or should be to discover relationships among outcomes, practices or treatments, and settings that will provide a basis for improvement of health care services. To achieve this purpose, data are needed on all domains.

I still have not discussed specifically what is to be evaluated; but before I do, I want to digress somewhat to try to clarify another issue.

CRITERIA AND STANDARDS

You may have noted that up to this point, I have not used the words, criteria or standards. This has not been an oversight on my part; it has been intentional.

In the literature on evaluation of quality, the terms, criteria and standards, are used interchangeably as synonyms. There are two concepts embedded in the terms, and these must be separated if progress is to be made in appraising quality. One concept relates to the *kind of variables* that is to be appraised, and the other relates to the *level of performance* that must be achieved in order to make the judgment that performance is at least adequate. It is the second concept, that is, the expected performance level to which the word, standard, should be attached.

Standards are absolutely necessary if we are to make final judgments about the quality of nursing care. After we obtain our data in an evaluation study, we want to be able to make a qualitative statement about the results, such as excellent, good, adequate, or inadequate. To do this, we must have a set of expectations against which we can compare the data that we have obtained.

The set of expectations represents the standards. But how are these to be set in such a complex field as nursing? First, we must understand that there is rarely an experimental or empirical method for establishing a standard. Standards can be established only by expert consensus, which means through discussion and argument.

Sometimes, these discussions lead to the setting of quite arbitrary levels of expectations. For example, consider the statement that the nurse should interview or observe the patient for assessment of problems within 12 hours of admission. The phrase, within 12 hours of admission, is an arbitrary standard. Since there is no experimental evidence to support it, its desirability as a level of expectation must be judged by experts in nursing.

Sometimes, experts set standards by using what is typically obtained in similar situations. For example, suppose we were going to evaluate the effects of nursing care on the number of days that patients with a particular diagnosis are hospitalized. We could gather data on the length of hospitalization for similar patients in similar settings and use the average number of days hospitalized as the standard.

This type of standard is a normative standard. It has certain advantages and disadvantages. Its advantages are that it is likely to be realistic and can be measured with a reasonable degree of precision. Its major disadvantage is that it represents the status quo and may not represent the best attainable level of performance that could be obtained by exerting a little more effort or by applying all of the knowledge that we presently have.

At present, the standards available for judging the practice of nursing or the effects of nursing practice are somewhat crude and at a low level of development. The professional organizations for nursing have made commendable efforts to develop standards for various kinds of nursing practice.

However, most of the standards presented are very general statements that are too ambiguous to provide an adequate frame of reference for judging the quality of nursing practice. For example, the statement, "The nurse supports and promotes normal physiological functioning of the older person," does indicate a dimension that should be appraised in judging the quality of geriatric nursing practice. It is, however, inadequate as a standard because it does not clearly indicate an expected level of performance on the variable.

Before we can set realistic and attainable standards, we must first identify clearly and specifically the variable or cluster of variables for which the standards are to be set. This is the reason that it is necessary to make a clear distinction between standards and variables.

The variables that are used as indicators of quality of care can be called criterion variables; the level of expected performance on each of these variables is the standard. For example, the number of days that a patient is hospitalized could be a criterion variable for evaluating the effects of nursing care. If we state that patients of a certain type should be hospitalized no more than 5 days if the nursing care is effective, then 5 days or fewer of hospitalization becomes our standard. Let me give you another example: The number of patients who require a medication for sleep is a variable. If we state that, with good quality of nursing care, 80 percent of the patients should be able to sleep without medication, then this becomes our standard.

The primary characteristic required of a criterion variable is that it be relevant to the universe or domain that we are evaluating; that is, that it be valid. As a rule, the relevance or validity of a criterion variable is judged by its content. For each variable, we ask the question: Does this variable belong to the domain? For all variables, we ask the question: Does the totality of variables adequately represent the domain? An evaluation can be invalid either because we have measured irrelevant variables or because we have failed to measure all aspects of the domain.

The latter comment should indicate to you that the number of variables in a domain are infinite and that all evaluations require that we sample from the domain. We need to establish that the particular sample of variables that we use for evaluation is valid. To do this, the domain needs to be defined very clearly and very explicitly, which brings us back to the point I had reached before I digressed.

DEFINING A DOMAIN

It would be impossible within the scope of a single paper to illustrate how we could define all of the possible domains of quality of nursing care. It is not even possible to illustrate the three domains that I mentioned earlier, namely: (1) the practices or interventions that constitute professional nursing, (2) the characteristics of the setting or conditions under which nursing care is delivered, and (3) the effects of nursing care on the patients or clients.

Let me try to illustrate by using the first domain, which I will call nursing practice. I have chosen this one, not because it is the easiest to define, but because most of the literature on quality of nursing care relates to this domain.

In the following illustration, I have shown three steps that must be taken in defining a domain. The examples I have given show how this major domain might be defined; they do not illustrate how it should be defined. There are no right or wrong definitions for the domain. Different definitions should be judged in terms of their usefulness in helping to determine validity, in terms of their logic, and in terms of their consistency with value systems of the identified group. As we go through the illustration, I will point out places where arguments can justifiably be made.

Illustration of Defining a Domain

Step 1: Identify the major domain and define (in general terms) its limits.

- Major domain: Nursing Practice
- Nursing practice is defined as: What experts in nursing think that nurses in hospitals should do for, to, and with patients and their families and visitors.

Note in *Step 1* that I have given a general definition of nursing practice. Although you may raise objections to my definition, it does have several elements that are necessary for a good definition. First it identifies whose values are being reflected, i.e., experts in nursing. Second, it delimits the setting where nursing practice is to be evaluated, i.e., hospitals. Third, it delimits the activities to be observed to those which the nurse does for, to, and with patients, their families, and their visitors.

Despite the inadequacies of the definition, it does permit us to exclude certain kinds of variables as being irrelevant to the domain as defined. For example, activities that physicians might think are important for nurses to do but which experts in nursing do not think nurses should do would be excluded. Variables that relate to nursing service organization, qualifications of the nurses, the number of hours of nursing service available and similar variables would be excluded, because they do not belong to the domain as defined. A well-defined domain should permit us to make this judgment with a high degree of confidence. The primary purpose of *Step 1* then is to set the limits or boundaries of the domain.

Step 2: Further define and explicate the major domain by identifying the major subdomains included:

Subdomains:
1. Nursing care plans.
2. Provisions for safe and comfortable patient environment.
3. Meeting physical needs of patients.
4. Meeting physiological needs of patients.
5. Meeting psychological, social, and religious needs of patients.
6. Implementing medical regimen for patients.
7. Teaching patients and/or family.
8. Keeping records of nursing care given to patients.
9. Evaluating the patient's responses to nursing interventions.

The purpose of *Step 2* of the process is primarily to identify more clearly the complexity of the domain so that we can obtain an adequate sample of all of the variables needed for a valid appraisal of the quality of nursing practice.

You may argue that the nine subdomains that I have listed are not enough or that there are other important subdomains of nursing practice. If you can logically defend that additional subdomains fit the general definition, then these should be added.

You will note that the scope of the subdomains varies tremendously. Numbers 1. and 8. are relatively narrow, but all of the others encompass a wide range of nursing activities. Perhaps you would want to divide some of the subdomains even more. *Step 2* of the process actually identifies categories of variables that we need to appraise.

Step 3: Analyze the subdomain in terms of the aspects that need to be appraised. These will be the criterion variables. Also, determine the level of performance expected on each criterion variable. These will be the standards.

Subdomain 1: Nursing Care Plans
A. Variables to be appraised
   1. Time when made.
   2. Completeness.
   3. Accuracy.
   4. Appropriateness to patient and situation.

B. Standards for judging adequacy
   1. ?
   2. ?
   3. ?
   4. ?

The purposes of *Step 3* of the process of defining a domain are: (1) to identify the specific variables within the subdomain on which we need to gather evaluation data and (2) to specify the standards by which we are going to judge the adequacy of performance.

The variables that are identified for a subdomain should have the following characteristics: (1) Each variable should be relevant to the subdomain, and (2) each variable should be amenable to observation. I have discussed the concept of relevance earlier.

The second characteristic, amenability to observation, needs some elaboration. The word, observation, as used here, means any method of eliciting data relevant to a particular variable. For example, a variable that focuses on the mental processes that a nurse uses to make decisions would be unsatisfactory because there is no way to observe mental processes; we can only observe the products of thinking. If a variable focuses on the appropriateness of the nurse's decision for a particular patient in a particular setting, then it is amenable to observation.

In the illustration, I have attempted to analyze the aspects of nursing care plans that might be important to appraise. You will note that I have listed four variables or aspects of nursing care plans to be appraised.

Again, you could raise legitimate questions as to whether I have identified all important aspects of nursing care plans or whether the ones I have listed are important or relevant in making the judgment of adequacy of nursing care plans. This is a matter which experts in nursing must discuss and about which they must arrive at an expert consensus as to what represents a valid appraisal.

You will note that I have not been brave enough to suggest standards for judging. Again, this is a task for experts in nursing, not a task for a neophyte like me.

I can illustrate the problem, though. Look at the variable, completeness. What represents completeness? What elements need to be present in a nursing care plan for it to be complete? How many of the nursing problems of the patient must be identified in order to say that performance is adequate? Do all have to be identified or only the important ones? If the latter, who makes the judgment as to which ones are most important? The questions raised about standards for this variable indicate that it needs to be reanalyzed.

There is another point that should be made about standards of performance, and this is a good place to make it. Not only does the evaluator face the task of judging whether the performance on each variable is adequate, but he also faces the task of making the judgment as to whether the performance in the subdomain is adequate.

Let us assume that the four variables that I have identified in *Subdomain 1* are adequate for appraisal of the subdomain, and let us assume that an evaluator finds that performance is adequate on three of the four variables but not on the other one. In this situation, would performance on the subdomain be judged to be adequate? The answer, of course, depends upon the standards which were set for the subdomain, and again we must depend upon expert consensus to set these.

I should also mention that if we want to make statements about the overall quality of nursing practice, we will have to set a summative standard, that is, a level of expected performance on the combined subdomains. In other words, standards may be needed at three levels: (1) for the individual variables within the subdomain, (2) for the subdomain, and (3) if desired, for all subdomains.

This discussion of defining a domain has touched on the crucial issues and problems that need resolution before we can determine what should be appraised when we evaluate nursing care.

At the risk of being repetitive and boring, I want to reiterate that different value systems and different priorities of values will lead to different definitions of a domain, to different sets of criterion variables, and to different standards or levels of expectation for judging the adequacy of performance in the domain. To search for *the* universal set of criterion variables or *the* universal set of standards is to search for an illusion, and this endeavor is doomed from the start.

The realities indicate also that the evaluator must communicate clearly to his audience the conceptual framework and definitions that he has used. He should avoid global and ambiguous labels, such as quality of nursing care, quality of health care, or quality of patient care.

If he uses a global label, he should use one that clearly reflects the criterion variables that he has appraised. For example, if he has appraised variables from the domain of what a nurse does for, to, and with patients, then he should use the label, quality of nursing practice—not quality of patient outcomes. If he has appraised variables like those outlined in the illustration, he has not appraised patient outcomes. Our knowledge about the relationships between nursing practices and patient outcomes is much too limited to permit us to make inferences about patient outcomes from knowledge about nursing practice.

An evaluator would communicate his results in a more meaningful way if he avoided the use of all global labels. As you can see from the illustration, the quality of nursing care is multidimensional. If the results of evaluation are to be used constructively to improve nursing practice, information is needed about each subdomain, at least, to determine where the strong and weak points are.

TARGET FOR EVALUATION

As stated earlier, the target for evaluation, that is, the persons or objects about whom data are to be collected, will be identified when the "what" of evaluation has been clearly identified. Nursing practice, as defined in the illustration, clearly identifies the target as nurses—all levels and all kinds of nurses. If the domain of patient outcomes is defined, then it will be quite clear that patients are the targets. Both of these two domains will have a single target.

However, if we start defining the domain of conditions and settings in which nursing services are delivered, we will find that this domain has multiple targets. For example, it will include things such as personnel policies, equipment, systems of organization, auxiliary services, policies concerning what different kinds of personnel can or cannot do, physical structure of the plant, medical and treatment policies.

In other words, the targets for evaluation in this domain are anything or everything that facilitates or hinders the delivery of nursing care to patients. The multiplicity of targets in this domain contributes to its complexity and to the difficulty of evaluating it—and raises the question of whether it should be treated as two or more domains.

With the target or targets for evaluation clear, the next issue that the evaluator must face is from whom or from where he is going to collect the actual data that he needs for each variable that he has identified as being relevant to the subdomains that he wants to appraise.

SOURCES OF DATA

If the would-be evaluator has done an adequate conceptual analysis of the domain and has identified unequivocally the target for evaluation, he should know the kinds of specific data, not categories of data, that he needs to collect.

For example, instead of being able to state only that he wants data on the continuity of care for the patient, he should be able to state that he needs data on things such as: (1) appropriateness of referrals, (2) whether initial contacts or actions required by the referrals have actually taken place, (3) whether the patient and/or his family has been given the specific information needed to follow the regimen, and (4) whether plans have been made to determine if a patient is following his health regimen. You can probably add to the list. We must be at least as specific as the illustration, to determine the appropriate source or sources of data.

Four characteristics are desirable in a data source: (1) validity, (2) freedom from bias, (3) reliability, and (4) practicality or convenience. The first three are the most important characteristics. Unfortunately, it has been the fourth characteristic, practicality or convenience, that has been used most frequently as the primary determinant of the data source.

A source of data may be either a direct or an indirect source. For example, if we observe what a nurse does when she cares for a patient, the observations are a direct source of data on her nursing practice. If, instead of observing, we ask the nurse to report to us what she has done, or ask the patient what the nurse has done, or use written records to determine what she has done, the reports of the nurse or patients or the written records are indirect sources of data. Indirect sources of data tend to be less reliable and to have more unknown biases than do direct sources; thus, they also tend to have lower validity.

Whether a source of data is direct or indirect depends entirely upon the nature of the data that are desired. A particular source of data can be an indirect source for one variable and a direct source for another variable. For example, records are indirect sources of data for the care that a nurse gives to a patient, but records are direct sources of data for determining how adequately the nurse keeps records.

Since it is almost impossible to talk about sources of data without talking about how to collect the data, I hope that you will forgive me for mixing the two in the remainder of this discussion.

In the evaluation of quality of nursing care (pardon my use of that global term for the moment), five major sources of data or methods of data collection have been used: (1) direct observation, (2) products, (3) reports of others, (4) self-reports, and (5) records. Occasionally, written or oral tests have been used when the evaluator wanted to determine the extent of knowledge that a patient has about his health status or his health regimen.

Let me discuss each of these sources or methods briefly. Systematic observation has not been used as extensively in evaluating health care as it should have been. There are many reasons why this is so. Observations are expensive, they are time-consuming to do and to analyze. The presence of an observer in a situation sometimes distorts or changes the practices that we want to observe; thus, the observer introduces a certain amount of unknown bias into the situation.

For these reasons, systematic observations should be reserved for situations in which there are no other valid or reliable methods for collecting data. For example, if in the evaluation of nursing practice, we want to obtain data on whether nurses suction patients correctly, direct observation of the process is the only valid method of obtaining the data. On the other hand, if we want to obtain data on whether the nurse uses the equipment for supplying supplementary oxygen properly (appropriate rate of O_2 flow, position of tubing, position of face mask, etc.), we do not have to observe the physical act of setting up the equipment. We have to observe only the final set-up, i.e., a patient receiving the supplementary oxygen. In this case, it is the final product that is important, rather than the process of setting up the equipment.

Whenever a final product is a valid and reliable source of data for a variable, the final product should be used instead of direct observation. The final product is a more or less permanent record that (1) can be evaluated at almost any time and (2) can be judged by more than one observer economically and practically, so that bias in one person's judgment can be reduced.

Many such products, that can be used as valid and reliable data sources, are available in nursing care settings. For example, nurse's records, IV setups, written nursing care plans, proper position of a patient in bed, and the proper use of supports for patients confined to bed are products of nursing care that can be observed.

The major disadvantage of evaluation of products is that the end product usually reveals little or nothing about the process used to produce the product. Sometimes, the process used is unimportant. For example, the quality of nursing care plans depends upon their containing all of the essential elements; it does not depend upon the mental processes used to prepare them. Suppose, however, that we want to evaluate whether a sterile dressing was applied properly. Examining a sterile dressing on a patient will not tell us whether a sterile field was maintained in applying the dressing. To determine this, we must observe nurses when they are applying dressings.

Direct observations of performance and products of nursing activities are usually direct sources of data for evaluation of nursing practice. The reports of others, self-reports, and records are usually indirect sources of data on nursing practice.

Suppose that we are interested in obtaining data on whether nurses explain treatments to patients. The direct source of data for this would be direct observation of nurses. Suppose, instead, that we asked patients whether the nurses had told them what they were going to do before some treatment was given. The patient would represent an indirect source of data.

Suppose that the patient responded to the question with a "no." Does this mean that no explanation was given? Or does it mean that the patient has forgotten the explanation or did not understand it?

Some people would argue that the important aspect of explanation to the patient is that he understand and remember the explanation; therefore, asking the patient would be the best way to obtain data. However, this argument indicates that the nature of the variable being evaluated by patient response is not whether or not nurses explain, but whether or not patients understand and remember the nurses' explanations. If the latter is what is intended, then the variable should be expressed in these terms.

Self-reports are indirect sources of data on nursing care activities and are subject to distortions of memory, social or professional desirability, and self-preservation. However, if we are interested in evaluating the feelings that patients have about the care they received, then self-reports of patients are the most valid and reliable sources of data. Self-reports are also useful when we are interested in evaluating the nurse's observance of social customs, such as courtesy. If we want to know whether nurses are courteous to patients and their families, only the patients and members of the family can make this judgment.

Self-reports are likely to reflect honest opinions when they are obtained at a time when the individual no longer feels the need to protect himself from possible recriminations. It is better to obtain self-reports either at the time of discharge, after discharge, or anonymously.

The last source of data that I want to discuss are records, not as products of nursing activities, but as historical records of what has happened.

Most of you are familiar with the nursing audit which is based entirely on existing records. Those of you who have done nursing audits know the weaknesses of records as a source of data.

First, existing records have usually been devised to serve some purpose other than evaluation. As a result, they frequently do not include the data we want or data in the form that we want. Second, since records are usually written, many entries in the record depend upon the verbal facility of the recorder. There are people who can do nothing, but who can write their "nothing" so well that it seems like a lot. There are other people who can and do accomplish a lot, but who write what they have done in such a way that it sounds like nothing.

Third, an omission on a record does not necessarily mean that an activity has not been done. Likewise, the presence of an activity on a record does not necessarily mean that it has been done. Fourth, a record tells little or nothing about how something was done. Fifth, entries on records sometimes require that the reader make inferences or assumptions about the meaning of the entry, which reduces the reliability of the appraisal. In other words, for some kinds of data, records are unreliable, biased, and invalid sources of data.

The primary advantage of records is that they are convenient to use. As compared with direct observation, evaluation by using records is much cheaper. If we are aware of the limitations of records, nursing audits may provide useful information. The data from an audit could provide information on the areas of nursing service that need further evaluation.

The most serious danger in using nursing audits is the tendency to use them as the only evaluation. They have too many sources of unreliability and bias to provide valid evaluations of the quality of nursing practice; they must be supplemented by other methods of evaluation.

SUMMARY

Before summarizing the major points that I have tried to make in this paper, I want to state explicitly a point that has only been implied. Evaluation of the type described in this paper focuses on program or system, not on the individual nurse or the individual patient.

We should be interested in determining whether nursing, as it is practiced in a unit or in a hospital, meets the expectations of the profession, not whether Nurse A meets these expectations. Although we should obtain data about individuals, or at least some individuals, we should be interested in finding what is typical or the average for all individuals.

Program or system evaluation requires sampling of individuals and settings; it does not require that each individual and each setting be measured for all variables.

The major point that I have tried to make in the paper is that the crucial basic problem in evaluating the quality of nursing practice, patient outcomes, or whatever is to conceptualize each of these major constructs adequately. A good conceptualization of nursing practice is comprehensive and reveals the interrelationships among the parts of what is called nursing process. Also, it is based on either knowledge about or hypotheses about the effects of nursing practice on the patients or clients. Thus, a good conceptualization of nursing practice should make it easier to conceptualize and define the domain of patient outcomes.

As we engage in these processes, we should remember the important and central role of values and value systems.

Above all, we must remember that evaluation, like nursing, is not a cut-and-dried science or technology. All of the answers to questions about evaluation cannot be found by locating the right book or article. Such books or articles do not exist. Evaluative research is in its infancy.

We must not be discouraged if our first efforts are not perfect. Hilmar* quotes a man named Chester Barnard as follows: "To try and fail is at least to learn; to fail to try is to suffer the inestimable loss of what might have been."

DISCUSSION OF DR. HAGEN'S PAPER

Dr. Kinsella: Are there questions or comments that you would like to address to Dr. Hagen?

Dr. Gortner: One of your last comments dealt with the illusion of a universal set of criteria or, at best, instrument set. As you know, some of the literature of the mid-sixties suggested very strongly that there is such a possibility, if we would just work hard enough at it. Could you comment on this?

Dr. Hagen: I think this is one of the very real issues in the type of complex evaluation that you are trying to do. In both the health field and in education, the concept of a "universal set of standards" and a "universal set of criteria" that would be applicable in every situation and in every setting is a very appealing idea. If such a set of criteria and standards could be devised, then everyone would appraise the same variables and judge the adequacy of a performance against a common set of standards. Evaluation data would then be comparable across settings.

The problem is to obtain enough agreement on what represents desirable nursing practice for every type of patient, no matter his condition, his status, or his location. I think it is impossible to have a national set of criteria that could be applied across the country.

I think that it is quite possible, within geographical regions or within similar agencies dealing with similar patient populations and similar goals, to have a set of criteria which has a hard core of commonality. Then, whatever is specific or unique to the particular agency could be added. I think it would be possible to get together groups of people to develop a common core of criteria and standards that would be universally applicable to particular, well-described patient settings.

We sometimes hear about efforts to achieve an overall index of quality. I think it is unreasonable to expect to obtain an overall index of quality that will serve as a useful measure. It is possible to get a number; you can get a number for anything. But to have the number mean anything is a different question entirely.

Ms. Kauffman: I wonder if we are really so far apart in our criteria. For example, skin care is a universal. Most of us accept the use of a sheep's pelt in skin care. None of us is surprised by the use of lotion. Maybe we might not be able to come up with universal criteria in all areas of nursing, but I think there are some areas where there is consensus.

---

*Hilmar, N. A., "Standards and criteria as health protection tools." *American Journal of Public Health* 59:1613–1617, September 1969.

Dr. Hagen: Think about the number of areas in which you have consensus. You may have consensus in a type of skin care. Do you have consensus in all types of skin care? Or only in the skin breakdown associated with prolonged pressure?

I think it is true that there are some kinds of things for which the treatment is very general and acceptable. However, if you start looking very intensively at this, you will find only a small cluster of these kinds of things.

This will be true particularly when you move away from something like skin care to, say, the types of interactions that the nurse has with patients to motivate and persuade a patient to follow a regimen after he leaves the hospital. I think you won't find as much commonality in the more complex types of nursing interventions.

Ms. Zimmer: Isn't it true that we are more likely to reach agreement on desirable health status than we are on how the patient arrives there?

Dr. Hagen: Yes. I think you will have more commonality and agreement if you try to identify the types of outcomes you want with patients, but not the methods of achieving them. There are many ways of achieving the same objective. You can find out whether the different ways achieved the desired objective, but you shouldn't say, "Since they haven't used my way, it isn't good." If you have the same outcome and you don't have unintended undesirable outcomes along with it, then people should be able to use their own ways of achieving objectives. This is the reason you run into serious problems when you talk about process in nursing.

Dr. Aydelotte: Isn't the decision to be made about the critical outcomes, or the critical indicators of outcomes in which nursing has an impact, one of our major problems? I am thinking, for example, that in a standardized educational test, you may have 100 items, but of those 100 items, 10 are really indicators and could give you the answer. I should like to have you speak to this point.

Dr. Hagen: At some point in time, one would like to be able to identify the effects that different nursing practices or interventions have on patients. To do this, you are going to have to be able to identify specific patient outcomes rather than very general outcomes and, of course, you are going to have to be able to measure these outcomes. I am not sure what you mean by critical indicators of outcome. It is true that, to determine quality of care, you do not have to measure all possible outcomes; you can sample. If you sample, you need to determine which ones and how many outcomes have to be measured to yield reliable and valid data.

Dr. Hegyvary: I would have to agree fully on trying to look at outcomes. We are confronted with certain patient situations, and we see there is a point, somewhere down the road, to which we want to help the patient arrive. Our big problem, as I see it, is how we go from here to there. What kinds of measures will we have to take to achieve a certain outcome? That, to me, is a critical research problem in nursing.

To some extent, I agree that everybody should be able to try their own ways of doing things. I prefer that we try that, in a research fashion, and compare data about which ways were successful under what circumstances and which were not. What we have found in our own study is that when you attempt to make specific criteria for certain institutions, personnel may refuse to accept the criteria and use existing hospital policies as the basis for their refusal.

If people were very objective about saying, "We don't wish to accept these criteria for evaluation because they are not in agreement with the procedure that we have developed for carrying out this function, this is unique to our institution, and we want to do it this way for a certain reason that we can justify to ourselves and to anyone who asks," then I would accept their decision.

Dr. Hagen: One point that I was trying to bring out, is that when you start looking at things and say, "This is the way I want to do it," your statement is like a set of objectives. You have to look at these objectives and place value judgments on them. For example, what you want to do may be known to be wrong or unwise. If it is, and you say, "But hospital policy permits me to do this," it is still wrong, and it doesn't make any difference whether or not hospital policy permits you to do it.

There is another thing about the outcome statements. If you look at the statements being used for nursing audit, I think you will notice it, too. Some of the outcomes for patients are stated in ways that cannot be appraised within the setting of the hospital. (I use the hospital here because if you are in a health agency, you go into the home and may be able to follow the person for a long period of time.) But when you are looking at outcomes and you know that you do not have money to go outside the hospital or institution to followup, then the kinds of outcomes you should focus on are those on which you can get data.

If you say, "But these other outcomes are so very important," then you have to find a way of following up on those outcomes. This, by the way, is one reason I would say that a consortium between a health agency and an acute care institution is probably helpful, because it gives you an opportunity to follow up some of these long-term objectives for your patients.

Ms. Reese: From a managerial standpoint, both in the use of manpower and funds, one of the things I think we stop short of very often is deciding when we have achieved our goal. It fits in with what was said earlier: When do we quit? This may be decided by the fact that the patient has left the hospital and no referral was made; thus, there is no followup. That ends it.

But in the home, we have a different problem. The nurse keeps thinking, "if I went back one more time, I might see something that I didn't do or that I ought to do." This becomes expensive, in more ways than one. I think that this is a research area that has tremendous implications. If we look at the wide range of health services that people need and at the time, effort, and cost, to both the patient and the health agency, of meeting these needs, we see that research is vitally necessary.

Dr. Hagen: Essentially, you are talking about a realistic approach to what can be accomplished. I think this is important, because it is unrealistic to think that some nursing objectives can be accomplished in the time that you have to interact with people, or with the resources that you have to support your interaction.

For example, when a patient has a short-term stay in a hospital and you have an objective which relates to changing the basic personality pattern of the person, that is unrealistic.

Ms. Reese: It is unrealistic in the home, too!

Dr. Hagen: When you are preparing objectives, you should be thinking about outcomes. You should ask yourself about the time schedule and exactly what types of changes you want to achieve. You should ask, "Are these realistic to expect in this period of time?"

Ms. Zimmer: I sense a need to sort out two more things. If I develop a list of priorities for evaluation in one column, I have one set of priorities. If I have another column for the things which should be researched to support quality assurance in nursing programs, I have a second set of priorities. One of the things that I find difficult to understand is: When is evaluation considered to be research?

Dr. Hagen: There is a great deal of research that we would like to do. Despite the difficulties, many of you have made efforts in evaluation of different kinds. If you would encourage people to document what has been done, it would be extremely helpful. You may say that the efforts have been too naive. But nothing is too naive if someone will write it, show what has been done, show what the results are, and communicate it clearly. From a pool of these reports, you could glean quite a bit of insight and quite a bit of help.

There are many things that I think could be researched. For example, you could do evaluative research in which you would try to control variables to rule out influences on what you are trying to study.

However, the problem that I was trying to address is not so much research, but the problem of how to obtain the data you need and want in attempting to improve the care that is being given to patients. I don't mind if you put a label of research on that, but I do wish people would be more systematic about collecting and sharing data.

People become very cautious about evaluation data. If it is good, they don't mind letting others see it. If it is not so good, they don't want others to see it. If you could encourage people to share their data, even in your own geographical areas, it is amazing how much you could get from that type of pooling.

Dr. Levine: I don't want to sound critical about the methodology for evaluation of care and quality assessment, but there is a certain element in it that is a statistician's nightmare.

To make my point, I would like to go back about 15 years. We were trying to develop a patient satisfaction instrument. We were looking around the country to see what kinds of instruments were in use, and we found that the American Hospital Association had been doing some work in the area. (In fact, I think this instrument is still being used today in some hospitals.)

This instrument consists of a series of hand-drawn faces, ranging from a face that looks very unhappy to a face that looks very happy. The patient is asked to cross out the face that best represents how he feels toward each of 20 or 30 items or factors; these are phrased very simply, such as "Food." It is a neat kind of instrument for people who have language problems, because it uses very little language. Such a patient satisfaction instrument sometimes gives trouble to people who are highly verbal.

Anyway, we explored the use of this instrument. I visited a hospital in Detroit and talked with a hospital administrator who had been using it. He said he was very happy about the instrument, because it kept a check on patient satisfaction and he felt that this is the best measure of the quality of care. He said, "After all, that is our product."

He was unhappy, though, about the results in his own hospital. When I asked him why, he said, "Well, we just received our report. Our hospital ranked as 96 percent satisfied." This indicated that 96 percent of the patients were satisfied with all aspects of care received.

Astounded, I asked him why he was unhappy with such high scores. He responded, "Well, the hospital next door had 97 percent."

The question that keeps turning over in my mind is: What is the basis for our comparison? What do we do with the statistics that we get from some of the measures that we use? We all realize that even if a hospital had a 50 percent score and another hospital had a 75 percent score, that does not mean that the one with the 75 percent is that much better. You have to look into the hospitals themselves.

For example, we know that many hospitals care for the more acutely ill type of patient. In complex settings, the number of things that can go wrong is much greater. A hospital that cares for a much less severely ill patient can more easily control the quality of care, as things can go much more smoothly. It relates to the old statistical concept of a population at risk. When you have a situation where many things can go wrong, then many more things might go wrong. Yet, at the same time, there may be more effort to control quality.

Basically, I am talking about this question of standardization. What do you use as a control? Do you use your own situation on a before and after basis? If you do, you run into a major problem. The instrument itself will influence the score. You alluded to this, the so-called Hawthorne effect. The minute a quality assurance program is instituted, the situation in the hospital is changed.

Dr. Hagen: Isn't that what you want to do?

Dr. Levine: Yes, but is it the instrument that is improving the quality? Or are there real changes in quality?

Dr. Hagen: You are asking about the reality of the change. That depends on the subtlety of your instrument. I think one of the reasons people are unhappy about the changes that occur with a CASH instrument is that you may achieve higher scores on things that many nurses do not believe represent the crucial parts of nursing. As soon as people see numbers (scores), they attribute to them a certain type of precision—a certain absoluteness—that the numbers usually don't possess.

If you are asking me to solve the problem, I can't do it. You are talking about a normative comparison. But when you start comparing things, such as the scores of this group versus the scores of this other group, it makes no sense to compare noncomparable groups. If you are going to use a comparison type base, then the range of scores must be obtained under similar conditions. Otherwise, it doesn't seem to me that they are very useful. What solution do you have?

Dr. Levine: It would be to go back to the previous question and look at some of the research models, where there is an attempt to control all of the so-called extraneous variables. I don't know, however, whether this is practicable.

Dr. Hagen: You can do that, but meanwhile, what are you going to do if you want to evaluate?

Dr. Levine: I think we have to pay more attention to the practical significance. Going back to the hospital administrator, even if there were some meaningful difference between 97 and 96 percent, what would it really mean in terms of some kind of outcome criteria?

Dr. Hagen: That's right.

Dr. Hegyvary: One point in regard to Dr. Levine's statement: I maintain there is some value in numbers in spite of all of the problems involved. We have had some problems, but we do find them useful. We have to have some way of indicating the quality of performance.

There is at least one value in comparison. When we started giving out scores and people saw that they were in the 30's, 40's, and 50's, with the average scores on the direct nursing care component then in the 40's and 50's in most hospitals, one nurse stated her reaction very well. She said, "If my son came home from school with a 50 percent on his report card, I would spank him." She was extremely upset with her own scores, because she was accustomed to seeing 95's. She knew, however, that her hospital was not doing 95 percent of the things she thought they should be doing.

So, I think the score is helpful. It is also true that it is dangerous to look at the scores of one hospital in comparison with those of another, without knowing all of the variables involved. But who can ever know all of them?

In our first year of data collection, we found that severe illness did not lead to lower scores. At a level of significance, the scores for complete and intensive care patients were higher than for the self-care or partial care patients. The scores achieved were based on separate criteria. Some of the criteria were the same, but the nursing care of the self-care patient is different from that of the sicker patient.

Dr. Hagen: I did not mean to imply that numbers are never of any value. Essentially, I am saying that I don't think you can give people numbers, without helping them to understand what these numbers mean. Too frequently, it is a matter of obtaining and giving numbers only.

Ms. Walton: I think Doctors Hegyvary and Levine have touched on something significant, that is, the sorting out of the measurements of the various agencies. Unless you can do this, you are comparing apples to oranges.

Some agencies have the mission of diagnosis or rescue of patients. Some have only the rehabilitative aspects of patient care. There is a continuum of care that goes on in all agencies, but by and large, some of the very acute hospitals are in the business of rescuing the patient and then sending him someplace else.

I think we ought to look at the mission of each agency and begin to match up groups of institutions. How many university hospitals are there that are so different from other institutions? Is their mission completely different from everybody else's mission? Can we look at them in comparison with a rehabilitative or long-term care agency?

Dr. Aydelotte: It makes me a little nervous when we start talking about comparisons and introduce the element of competitiveness. I go back to the question: What is the purpose of doing this in the first place? I think each institution must ask itself this question. What is the purpose of doing evaluations? How does it relate to the mission of the institution?

If we want to compare ourselves, and those of us in the UATC hospitals have a difficult time trying to obtain comparable data, I think the question which all of us must ask concerns the purpose of the exercise. The purpose must be understood by our staff, because the purpose is going to determine the kinds of data we obtain and their use.

Ms. Paulson: Not only do we have to be careful about comparing institution to institution, even though their missions appear to be the same, but also we have to be careful about comparing data from unit to unit within the same institution.

Our hospital has 35 units, and every one of these has a different mission — different purposes and objectives. The evaluation and assessment procedures that we are using are really so specific to these units that we do not make comparisons between them. The problem is serious for the nursing service administrator, as she seeks an overall judgment about quality assessment for the entire institution.

The mission of one of our largest areas of work, at present, is in the chemical dependency unit. We have 70 inpatient beds, and 70 halfway house beds. There is also a very large outpatient program, where we are able to do some followup. One problem is that 80 percent of the time, the nurse is not primary; she is secondary. How do you evaluate that?

Ms. Szukalla: I have one problem with this whole business of outcomes. In other discussions we have had, I have never heard anyone identify the input from a patient in determining how far he wants to go in his recovery. As we get into more and more care of critical conditions, and I am sure all of us have seen this, we have seen patients kept alive who did not want to be kept alive. I think we get into a social issue here that is becoming very critical at present. But we don't talk about it. How does a patient's desires fit into the objectives that are set for him?

Dr. Hagen: Are you asking me as a potential patient? I would say that patients should have a very real input. One of the things that bothers me (and I am speaking now as a potential patient, not as an evaluator) is the setting of certain kinds of goals or objectives for patients. Let's say that you want to maintain the patient at a particular level of function, and you think that this is all he can achieve. Conceivably, you would be giving excellent nursing care by keeping him there. Suppose, however, that I, as a patient, do not want to stay there. Could we still consider your nursing care to be excellent?

Ms. Hauer: I have heard no one mention anything about costs. In terms of variables, I feel that we really should do the assessment within our own institutions—and not make comparisons between institutions. I think there are too many variables to make comparison useful. The cost of health care in one institution can be very different from that in another. I think we have to set our own objectives and try to meet those objectives within the nursing service philosophy of our institution and based on the budget that the director of nursing has.

Dr. Hagen: The thing that interests me about that statement is that it is very close to the kinds of statements being made in education today, in situations of trying to assess the quality of education across a State which is heterogeneous. Most of the States that have been successful in this have approached it by saying to each school, "Set your objectives for each one of these, and then we will supply you with ways of appraising the extent to which you have achieved those objectives."

Ms. Hauer: Of course, another aspect is the cost to the patient; that is another variable.

Dr. Hagen: That's right.

Dr. Gortner: If we could follow through with Mrs. Hauer's thoughts, they are very important from the consumer's point of view. It is particularly critical that the mission of an institution, where it gets its priorities, how much it costs, how many board-certified men are on the roster, who gives the anesthesia, etc., be recorded in such form that it is available for public review at least on elective admission. Precipitous admissions through emergency rooms are a different matter. But I think that if we assume that hospitals are noncomparable and accept that they do have different objectives, budgets, and emphases, then it is only right that those differences be made quite explicit.

Dr. Hagen: Another aspect is that you must be prepared for an evaluation of the objectives of your institution, that is, evaluation of what you are *trying* to do. You see, there is evaluation at that point, as well as at other points along the line.

Ms. Fine: I want to go back to the question of involving the patient. I think that most of us have tried to, or are, involving the patient in contracting in psychiatry. We are presently trying to involve the patient through verbal contracts in other areas of the hospital, because there are many areas in which we can have agreement with the patient before we start to work with him. If we interpret this as a contract between the patient and the nursing service, it seems to work a lot better, and patients understand what we are trying to say. While psychiatry has been the pioneer in the use of the contract approach, I think we have been fairly successful in using this in areas other than psychiatry.

Ms. Alfano: I am relatively naive about research, so I would like to ask a couple of questions in relation to outcomes and patient involvement. Is it conceivable that one of the criterion outcomes could be that the patient achieves his desired status? It seems to me that a definition of quality should be determined by recipients, not by deliverers.

Dr. Hagen: The thing is that both recipients and deliverers are judges. But the judgments may be different.

Dr. Levine: Related to that, and to Ms. Szukalla's point, is the matter of whether the service is really needed. We see this in the criticism leveled against the medical profession in regard to so-called unnecessary surgery. We have to think of the concept of efficacy, that is: Does the recipient really need what he gets? For example, a hysterectomy could be performed and, by every standard of surgical care, done perfectly. But, was it needed in the first place?

If we look at our national statistics on surgery, we see that we exceed England and Wales by two or three times; a much higher mortality rate is correlated with that. For example, a recent article shows that the prostatectomy rate in this country is three times that of England and Wales. Deaths from gall bladder disease are three times greater. Nobody has been able to prove that people in this country have a great inclination toward gall bladder disease, especially fatal gall bladder disease.

I think there is a relationship between this and nursing. We could do a beautiful job of caring for the patient, but does he really need the service in the first place?

Dr. Hagen: I was thinking a little bit about that when various people were talking, because we were talking about psychiatric patients. We were talking about patients who have some kind of chronic condition that they will have to live with. The kinds of services they need are quite different from, let's say, a patient with acute appendicitis. A few days after the appendectomy, the patient is fully recovered, and long-term care just doesn't apply. If you started to speculate on the kind of therapy this patient *might* need, again, it might mean unnecessary kinds of outcomes as far as he is concerned.

SUMMARY

While concern for the quality of health care has probably existed since the beginning of time, the need for systematic assessment has never been greater than it is at present. The primary purpose of such program evaluation is not to justify what presently exists, but to provide descriptive data on the current status to assist in future decision-making as to what should be kept and what should be changed.

The problems and issues in evaluation arise when attention is focused on the *who*, the *what*, and the *how* of evaluation.

Who: There are many stakeholders or groups who have an interest in health care programs and systems. The various groups may have different values which may be divergent or, at times, conflicting. Therefore, there may be controversy in regard to the questions: Who shall determine what shall be evaluated? On whom shall data be collected? Who shall make the final judgments on the adequacy of the results? Whose values shall dominate?

What: For successful evaluation, there is a need for a conceptual framework for a clear definition of the universe of variables, or domains to be examined. An essential requirement of a conceptual framework is the explicit identification of the group whose values are being reflected.

In appraising quality, there are two concepts which must be differentiated, i.e., criteria and standards. While much of the literature fails to distinguish between criteria and standards, it is important for one who is looking at programs of health care and nursing practice to distinguish clearly between them.

A criterion is a variable which is to be appraised, while a standard is a value judgment which indicates the level of performance to be attained on the criterion variable under study. A standard implies some degree of expert consensus as to what constitutes an adequate or acceptable level of performance.

To be useful, standards must have five identifiable characteristics: (1) they are relevant to the domain under consideration; (2) they are realistic and attainable, considering the state of the art and the resource available; (3) attainment should be measurable with some precision; (4) they are aggressive, pushing toward maximum potential; and (5) they are dichotomous, serving as a cutting point to distinguish satisfactory from unsatisfactory performance.

How: When the decisions have been made as to the domains (and subdomains) to be studied, the targets for evaluation become clear. Then a choice of method for securing the data must be made in light of the time available, the cost, and the outcomes to be attained. Generally, the methods involve a study of the process by which the service is rendered or of the outcome which is achieved. The data sources must be very specific and have validity, reliability, freedom from bias, and a practical availability.

In evaluating the quality of nursing practice or patient outcomes, a good conceptualization of these domains is essential. Such a conceptualization is comprehensive and reveals the many components of nursing process, giving evidence of the results of nursing practice on patient outcomes.

There is an urgent need for evaluative research in nursing. Studies, however primitive, should be documented and reported to the profession to serve as a pool of data for more systematic studies.

HUMANISTIC EXERCISES

PART I
METHODS OF THE
NURSING PROCESS

EXERCISE 1
Personalized Care Plan

PURPOSES

1. To learn the steps of the nursing process.
2. To explore all the personal aspects of self that make up one's existence.
3. To develop an awareness of one's needs in relation to goal accomplishment.
4. To isolate problem areas in individual goal accomplishment related to one's own life.
5. To brainstorm how one's needs can be met.

FACILITY

A large room with a table where participants will be able to sit in a circle and write.

MATERIALS

Paper, writing materials, posterboard, construction paper, or work sheets may be used, plus blackboard or newsprint and magic markers.

TIME REQUIRED

Three to four hours +.

GROUP SIZE

Unlimited groups of four.

NEEDS SCHEME

1. comfort
2. nutrition
3. exercise
4. diversional activities
5. dependency
6. independency
7. socializing
8. security
9. self-esteem
10. self-actualization
11. to be appreciated
12. to be loved
13. safety
14. environmental considerations
15. teaching
16. prevention of complications
17. skills and competencies
    a. organizational skills
    b. technical skills
    c. interpersonal skills
    d. decision-making skills
    e. communication skills
    f. teaching skills
18. others (may be decided by individual members or groups)

SOURCE: This exercise, the PELLEM Pentagram (Chapter 20), and exercises contained in Part V were jointly created and designed by Eunice M. Parisi and Elaine L. La Monica at the University of Massachusetts, 1975–1976.

Eunice Parisi received her doctorate from the University of Massachusetts in 1972 in the behavioral sciences. As a counseling psychologist, a member of the International Association of Applied Social Scientists, and a member of the National Training Laboratories, she has done extensive consulting in the area of interpersonal dynamics, staff development, and organizational development. Currently, she is the director of a specialist degree program in group dynamics and leadership at the University of Hartford in Connecticut. The focus of this post-masters degree program is on personal and organizational development.

DESIGN

1. The purposes of the exercise should be explained to the participants, expanding on the fact the nurses are involved with writing care plans for their clients every day. Since nurses are individuals, too, it might be helpful for participants to look at themselves, their needs, and ways of meeting them. Participants will actually be confronting and exploring their own selves, then receiving feedback on care plans with the intent of expanding the data and ideas. In a sense, each participant will lead and be the subject of a team conference.

2. **Data base.** Each member should start with a piece of paper (or Work Sheet A from this book) and add sheets as necessary since this part may be lengthy. Divide the paper into three columns titled: Psychologic, Physiologic, and Social. Under these headings, the participants place all the facts about themselves that come to mind. An example of each would be the following:

PSYCHOLOGIC	PHYSIOLOGIC	SOCIAL
1 needs to be independent	3 small-framed	5 married
	4 blond	6 two children
2 fears authority		7 likes to have people near

3. After participants have filled in their data bases, they then share these in groups of four (approximately 20 minutes).

4. After sharing, the participants are asked to go back and individually rethink and expand their data base by writing down any personal facts that were not mentioned during the sharing and not included presently. Following this, participants should number the data base as shown above.

5. Referring to the needs schema, which may be listed on a blackboard or Xeroxed for each member (Work Sheet B), individuals should jot the needs down on paper and indicate what numbers from their data base apply or are important in considering those stated needs. An example would be the need for dependency. The following numbers might be placed after it from the data base information: 1, 2, 3, 5, 6, 7. There are no absolutes in this section; participants should just think about the data and if it may be pertinent to the needs in some way, place the need number beside it. The purpose of this step is to provide an individualized picture of each person in relation to stated needs.

159

6. From the needs schema, individuals should pick the ten top priority needs that they feel they have. Place a star next to them.
7. Numbering from 1 to 10, highest priority to lowest, members arrange in order these ten priority needs.
8. Looking at the highest priority down, personal diagnoses should be made concerning each need relevant to the pertinent data. Write these on a piece of paper lengthwise with columns. Leave a space between diagnoses (Work Sheet C).

PERSONAL DIAGNOSES	RATIONALE	PERSONAL ORDERS	AREAS OF CONCERN
1.			
2.			
(etc.)			

9. Use the following formula for writing each nursing diagnosis, filling in the blanks:
I feel that I need _____
because _____

The first blank becomes the diagnosis, the second is the rationale. Emphasis at this point is that thoughts are important rather than semantics. Members may have more than one diagnosis for each of the 10 priority items on the needs schema.
10. After individuals have written their diagnoses and recorded them, the next step is to individually brain-storm ways that the diagnoses (needs) can be met. Write these in the Personal Orders Column and number them. While completing this, participants ask themselves, "If I had everything in any way I wanted it, what would be done to meet these needs?"
11. Members should now have a number of sheets of paper which include at least ten diagnoses and rationales and several personal orders under each. Participants regroup into fours and share these. Members should provide feedback for each other on each of the areas and offer additional suggestions for orders.

12. Following the sharing section, individuals next extrapolate from each diagnosis and orders; they note issues or areas of specific concern; that is, aggression, assertion, etc. They may ask themselves, "Of all this material, what is the central issue I need to work on?"
13. Regrouping into fours, participants share these central issues and write them on a separate sheet including everyone's individual issues and the number of times issues are mentioned by individuals.
14. A large group is formed and all of the issues are written on a blackboard or newsprint; rate priorities of needs according to the number of times issues are mentioned by groups. This list provides a lead-in for focusing on issues of concern to the group.
15. Discuss the experience.

VARIATIONS

This may be done in part by assignments at home or may be divided into concurrent sessions.
An added dimension would be for individuals to look at the needs not in top priority and suggest when it is anticipated that this need would emerge for action.

DISCUSSION

The central issues obtained from the participants can form the basis for further work in the group. The nursing orders can be utilized in action steps. What is intended to be gained is a picture of one's life in relation to individual needs followed by a plan on how needs can be met. Looking at oneself in such a manner often makes consciousness reachable. The steps followed in this Personal Care Plan are analogous to those in the nursing process.

DATA BASE

Psychologic	Physiologic	Social

NEEDS SCHEMA

1. comfort
2. nutrition
3. exercise
4. diversional activities
5. dependency
6. independency
7. socializing
8. security
9. self-esteem
10. self-actualization
11. to be appreciated
12. to be loved
13. safety
14. environmental considerations
15. teaching
16. prevention of complications
17. skills and competencies
    a. organizational skills
    b. technical skills
    c. interpersonal skills
    d. decision-making skills
    e. communication skills
    f. teaching skills
18. other _____
19. _____
20. _____

EXERCISE 1
WORK SHEET C

PERSONAL CARE PLAN

Personal Diagnoses	Rationale	Personal Orders	Areas of Concern

EXERCISE 2
Nursing History Interview Format

PURPOSES
1. To develop a personal nursing history interview format based on one's individual philosophy of practice.
2. To experience using the format with peers.

FACILITY
A large room where participants can form dyads and interview one another.

MATERIALS
Paper and other writing materials.

TIME REQUIRED
One hour.

GROUP SIZE
Unlimited dyads.

DESIGN
1. As a homework assignment, have participants read Part I, plus Chapters 7, 8, and 9 of Part II and other nursing history articles and written materials.
2. With the information gleaned from the above, request that each student bring to class a nursing history interview format that is based on individual beliefs concerning this area. Interview techniques to be used should be explained and should reflect the individual's experience and needs concerning this skill.
3. Request members to form into dyads and use their nursing history formats on each other. The student being interviewed should provide feedback, if requested by the interviewer (see Chapter 12 for guidelines in giving feedback).
4. Personal reactions of the interviewer and interviewee may be shared.
5. Nursing history interview formats can now be re-evaluated and changed by the interviewer, based on the results of this experience.
6. Reform into a total group and discuss the experience.

VARIATIONS
This exercise can be done completely as a homework assignment. Further, learners may use their formats in the clinical laboratory or with their clients.

EXERCISE 3
Project: The Nursing Process

PURPOSES

1. To carry out the steps of the nursing process with a patient in a clinical setting.
2. To formally report the results of the method.

FACILITY

A clinical setting where each student can choose and work with a client family.

MATERIALS

Paper, construction paper, poster boards, scrolls, or any other media desired by the learner on which report can be made.

TIME REQUIRED

Variable, but generally long-range.

GROUP SIZE

Not applicable.

DESIGN

Term / Course / Module Assignment
1. Use a client and/or family and/or community as the focus of the project.
2. The project is to include the following parts:
   a. Brief overview of client; include the time period covered by the paper relative to client's stage of illness/wellness and the reason(s) for care.
   b. Data—include sources for data collection.
   c. Data processing relevant to needs.
   d. Diagnosis.
      1) determination of need.
      2) priority arrangement.
   e. Action.
   f. Responses (actual).
   g. Action(s) which would have been more effective.
3. Steps:
   a. Gather all available data—itemize and organize.
   b. For each of the needs listed below, indicate which combination(s) of data are relevant to determining the specifics of this patient's need.
   c. Write nursing diagnoses for patient's needs.
   d. Pick the top ten priority diagnoses of this patient or family and indicate order of priority.
   e. Write nursing orders for each of the ten priority needs.

SOURCE: This exercise is an adaptation of one used by Virginia Earles, University of Massachusetts, Division of Nursing, 1975.

f. For each of the diagnoses not in top ten priority, suggest when you anticipate this need would emerge for action.
  g. Indicate what was actually done relevant to each need.
  h. Evaluate each response in relation to its effectiveness.
4. Needs Schema
    1) comfort
    2) nutrition
    3) exercise
    4) hygiene
    5) sleep, rest patterns
    6) diversional activities
    7) socializing
    8) elimination
    9) safety
    10) environmental consideration
    11) teaching
    12) spiritual
    13) prevention of complications
    14) assurance of physiologic status
    15) emotional support, counseling

VARIATIONS   Reports of project can be made in class, thus giving the opportunity for teaching and learning experience to the reporter.

EXERCISE 4
The Nursing Care Plan

PURPOSES 1. To practice developing rationally-based nursing diagnoses and orders using case material.
2. To develop succinctness and clarity in writing comprehensive nursing care plans.

FACILITY Writing space and areas where groups of four can share.

MATERIALS Paper and pencils.

TIME REQUIRED One hour.

GROUP SIZE Unlimited groups of four.

PHYSIOLOGIC DATA
42 years old
male
c/o occipital lobe headaches
dizziness
excess thirst
frequent urination
malaise—symptoms 6 months
   duration
gained 20 lbs
(5'6", 200 lb)
tonsillectomy at age 12 in S. Car.
allergic to Penicillin
tetanus booster—1972
polio booster—1968
regular diet

PSYCHOLOGIC DATA
Pt feels he has blood pressure
   problems
feels healthy
pressure on job (auto assembly-
   line foreman)
difficulty sleeping
feels anxious (smoking 1 to 3
   packs/day; liquor intake is
   moderate)
eats and smokes when "uptight"
has no hobbies except keeping
   house and yard up
feels pressured to get better
   and go back to work

DOCTOR'S ADMISSION ORDERS

admit to Ward B
height and weight
TPR B.I.D. for 3 days
x-ray of chest
CBC
urinalysis
fasting blood sugar
BUN
VDRL serology test
consultation with podiatrist
routine recreational outing
  privileges—accompanied
FBS
BRP
1800 cal low-salt diet
Dalmane 30 mg PO, HS PRN
  for sleep
BP Q4h when awake

SOCIOLOGIC DATA

married
no previous hospitalizations
five children (ages 16, 12, 10, 8,
  6—3 boys, 2 girls)
bills all over—unable to pay
protestant
served four years in the army
works 40 hours/week
owns home—1 bath, 3 bedrooms
lives in suburbia
high school education
income $8500/year
oldest child of three siblings
brother—age 40—L & W—S.C.
sister—38—diabetes since age 12
brother—30—ok
father—68 c heart disease and
  hypertension
mother—64—L & W
wife prepares food
gets up at 5:30 a.m. and has four
  cups coffee
eats no breakfast or lunch
has two cups coffee for lunch
eats large supper at 6:30 p.m.

DESIGN

1. Using the above data base, learners should individually develop a nursing care plan using Work Sheet A.
2. Following the above step, have each participant share his or her care plan with the other members of the group of four. Each person should have this opportunity.
3. Participants should pay particular attention to the differences and similarities of the care plans. Since everyone started with the same data base, similarities increase the reliability of perceptions and differences underscore the individuality of perceptual fields. The latter should especially be looked at.
4. If time permits, the group can devise a nursing care plan that reflects their combined beliefs.

VARIATIONS

This excercise can be a homework assignment.

EXERCISE 4
WORK SHEET A

NURSING CARE PLAN

Nursing Diagnosis	Rationale	Nursing Orders

PART II

SKILLS AND COMPETENCIES

7

Observation and Listening

The purpose of Part II of this book is to discuss the skills and competencies needed to carry out the steps of the nursing process—assessment, planning, implementation, and evaluation—as described in Part I. Once again, the discussion moves from simple to complex, beginning with skills of observation and listening. Building on this base, the skills discussed become more complex, more interrelated, and more dependent on other skills.

The chapter topics are not meant to be all-inclusive, but rather should reflect basic skill areas which the practitioner can expand through experience and continued education.

This chapter begins to build the foundation of skills with a discussion of observation and listening. Observation and listening are key skills that are used by the nurse in every facet of work. Because they appear to be such simple skills, observation and listening are sometimes quickly discounted. Yet these two skills are vital tools in providing health care—particularly in providing individualized, humanistic health care.

Observation and listening can be thought of as lifeline skills, for it is through use of these tools that the care-giver can determine clients' physiologic and emotional status, as well as changes in clients' status.

Observation and listening are continuous, formal and informal, and have ever-changing results. These skills are essential in all phases of the nursing process, but are particularly valuable in assessment and evaluation.

Observation involves constant, alert interest and attention paid to all the various systems and changes in systems. Listening involves more than hearing; it includes the ability to be attuned to people and the environment and to the meanings of things that are spoken or unspoken. Both are very human skills and at times are very difficult.

A conceptual framework for understanding these concepts involves a study of perception and empathy. Following the discussion of concepts, the chapter delineates the physical and emotional factors in nursing care that mandate uses of these skills. Feedback as a means of validating observation and listening concludes Chapter 7.

CONCEPTUAL FRAMEWORK

The framework founding and guiding the understanding of observation and listening predominantly includes concepts of perception and empathy. These behavior patterns are important facets of a care-giver's humanistic skills.

Perception

Perception is that organizing process by which one comes to know objects in their appropriate identity (Garrett, 1955). It means recognizing something, having insight into it, understanding it, and being able to interpret and explain it. An object, place, person, or event is recognized and perceived by the use of receptors (receivers): exteroceptors, interoceptors, and proprioceptors. Langley, Cheraskin, and Sleeper (1958) very early defined *exteroceptors* as those sensitive to stimuli outside of the body and *interoceptors* as those sensitive inside the body. Those receptors focusing on movements of the body are called *proprioceptors.*

In order to perceive, one must always observe first, and the time interval between observing and perceiving seldom is noticed (Smeltzer, 1962). One pays attention in three ways: voluntarily, involuntarily, and habitually (Smeltzer, 1962) with perceptions being the interpretations given to sensory experience within oneself. Since physical organisms are capable of receiving a broad range of sensory experiences, it follows that people are capable of developing a broad range of perceptions. Perception is, therefore, a dynamic and learned process (Hilgard, Atkinson, and Atkinson, 1975). It involves comprehending a present situation in the light of past experience, always within the unique world of the observer.

One's awareness of self and the world around depends on sense organs and the stimuli which excite them. The sense organs are commonly referred to as eyes, ears, nose, mouth, and skin (seeing, hearing, smelling, tasting, and touching) with Kelley (1947) designating vision as the most important. Using all of one's sense organs, the world is constructed and reconstructed in accordance with how one perceives and knows it.

Perception is selective. And since one selects what one perceives, the perceptual field of each individual is unique. Sense organs are constantly bombarded with stimuli, some of which are perceived and others of which are blocked. Much of what is allowed to enter depends upon *mental set,* that is, on what one is geared to perceive. Jarvis and Gibson (1965, p. 36) state that "reception of stimuli in consciousness can be cut out." A sudden stimulus, however, might make one attend to a stimulus involuntarily. This is termed "attention getting factors in the stimulus (Garrett, 1955, p. 157)." Mental sets and, therefore, perception are influenced by past experience. Interest and training can lead one individual to perceive aspects and details that escape others (Hilgard, Atkinson, and Atkinson, 1975). Jarvis and Gibson (1965) further explain this point by saying that the way one sees is learned. Sociologic factors, therefore, play a primary role in one's perceptual field.

Factors Governing Perception   Research has shown that there are many external factors governing what one attends to and hence, what is perceived. Intensity and size affect what is perceived (Matheson, 1975). If two stimuli are competing for attention, the most intense or largest will be the first one noticed. Change causes one to shift attention (Smeltzer, 1962) and repetition of a certain stimulus can increase sensitivity or alertness to it (Matheson, 1975). Human beings are quite sensitive to objects that move in their field of vision (Smeltzer, 1962) with anything unusual or novel catching one's attention. It has been noted that perception can be determined by direct or subtle suggestions as well as curiosity. One also views objects as members of a common group when they are similar though not identical; gestalt psychologists term this phenomenon *similarity* (Matheson, 1975). Individual needs and values strongly influence what is perceived.

Since needs and values (motivation) affect perceptual intake, Maslow's (1954) hierarchy of needs can be applied in understanding perception. If one is hungry (physical needs), the sights, sounds, and smells of food become priority items to the exclusion of other items.

Another factor governing what is perceived is *closure;* closure is the tendency to fill in gaps of stimulation so that the whole is perceived rather than parts (Matheson, 1975).

Perceptual organization also encompasses the gestalt term called *figure-ground* relationship. When a simple, definite object is placed on a background, it is immediately perceived as a figure even though it may not be recognized or identified (Matheson, 1975). Another example is that letters on a textbook page are perceived as black letters on a white background. It is not common to think of a black background with white letter frames.

Shape, size, and color are *perceptual constancies* (Jarvis and Gibson, 1965). This is a phenomenon in which objects are perceived as they really are rather than according to the stimulation received from them. In shape constancy, there is a strong tendency for the perceived shape of familiar objects to remain the same irrespective of their positions or the conditions in which viewed. If cues of depth perception are operative, an image will look smaller in a positive relationship to its distance; this is termed size constancy.

Color is usually constant regardless of any abnormal condition present in the object (Matheson, 1975).

Visual cues are usually threefold: *monocular* cues are depth cues when one eye is looking; *binocular* depends on two eyes; and kinesthetic impulses from eye muscles signalling the brain regarding their position and tension form the third visual cue commonly referred to as *accommodation* (Matheson, 1975).

Tools of Perception Words, signs, symbols, and functions of objects are called tools of perception (Smeltzer, 1962). A considerable part of life's learning time is devoted to the names of objects. Signs and symbols are used to shorten the stimulus presentation for perceptual processes. Moreover, the functions and uses of objects usually comprise the largest area of perceptual tools. Giving attention to something is most often followed by interpretation of what it is for, what it will do, and how it works (Smeltzer, 1962).

Anomalies of Perception Illusions, hallucinations, and delusions are seen as anomalies (deviations) of perception. An *illusion* is a common misinterpretation of a stimulus. Sensory experiences minus relevant or adequate sensory impulses are called *hallucinations. Delusions* are false opinions or beliefs that cannot be shaken by reason (Matheson, 1975); hallucinations and delusions are often evident in psychotic behaviors.

Extrasensory Perception Extrasensory perception (ESP) is a rapidly growing science that involves one's ability to obtain information about an object or person when sensory input (as far as we know) is nonexistent. It may involve intuition, precognition, clairvoyance, and/or telepathy. With expanding affirmative documentation of a reality-base (Ostrander and Schroeder, 1970; Rao, 1966), this area of perception must be noted and considered.

Theoretical Model of Perception Over two decades ago, Ittelson and Cantril (1954) developed a theoretical model for perception composed of three major features. It is seen as useful for actualizing the concept of perception.

The first feature of the perception model is the concept of *transactions.* According to Ittelson and Cantril, "the facts of perception always present themselves through concrete individuals dealing with concrete situations. They can be studied only in terms of the 'transactions' in which they can be observed (Ittelson and Cantril, 1954, p. 2)." It is impossible to isolate and study a perception without seriously distorting its meaning. Since no perception stands alone, it follows that it must be studied in terms of the situation in which the phenomenon takes place. This requires utilization of a systems approach as well as sociologic perspective for studying perceptions. The term *transaction* is applied to indicate that all parts of a situation have an active role in affecting perception and perception owes its existence to this active participation; neither the parts of a situation nor perception exist separately.

The second feature of the theoretical model is the *personal behavior center*. Each person gives and takes personal experiences out of a given situation with each party engrossed in a situation reflective of his own personal experience (Ittelson and Cantril, 1954). Two people in different professions may have varied perceptions and experiences relative to a given object or phenomenon. In contrast, two people in the same profession may have common experiences and perceptions. This point is the basis for all social activity. Nevertheless, each person's perceptions are still unique to the individual observer.

The last feature of the model is *externalization*. This is the actual means by which a person puts together a transaction (Ittelson and Cantril, 1954). The experience of perception is externally oriented—the things heard, tasted, seen, and touched are experiences outside of self. Yet, they possess for themselves the characteristics that one individually creates, in light of past experience and one's personal world of objects and events.

Application to Nursing   Why is it important in nursing to understand the theories of perception? It is known that one's perceptions are comprised, formed, and realized individually and that these are based on thoughts, feelings, philosophies, values, desires, behaviors, and experiences (PELLEM Pentagram, Chapter 20). If one desires to observe and listen for client information to plan individualized nursing care, how can one get past one's own selective motivations to perceive in order to have truly a clean slate and pick up what is important in the client's world? The absolute answer to this question is that it is an impossible event, for one cannot disengage self from self for others. The nurse must move from a deterministic model to a probabilistic model and pose the question: how can one move closer to another's world? How can one gain greater insight into another perceptual field while realizing self exists? These questions can be answered and involve three components: (1) awareness of one's own perceptual motivations facilitated by the consciousness-raising activities of the PELLEM Pentagram*; (2) establishing reliability for perceptions by checking them with others to note similarities and differences (feedback); and (3) having empathy.

Empathy

This concept, empathy (discussed more fully in Chapter 18), is generally viewed as an ability to place oneself mentally and emotionally into the world

---

*Chapter 20 provides a discussion of this model.

of the person with whom one is interacting (Rogers, 1961). It is necessary to free one's mind of self to accomplish this task. Logical reasoning dictates the impossibility of freeing oneself from anything unless one is aware of what is to be freed (in other words, "I cannot put away what I do not know I have!"). This point emphasizes the need for self-awareness. It also frees one to perceive another and this is best done when the perceiver takes all information known about another and constructs a fantasy. The guiding questions asked of self are: Given the points known and what has been said, how would I feel in this situation? What would I feel if in the other's shoes? What would I want, need, and think? What would be helpful to me? This process involves understanding and interpreting self-perceptions with emphasis on another's world. It also involves using self purposefully and with awareness rather than attempting to repress or blot out one's own perceptual system with the delusion that one can disengage self from the other. Involved is an owning or meeting of oneself as a means to understand others. If one knows self, there is greater probability that one can move closer to knowing and understanding another since the art of exploring self is similar to exploring another's individuality and perceptual field. Conversely, when one is unable to look at oneself for whatever reason, how could one ever truly perceive an array of aspects in another without being oppressed in selected areas? Massarik and Wechsler (1959) term this process *interpersonal perception* (subtitled *empathy revisited*); it is the process of understanding people.

The conceptual framework involving perception and empathy has been discussed. Observation and listening as skills necessary in nursing will be shown in operation in the following portions of Chapter 7; the discussion is reflective of the theories described.

OBSERVATION AND LISTENING IN OPERATION

Perhaps the most succinct and articulate definitions of the observation and listening skills are by Webster (1971). This source views observation as the act of perceiving, noticing, and watching attentively. Listening is attending closely, with the sense organ being the ear; it means making a conscious effort to hear. Looking at the organs of perception, the following becomes evident in terms of these skills: observing involves the senses of sight, touch, and smell; listening involves the sense of hearing.

The act of talking becomes important when providing feedback or seeking clarification or affirmation on what has been observed and heard. Logic tells one, therefore, that observation and listening come first; talking second— unless, of course, one wishes to be observed and heard first; this type of behavior implies one's own agenda is more important and the client is only secondary. However, when seeking to discover priorities in the client's world to uncover areas needing assistance, a helping nurse must place the client's agenda—what the client needs to have taken care of—in the foreground. In later stages of the nursing process, and in line with the model presented in Chapter 5 for implementing nursing care, the agenda of the nurse may be foremost at times, but certainly not always. Of course, the nurse often initiates the observation and listening process by talking and asking leading questions to elicit information requiring further observation and needing to be heard. But it is important to remember that professional expertise is only a guide to giving care; it should not be an end in itself. An individual client's agenda is paramount.

Categorically speaking, there can be two basic divisions of data regarding a client that must be observed: physical aspects and emotional aspects.

Physical Aspects

The area of physical aspects refers primarily to the physiologic signs and symptoms that a professional nurse should be alert for and accurately report so as to facilitate understanding with a variety of health personnel. The list of signs and symptoms provided in Table 7-1 is not meant to be exhaustive, but rather provides a framework. Physical assessment skills are necessary in many areas.

Emotional Aspects

The nurse is constantly listening for and observing emotional aspects of the client. These are feelings of the individual. Perception of his feelings is closely entwined with verbal and nonverbal communications of the client, an area covered in the next chapter. For purposes here, it is necessary to look broadly at the perception of feelings. Gazda, et al (1977) have divided feelings into two dimensions: surface and underlying. Surface feelings are those that are explicitly expressed by the client; they are obvious by the words or way a person says something.

Example: (Pale, listless client to nurse in weak voice) "I am not feeling like my usual self—my energy seems gone."
Feelings expressed: weak, listless, lacks energy, sick, unhappy, down.

Gazda, et al (1977) further explicated underlying feelings as a content interpretation of what a client says; these feelings may not have been overtly verbalized, but a nurse can read between the lines, also considering feelings in relation to previous observed data.

(Text continues on page 182)

TABLE 7-1
PHYSICAL SYMPTOMS TO BE OBSERVED
AND TERMS TO USE IN REPORTING THEM

	OBSERVATION	TERM TO USE
Abdomen	1. Hard, boardlike 2. Soft, flabby 3. Appears swollen, rounded 4. Hurts when touched 5. Filled with gas 6. Note area of abdomen observed	1. Hard, rigid 2. Relaxed, flaccid, soft 3. Protuberant 4. Sensitive to touch 5. Distended, tympanites
Areas		1. Epigastric 2. Right lumbar 3. Umbilical 4. Left lumbar 5. Right iliac 6. Hypogastric 7. Left ilias
Belch	Belching	Eructation
Bleeding	1. Spurting of blood 2. Very little 3. Nosebleed 4. Blood in vomitus 5. Blood in urine 6. Spitting of blood 7. When bleeding is stopped 8. Color	1. In spurts 2. Oozing 3. Epistaxis 4. Hematemesis 5. Hematuria 6. Hemoptysis 7. Hemorrhage controlled 8. Bright red, dark red, frothy
Breathing	1. Breathing 2. Act of inhaling 3. Act of exhaling 4. Difficult breathing 5. Short periods when breathing has ceased 6. Inability to breathe lying down 7. Normal breathing 8. Rapid breathing 9. Increasing dyspnea with periods of apnea 10. Snorting breathing 11. Large volume of air inspired or expired 12. Small volume of air inspired or expired 13. Abnormal variation in rhythm	1. Respiration 2. Inspiration 3. Expiration 4. Dyspnea 5. Apnea 6. Orthpnea 7. Eupnea 8. Hyperpnea 9. Cheyne-Stokes respiration 10. Stertorous breathing 11. Deep breathing 12. Shallow breathing 13. Irregular respiration
Chill	1. Blanket applied to help warm the patient 2. Type as to severity 3. Duration	1. External heat applied 2. Severe, moderate, slight 3. Lasting number of minutes
Coma	1. Partly in coma 2. Deep in coma	1. Partially comatose 2. Profound coma
Convulsion	1. Continuous shaking 2. Shaking with intervals of rest 3. Begin without warning	1. Duration and description 2. Duration and description 3. Sudden onset
Cough	1. Coughs at all times 2. Coughing over a long period of time 3. Coughs up material 4. Short, hard cough	1. Continuous cough 2. Persistent cough 3. Productive cough, describe 4. Hacking cough

(Table 7-1 continues)

TABLE 7-1 (continued)

	OBSERVATION	TERM TO USE
Defecation	1. Bowel movement material 2. Bowel movement (act of) 3. Excessive defecation 4. Gray colored stool 5. Dark brown liquid 6. Formed, yet soft stool 7. Formed, yet hardened stool 8. Infrequent bowel movements 9. Black stool	1. Feces, stool 2. Defecation 3. Diarrhea, describe 4. Clay colored liquid stool 5. Highly colored liquid stool 6. Soft formed stool 7. Hard formed stool 8. Constipation 9. Black, tarry stool
Dizziness	Dizziness	Vertigo
Drainage	1. Watery, from nose 2. Containing pus 3. Bloody 4. Consists of feces 5. Of serous fluid 6. Containing mucus and pus 7. Tough, sticky 8. From vagina (after delivery)	1. Coryza 2. Purulent 3. Sanguinous 4. Fecal 5. Serous 6. Mucopurulent 7. Tenacious 8. Lochia
Dressings	1. A second dressing added to the first 2. Dressing removed, another applied 3. Drain tubes cut off 4. Drain taken out	1. Dressing reinforced 2. Redressed 3. Drain tubes shortened (number of inches) 4. Drain removed
Emesis	1. Produced by effort of patient 2. Ejected to a few feet distant 3. If blood is only noticeable 4. Material vomited 5. Contents	1. Induced 2. Projectile 3. Blood tinged 4. Vomitus, emesis 5. Describe color, odor, appearance, consistency
Eyes	1. Sharpness of vision 2. Yellow in color 3. Puffy 4. Motionless 5. Sensitive to light 6. Double vision 7. Squinting 8. Abnormal protrusion of eyeball 9. Inflammation of conjunctiva	1. Visual acuity 2. Jaundiced 3. Edematous 4. Staring 5. Photophobia 6. Diplopia 7. Strabismus 8. Exophthalmus 9. Conjunctivitis
Faint	Fainting	Syncope
Fever	1. Without fever 2. Temperature above normal 3. Temperature greatly above normal 4. Temperature suddenly returns to normal 5. Temperature gradually returns to normal	1. Afebrile 2. Pyrexia 3. Hyperpyrexia 4. Crisis 5. Lysis
Gas	1. Gas in the digestive tract 2. Having gas in the digestive tract 3. Swelling of abdomen	1. Flatus 2. Flatulence 3. Distention
Hallucination	1. Of hearing 2. Of sight 3. Of smell 4. Of taste	1. Auditory hallucination 2. Visual hallucination 3. Olfactory hallucination 4. Gustatory hallucination

TABLE 7-1 (continued)

	OBSERVATION	TERM TO USE
Head	1. Forehead 2. Region over temple 3. Back of head 4. Base of skull	1. Frontal region 2. Temporal region 3. Occipital region 4. Basilar region
Joints	1. Bending 2. To straighten 3. Turn inward 4. Turn outward 5. Revolve around 6. Move away from median line 7. Move toward median line	1. Flexion 2. Extension 3. Inversion 4. Eversion 5. Rotation 6. Abduction 7. Adduction
Lice	1. Head, body, pubic 2. Condition of lousiness	1. Pediculi 2. Pediculosis
Nourishment	1. Very small amount of water 2. Small pieces of ice 3. Drink of water 4. Given through tube into stomach 5. Given by enema	1. Sips water 2. Chipped ice 3. Water (number of cc) 4. Lavage 5. Nutritive enema, fluid and amount
Odor	1. Not unpleasant 2. Like fruit 3. Very unpleasant 4. Belonging to a particular drug, etc. 5. Like feces	1. Aromatic 2. Fruity 3. Offensive 4. Characteristic 5. Fecal
Pain	1. Great pain 2. Little 3. Spasmodic; period of great pain followed by period of little or no pain 4. Spreads to distant areas 5. Started all at once 6. Hurts worse when moving	1. Severe 2. Slight 3. Paroxysmal 4. Radiating 5. Sudden onset 6. Increased by movement
Paralysis	1. Of the muscles of the face 2. Of the legs 3. Of one side of the body 4. Of a single limb 5. Both arms and legs	1. Facial 2. Paraplegia 3. Hemiplegia 4. Monoplegia 5. Quadriplegia
Perspiration	1. Large amount 2. Small amount	1. Profuse diaphoresis 2. Scanty
Pulse	1. Number of beats per minute 2. Rhythm 3. Beats missed at intervals 4. Over 100 beats per minute 5. Very rapid, beats indistinct 6. Slow in rate 7. One scarcely perceptible 8. Small, rapid and tense	1. Rate 2. Regular or irregular 3. Intermittent 4. Rapid 5. Running 6. Slow 7. Thready 8. Wiry
Skin	1. Normal 2. Pink, hot 3. Blue in color 4. Very white 5. Shines 6. Raw surface 7. Yellow in color 8. Torn 9. Containing colored areas 10. Wet 11. Scraped 12. Black and blue mark 13. Cold, clammy	1. Healthy 2. Flushed 3. Cyanotic 4. Extreme pallor 5. Glossy 6. Excoriation 7. Jaundiced 8. Lacerated 9. Pigmented 10. Moist 11. Abraded 12. Ecchymosis 13. Cold, clammy

(Table 7-1 continues)

TABLE 7-1 (continued)

	OBSERVATION	TERM TO USE
Unconscious-ness	1. Complete unconsciousness 2. Partial unconsciousness 3. Pretended unconsciousness	1. In comatose condition 2. In stuporous condition 3. Feigned unconsciousness
Urination	1. To urinate 2. No control over urination 3. Burning when voiding 4. Large amount of urine voided 5. Total suppression of urine 6. Frequent voiding at night 7. Painful urination 8. Pus in urine 9. Blood in urine 10. Hemoglobin in urine 11. Glucose in urine 12. Albumin in urine 13. Acetone in urine 14. Bile in urine 15. Scantiness of urine 16. Sugar in urine	1. Void, urinate 2. Involuntary, incontinent 3. Burning sensation on urination 4. Polyuria 5. Anuria 6. Nocturia 7. Dysuria 8. Pyuria 9. Hematuria 10. Hemoglobinuria 11. Glucosuria 12. Albuminuria 13. Acetonuria 14. Choluria 15. Oliguria 16. Glycosuria
Weight	1. Overweight 2. Thin, underweight	1. Obese 2. Emaciated
Wounds	1. Deep 2. Slight, surface only 3. Not infected 4. Discharging pus 5. Infected 6. Torn	1. Deep 2. Superficial 3. Clean 4. Suppurating 5. Infected 6. Lacerated

SOURCE: These descriptions were derived from materials compiled by an anonymous source.

Same example (plus the following information): The nurse knows the client is one day postoperative of abdominal surgery.

Underlying feelings: washed-out, sicker than she thought she'd feel, wondering if feelings are normal.

It is important to note that verbal ability and appropriate use of the language can facilitate accuracy in responding to surface and underlying feelings. Included in the suggested reading portion of this chapter is an article by Moorhead (1972) containing a list of words used to describe feelings. Gazda, et al (1977) also contains an appendix of affective adjectives. Reference to these sources may be helpful.

Feedback

It follows that after one perceives the physical and emotional dimensions of the client, it is necessary to establish validity of same because one's perceptual field is guided by self. Empathic responses must be perceived by the receiver. This process involves feedback—to the client and colleagues.

Knowledge and experience enable the nurse to rest with more security on perceptions of physical signs and symptoms. If unsure, it becomes the nurse's responsibility to check findings with one more experienced. This process usually involves asking another for an opinion or consultation. It parallels what physicians do when they request expert consultation. When two people agree, the perception is more reliable; conversely, if disagreement occurs, clarification and discussion becomes necessary.

This same process is carried into the client's emotional domain, but consultation with the client is necessary. Orlando (1961, p. 1) described the task of the nurse as distinguishing "between the understanding of general principles and the meanings which she must discover in the immediate nursing situation in order to help the patient." In order to accomplish this, the nurse must understand the meanings in the client's world and then exercise his or her professional functions with relation to the client's needs. In essence, this involves perceiving feelings and validating them with the client.

Validation requires stating what was heard from the client reflectively and in one's own natural words. It means building a response to the client conveying that one heard the expressed feelings and understands underlying feelings, all of which personifies empathy. Cash, Scherba, and Mills (1975) proposed five steps meant to assist the helper in the aforementioned process of building empathic responses:

1. Identify mood.
2. Specify feelings—surface and underlying.
3. Decide intensity level of feeling—high, low, moderate.
4. Select words that are analogous with expressed feelings.
5. Verbalize a sentence incorporating perception of items 1–4.

Gazda, et al (1977) further pointed out guidelines for building responses:

1. Verbal and nonverbal behavior should be the focus of the helper.
2. The helper should formulate responses of empathy in a language and manner that is most easily understood by the helpee.
3. The tone of the helper's response should be analogous to that of the helpee.
4. The helper should actively use empathy in responding to the helpee.
5. The helper should concentrate on what the helpee is expressing, and also be aware of what is not being expressed.
6. The helper must accurately interpret responses to the helpee and use them as a guide in developing future responses.

Using the same example previously explicated, a natural response that incorporates these guidelines would be:

Natural response of the nurse: "You sound like you are feeling extremely weak and exhausted, possibly even wondering if you will ever feel like yourself again."

In this example, the nurse has communicated that the nurse heard what the client expressed and also has understanding of what the client did not express. The nurse also is communicating interest in and concern for the client and has granted the client permission to express personal feelings. This factor alone is paramount in building a trusting nurse/client relationship. It opens the door for further client-centered communication.

Validation of perceptions by the client is possible because the client has an avenue through which to respond, knowing that the nurse cares and will listen. Because the nurse did not ask questions at this time (nurse's agenda), the client has freedom to respond with her own and the nurse can then obtain client-centered data. Closure of the interaction is predominantly guided by the client.

SUMMARY

The skills of observation and listening were presented using a conceptual framework involving perception and empathy. Physical and emotional dimensions were discussed and the use of feedback was presented as a method for validating perceptions.

REFERENCES

Cash, R., Scherba, D., and Mills, S. *Human resources development: A competency based training program.* (Trainer's Manual) Long Beach, Calif.: The Authors, 1975.

Garrett, H. *General psychology.* New York: American Book Company, 1955.

Gazda, G., Asbury, F., Balzer, F., Childers, W., and Walters, R. *Human relations development: A manual for educators.* Boston: Allyn and Bacon, 1977.

Hilgard, E., Atkinson, R., and Atkinson, R. *Introduction to psychology.* New York: Harcourt, Brace, and Co., 1975.

Ittelson, W., and Cantril, H. *Perception: A transactional approach.* Garden City, N.Y.: Doubleday, 1954.

Jarvis, J., and Gibson, J. *Psychology for nurses.* Oxford, England: Blackwell Scientific Publications, Ltd., 1965.

Kelley, E. *Education of what is real.* New York: Harper and Brothers, 1947.

Langley, L., Cheraskin, E., and Sleeper, R. *Dynamic anatomy and physiology.* New York: McGraw-Hill Books, Inc., 1958.

Maslow, A. *Motivation and personality.* New York: Harper and Row, 1954.

Masserik, F., and Wechsler, I. *Interpersonal perception. California Management Review* 1:36–46, 1959.

Matheson, D. *Introductory psychology: The modern view.* Hinsdale, Ill.: Dryden Press, 1975.

Moorhead, T., Jr. *Communication for educational problem-solving.* Melbourne, Fla.: Human Dynamics, Inc., 1972.

Orlando, I. *The dynamic nurse-patient relationship.* New York: G. P. Putnam's Sons, 1961.

Ostrander, S., and Schroeder, L. *Psychic discoveries behind the Iron Curtain.* Englewood Cliffs, N.J.: Prentice-Hall, 1970.

Rao, K. *Experimental parapsychology.* Springfield, Illinois: Charles C. Thomas, 1966.

Rogers, C. *On becoming a person.* Boston: Houghton-Mifflin, 1961.

Smeltzer, C. *Psychology for student nurses.* New York: Macmillan, 1962.

Webster's Third International Dictionary. Springfield, Mass.: G. and C. Merriam Company, 1971.

SELECTED READING

The article by Moorhead (1972) provides a rich discussion of the communication process. Examples are given for listening, validating perceptions, and giving information (describing behavior and feelings to others). The author includes a word list that is helpful in building responses that can accurately reflect feelings of others.

Communication for Educational Problem-Solving

Ted B. Moorhead, Jr.

Communication is from the Latin *communis*, common. When we communicate we are trying to get something in common between us. You may know a fact which I do not know. In some way you make that fact known to me, then you and I both know that fact: We have it in common.

So, through communication processes we share facts, ideas, attitudes, opinions, and feelings. Thus we learn from each other and come to understand one another, if communication is effective. If it is ineffective, learning is blocked and misunderstandings occur.

We tend to assume we communicate well. If we are misunderstood, it's because someone else is stupid. We also tend to assume we receive and understand the communications of others well. If we don't understand someone, it's because he can't talk straight.

Actually, communication is a very complicated process. There are many points in this process at which breakdowns can occur, even between highly intelligent persons. Also, few of us have opportunity to develop and check out our communication skills in a structured program. The purpose of these sessions is to give you such an opportunity.

Let's look at communication between two persons:

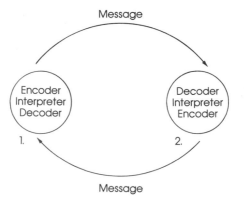

Suppose person 1 initiates communication. He must decide what it is he wants to communicate, how to do it, and how it is likely to be received by person 2. Let's say person 1 communicates a message with words (including vocal inflections, tones, and volume), facial expressions, hand gestures, and body position. Person 2 must receive all this data, decode the symbols, interpret what the total message means, decide on a response, encode that response, and send the message.

This is actually a simplified diagram. It does not take into account the interplay of the emotional and rational processes within an individual which influence his communication. But it should be clear that the communication process we often take for granted is indeed intricate. And it requires maintenance if it is to be kept intact.

Communication can break down at any point in the process. Person 1 may not understand himself well, or what he wants to communicate, or what kind of response he is trying to get from person number 2. In this case, he stands a strong chance of putting his foot in his mouth.

Then there is the problem of semantics. A word may mean one thing to person 1 but something entirely different to person 2. So the decoder doesn't match the encoder.

And any of the other communication symbols can be misinterpreted. Some people "sound" angry all the time. Others "sound" happy all the time. Until you get to know them and can pick up other clues, it is difficult to understand their feelings.

When a message is sent and another is sent back, the return process is called *feedback*. By paying close attention to our feedback, we can learn a lot about how our messages are being received and interpreted. And we can make adjustments and develop our communication skills.

COMMUNICATION FOR SOLVING PROBLEMS

All of life can be viewed as a series of problems to be solved. The word "problem" is used here not in a negative sense of situations to be avoided, but in a positive sense as the very process of life. My basic problems are how to get the food, air, water, and affection I need to survive. As an infant, I communicated these needs by crying, squirming, and cuddling. My mother and other meaningful persons helped me solve these problems by responding to my communication. Sometimes they became confused as to what my problem was and how they could help, because my communication was not clear. We have a better chance of solving problems when communication is clear.

Educational processes are also a series of problems to be solved. A person needs to learn to perceive himself, others, and life situations accurately. He needs to learn behavior which will enable him to function responsibly and productively in meeting his own needs and as a member of society.

Communication is the key to solving these and other problems. And by communication I mean action as well as words, for we communicate by what we do and by what we say.

Through communication *helping relationships* are built. These are relationships in which each helps the other to solve problems of mutual concern.

This is an ideal teacher–pupil relationship. A pupil has a problem: He needs to improve his reading skill. The problem is of concern to the teacher: He has responsibility for helping pupils improve reading skill, feels for the pupil in his need, and wants to help. So the teacher does what he can do to help the pupil solve the problem.

In a helping relationship, each person must help the other. The problem may be identified as primarily belonging to the pupil. And the teacher may see the pupil as the one receiving help, and himself giving. But unless the teacher also receives help from the pupil, he cannot give help to the pupil. The pupil must help the teacher understand what the problem is. The teacher needs to receive information from the pupil, without which the teacher will be unable to give help. Also the pupil must help the teacher by cooperating with whatever strategy is developed to solve the problem.

So two-way communication is essential to the educational problem-solving process. And the more effective this communication is in bringing about sharing of information relevant to a problem, the better the chance of solution.

Let's say a child is behaving disruptively. This is a problem for the child (hindering his learning and socialization), for the teacher (hindering his efforts to maintain a climate for learning), and the class (hindering their learning and socialization). In order to help solve the problem, the teacher must understand the nature of the problem. Is the child bored, confused, restless, frustrated, hostile, desiring attention, or what? He must decode and interpret the message sent by the child in his behavior and respond helpfully. That response must be a message which is clear enough to be decoded and interpreted accurately by the child.

So in the educational problem-solving process, clarity and accuracy of two-way communication is important.

Also vital is an openness of communication lines between persons so that the necessary information can be exchanged. If the child feels constrained in communicating with a teacher, through fear of rejection or punishment, the teacher is not likely to get much needed information from the child.

Let's say Johnny is struggling with his reading. Teacher says, "Johnny, I see you are having a hard time in reading. What's the problem?" Johnny says, "I don't know. I just don't like to read." This is a crucial point at which a helping relationship can either grow or be squelched. The teacher can react defensively: "Well, you'd better learn to like to read because there's plenty of it all the way through school." Interpreted by Johnny, this means his feelings don't matter; school must be accepted as hateful work because that's the way it is. And he is not likely again to give this teacher such information about how he feels. But on the other hand, the teacher can respond openly: "I'm sorry you aren't enjoying reading. I'd like to help. Tell me more about how you feel when you read." This opens the way for a further exchange of information and a possible revelation of the root of the problem.

There are certain communication skills which can facilitate a maximum exchange of information needed to solve problems. These skills are not common. The lack of their use hinders classroom communication and problem solving. But these skills can be learned and used by teachers, pupils, and administrators. The result is a cultural change away from destructive game-playing and toward the problem-solving communication of helping relationships.

SKILLS IN RECEIVING INFORMATION

Reflective Listening

Listening is a vital skill for building helping relationships between persons. Perhaps the most vital.

Reflective listening is a method for verifying and clarifying what one hears. It can facilitate effective communication and can help ensure accuracy of understanding.

Also, this can be supportive and affirmative to the person who is talking. It says you care enough about him to listen to what he says and to make sure you understand. It communicates acceptance of him as a person, whether or not you agree with what he says.

Furthermore, this style of listening opens the way for maximum reception of needed information. The person sending information tests, consciously or unconsciously, to see how he is being heard. He sends a message. If the response indicates misinterpretation by the receiver, he may try again or give up. If the receiver indicates indifference to the message, the communication line is damaged. If the receiver gives back defensiveness, communication is blocked. But if the receiver is interested and open, giving out data indicating he is hearing and understanding or wants to understand, the sender is reinforced in giving more data.

Look at an example: Mary, who is making poor grades, has her head on the desk while teacher is giving an assignment.

> Teacher: "Mary, will you look up please. You are missing an important assignment."
> Mary: "Aw, I'm tired of this class."
> Teacher: "Your problem, Mary, is you're lazy. Now sit up and listen."

What did Mary communicate? She could have meant she was tired at this moment in time. Past data (grades) would indicate the problem is more chronic. But does she see the subject matter as irrelevant, herself incompetent, the teacher incompetent, or what? The teacher will not learn for sure what the problem is—he has already assumed it is Mary's laziness. By pinning this label on her, he confirms his negative perception of her, which may be also a confirmation of her own low self-esteem. This transaction is not likely to be helpful. If I see myself as lazy and no-good and you tell me I am lazy and no-good, I am likely to act out our mutual perception in an interpersonal relationship.

Now look at another way the transaction could have occurred:

Mary: "Aw, I'm tired of this class."
Teacher: "Do you mean you're not interested in what we are doing?"
Mary: "Yeah, I don't see any sense in all this work we're doing. It doesn't mean anything to me."
Teacher: "You mean you don't see any way that what we're studying applies to your life right now?"
Mary: "Yeah, that's it."
Teacher: "Perhaps some others have this same problem. I'd like to know how some of the rest of you feel about this."

This opens the way for others as well as Mary to give the teacher information vitally needed to solve problems. One result could be modification of curriculum or teaching methods to make the learning process more relevant. Another result could be the disclosure of reasons why the present material is relevant—reasons which would have special appeal to Mary, coming from her peers. Or additional discussion could reveal hidden problems, such as interpersonal conflicts, which were behind Mary's disinterest.

At any rate, Mary has been heard rather than cut off. This in itself affirms her and supports her self-esteem. Being heard may in itself motivate her to do better work. It gives her a feeling of being a more valuable person, one whose opinions are worth listening to. And it gives her a perception of the teacher as a person who cares enough to listen.

Some teachers say they do not have time for this kind of discussion or individual attention in a classroom. This reflects the condition of getting so locked into content that the process of instruction cannot be dealt with. When process is ignored, content will inevitably get bogged down. The task as well as interpersonal relationship will suffer. It would pay in the long run to take the time necessary to do "processing," as in the above example between the teacher and Mary.

Also remember that when you are engaged in a meaningful exchange with one person others are also learning. Others, as well as Mary, were learning something about the relevance of the curriculum. They were learning about the teacher as a helping person, and about themselves as being able to communicate with this adult. Most of all, they were learning they could participate in making decisions and solving problems. They could share in educational responsibilities, rather than having these all handled exclusively by the teacher. Thus, they could begin to see themselves as responsible persons, and behave accordingly.

The key to true "reflective listening" is empathy. Put yourself mentally and emotionally into the place of the person to whom you are listening. Think with him and feel with him until you understand what he is thinking and feeling.

Another important element is suspension of evaluation or judgment of what is being said until understanding has occurred. Carl Rogers said, ". . . the major barrier to mutual interpersonal communication is our very natural tendency to judge, to evaluate, to approve or disapprove, the statement of the other person, or the other group."* Our listening pattern is typically to judge first and to clarify understanding second, if at all. This pattern must be reversed in order to practice "reflective listening" and to facilitate understanding.

Note that there is a difference between understanding and agreement. I may listen to your opinion and check my interpretation of what you are saying until I fully understand, yet still disagree with you. Agreement is much more likely when this quality of communication is taking place. But understanding is the essential goal. Two persons may have a mutual helping relationship and yet disagree in many areas. But they cannot have such a relationship without understanding each other.

There are several techniques which may be employed in "reflective listening."

One way to make sure you received a message clearly is to repeat it word for word: "I do not like what is happening." — "I heard you say 'I do not like what is happening'." The sender has a chance to confirm or correct what you heard. And he knows you are listening. But he does not know how you are *interpreting* his message. You have verified the words you heard, but not your understanding of the words.

Another response could be, "What do you mean by that?" This puts the entire burden of clarification on the sender, and may draw a defensive reaction. It implies that you have no idea of what he is trying to communicate and that he is failing completely to get through to you. A better response, if indeed you have no comprehension of what is being said, is to admit you are having a problem understanding and ask the person to repeat the message. If the communication is vague, ask for an example.

An excellent technique for "reflective listening" is to *paraphrase* what you think the person means. Reflect back your interpretation of his message, putting what he said in your words: "I do not like what is happening." — "Do you mean you are uncomfortable with what we are doing?" This gives the sender an opportunity to hear how you interpret what he says and to decide whether or not you understand. Also, this opens the way for him to confirm or correct and increase your understanding of his message by further communication.

"Do you mean...?" is a good preface to paraphrase. Others are, "Are you saying...?", "Let me check my understanding...", "You mean...?", "This means...?", and "In other words...?"

A paraphrase may be quite direct, with only a key word or two changed: "I am happy we solved that problem." — "You mean you are happy we worked that out?" This is a safe reflection and can frequently open the way for further communication. It is not likely to get a "no" response. However, it does not give back much data on the depth of your understanding. So the direct paraphrase is useful, but limited.

An amplified paraphrase contains more interpretation of the message: "I am happy we solved that problem." — "Do you mean you are relieved and

*Carl R. Rogers, *On Becoming a Person* (New York: Houghton Mifflin), p. 330.

glad that a difficult problem is solved?" Such an amplification could be based on data in addition to the words spoken. The listener may be aware of background information which gives clues to meaning. Non-verbal and verbal signals provide data on the intensity of feelings, which can be reflected in the paraphrase. Facial expressions, gestures, body positions give impressions. And tone, volume, and velocity of voice are all a part of the message. The amplified paraphrase gives back much data on your understanding. It is more difficult to do, and more frequently subject to challenge since it is more subjective.

A reverse paraphrase can help clarify understanding: "I am happy we solved that problem." — "Do you mean that problem was bothering you quite a bit?" Here both sender and receiver can take a look at a communication from another perspective: A positive statement can be restated negatively, or a negative statement can be restated positively. Either way could be helpful: "If only we could work together, things would go better." — "Do you mean there are ways we are not working together which are preventing things from going better?" "Things are going terribly." — "Do you mean you would like for things to go better?"

An "alternatives" paraphrase can help differentiate between two or more possible meanings: "I don't like this course." — "Do you mean you are dissatisfied with the content or the method of presentation?"

The type of paraphrase to use can usually be played by ear so long as the listener is effectively practicing empathy and suspending evaluation.

Obviously, one need not paraphrase every incoming message. This method is especially helpful in these conditions:

1. When there is a possibility of misunderstanding, and to understand is important.
2. When the other person may be helped by the assurance he is understood (by feeling accepted as a person and cared for).
3. When an incoming message carries heavy emotional weight (such as in a conflict).

"Reflective listening" has benefits beyond simple verification and clarification of communication. It can help remove blocks to understanding in heavy emotional situations. Frequently, in conflict persons become so intent on defending a position that neither one is actually hearing the other. Paraphrasing requires listening to each other and breaks through such blocks. Thus, it is an important skill in conflict resolution.

Also, it can help a person understand himself. As he hears his communication reflected back as interpreted by another, he clarifies his own understanding of what he means. Often one will find his feelings about a matter moderating as another listens receptively. He hears irrational elements in his message as it is reflected back. If the receiver is not defensive, the sender's need to be defensive is minimized. Faulty opinions are more likely to be changed under these conditions.

And, most helpfully, "reflective listening" to a person can facilitate his self-acceptance and self-esteem. When someone listens, understands, and accepts his feelings, a person can better accept himself. When someone values him as a person enough to listen and understand his communication, a person can better see himself as having worth. Such self-acceptance and self-esteem are basic essentials to growth and actualization of one's potential as a person.

Carl Rogers describes the "helping relationship" which can occur when communication skills such as "reflective listening" are used effectively. He says the following:

> I am by no means always able to achieve this kind of relationship with another, and sometimes, even when I feel I have achieved it in myself, he may be too frightened to perceive what is being offered to him. But I would say that when I hold in myself the kind of attitudes I have described, and when the other person can to some degree experience these attitudes, then I believe that change and constructive personal development will *invariably* occur—and I include the word 'invariably" only after long and careful consideration.*

Perception Check

A "perception check" is another way to verify information received. This is a question by which you check your perception of the feelings of another person. It is useful when a person is sending verbal and/or non-verbal signals about his feelings which are not completely clear or direct. Also, the "perception check" can help a person become conscious of feelings which he is communicating but which are beneath his level of awareness.

Let's say Johnny is scratching his head, frowning, and not writing when the class is supposed to be working on a written assignment. Teacher, picking up these non-verbal signals, says, "Johnny, are you having difficulty with the assignment?" (perception check). This tells Johnny you are aware of his having a problem, but that you aren't making assumptions about the nature of the problem without checking with him. It opens the way for Johnny to help teacher understand the nature of his problem so as to be helpful to him.

Mary says, "This is a stupid course." She is not talking about her feelings. She is giving an evaluation of the course. But feelings are evident in her voice and body expressions. Teacher picks this up, and says, "Mary, are you feeling angry about having to do this work?" (perception check).

Mary: "Yes, I think it's stupid and I don't like it."
Teacher: "You mean you don't understand the purpose of what we are doing and get tired of doing it?" (reflective listening)
Mary: "Yes."
Teacher: "I'm sorry you're having problems with it. I want to help you. Can we work on it?" (description of feelings and offer to help solve problem)

Helping relationships are built as persons communicate on a "feeling" as well as intellectual level. Teacher could have had an intellectual debate with Mary on the merits of the course and accomplished nothing. By being aware of

*Ibid., p. 35.

and checking out what Mary was feeling, accepting her feelings, and going on to share her own feelings and an offer to help, teacher practiced effective problem-solving communication.

In making a "perception check," it may be more helpful to actually check your perception with a question rather than assume your perception is accurate and make a statement about it.

You see someone getting red-faced and talking loudly. NOT — "You are getting angry. What's wrong with you?" BUT — "*Are* you getting angry with me?"

It is helpful in making a "perception check" to pinpoint the object of feelings, like, "Are you getting angry *with me?*" The person could be angry with someone else or about something apart from you. Clarification could result from such a check.

After making a "perception check," communicate acceptance rather than judgment toward the feelings. NOT — "Are you getting angry with me?" "Yes." "Well, that's too bad. You better cool off." BUT — "Are you getting angry with me?" "Yes." "I see. Can we work on the problem? What's bothering you?"

A pupil needs to learn to be aware of, accept, own, and describe his feelings. He needs to learn that feelings are internal to himself, not out in the external environment where he may tend to project them. The fact is not that the course is stupid. That is an opinion. But the fact is Mary is feeling disturbed in the course. Mary needs to learn to differentiate between an opinion she has of the course and her disturbed feelings, which are a more vital component of the problem. Teacher's perception check can help her learn this differentiation and how to accept and cope with negative feelings—an important element of emotional development.

So far, checking perception of negative feelings has been discussed. Also valuable is the "perception check" of positive feelings. Johnny, who has been struggling in language arts, comes up to teacher with face aglow and says, "I got a B on my test!" NOT — "I know, I graded it." BUT — "Say, you're happy about that, aren't you?"

The "perception check," as well as verifying perceptions of others' feelings, says you care and are aware of how they feel—that you feel with them in their pain and joy. With this, you come through a real person and a sincere helper. You can give the kind of emotional support and aid to effective development needed by many children.

SKILLS IN GIVING INFORMATION

So far we have focused on listening and checking perceptions. Now we look at the sending side of the communication cycle.

How can you be sure the messages you send are clear and accurate? How can you assure a congruent signal, readily understood, rather than mixed messages, which can be confusing? How can you differentiate between facts and opinions, and communicate objective observations rather than inferences, when this is important? How can you cope with and communicate your own emotional feelings, both positive and negative, to pupils?

These are vitally needed kinds of communication to be exchanged in the helping relationship of a classroom. But unusual communication skills are required for such transactions. Skills of giving information so as to maximize the reception and effectiveness of such information can be developed.

Describing Behavior

In order to have satisfactory relationships, people must consider how their behavior affects other people. If someone is doing something that damages the relationship between you and him, he must know what that action is if he is to consider changing it. On the other hand, if someone's behavior is enhancing the relationship, it is more likely to continue if identified and affirmed.

But many people do not describe behavior clearly enough for others to know what they mean. Instead of describing behavior, often inferences are made about feelings, motivations, and attitudes. Also, a lot of value judgments are passed off instead of behavior descriptions.

Example Behavior description, combined with description of feelings and establishment of authority: "Johnny, you threw a paper wad. I am angry because this disrupted the class. You must not do such a thing again."

Value judgment and inference: "Johnny, you are a bad boy. You are trying to show off for the whole class."

The skill of behavior description depends on accurate, objective observation. It requires being able to distinguish between an objective observation of fact (what you actually saw and heard) and inferences you may have drawn from the observation. People often become so accustomed to making inferences they are unaware of the actual behavior from which the inference was drawn.

Example "Hey, why are you so gloomy?" "What makes you think I'm gloomy?" "I don't know, you just seemed gloomy." "No, I'm just tired."

Also, an objective behavior description is nonevaluative. It does not imply that what happened was good or bad, right or wrong.

Examples

Behavior descriptions	Evaluative or inferential statements
"Mary, you interrupted Joan while she was talking."	"Mary is rude." "Mary wasn't interested in what Joan was saying."
"Larry, you did not complete your assignment."	"Larry, you work too slowly." "Larry, you are playing when you should be working."

Now let's see what difference the use of this skill can make in communication.

Suppose you see me do something and you say to me, "You are acting bad. Stop it." I may not know specifically what the behavior is that you are talking about. Furthermore, I may not agree with the opinion that what I was doing was bad. I may stop it so as not to incur your wrath, but there has been minimal learning and our relationship may have been damaged, and has not been helped by this transaction. There is no basis for increased understanding.

But suppose you tell me, "You are talking when I am talking. Stop it." I know exactly what I am doing that drew your reaction. There is no question of whether it was good or bad. It obviously affected you adversely and you wanted it stopped. If I care about you as a person, I am responsive to this kind of communication. At any rate, you have given me clearer data on my behavior, which gives me a better chance to learn and change my behavior.

So, in order to develop skill in describing behavior you must sharpen your observation of what actually occurs and carefully distinguish this from inferences and value judgments. As you practice this you may discover how much your own feelings affect the way you react to others. You may discover persons who have no observable behavior patterns which should affect you. But, for some reason you do not like them. This could indicate that you are stereotyping people and projecting your own feelings and motives onto them.

Description of behavior can be helpful in educational problem-solving, particularly when combined with other communication skills.

> Teacher: "Johnny, you have not turned in your work for three successive days." (Description of behavior, rather than an inference, such as, "You are getting quite lazy about your work.") "I am wondering if you are having a problem."
>
> Johnny: "I don't understand this work you have assigned us."
>
> Teacher: "Do you mean you don't know how to do the work?" (Reflective feedback.)
>
> Johnny: "Yes."
>
> Teacher: "Would you like to work with someone who is getting it?"
>
> Johnny: "OK."
>
> Teacher: "If you continue to have problems or if something like this happens again, please let me know. I want to help. And I like for you to keep up in your work. OK?" (Suggestion of alternate behavior, description of own feelings, clarification of expectations and check for commitment.)

Skill in behavior descriptions can help solve problems in these ways:

1. It can give persons more specific data on behavior which affects you and increase the possibility of change.
2. It can prevent your drawing hasty and unfounded inferences about people's behavior.
3. It can prevent your projecting your feelings and value-judgments on the behavior of others.
4. Particularly when combined with a description of your feelings it constitutes an effective message with high learning potential for the receiver. He is getting clear feedback on his behavior and the way it is affecting you.

5. Particularly when combined with a description of alternate behavior and request for commitment to try alternate behavior, it helps pupils to learn more responsible and productive behavior.
6. It helps pupils differentiate between behaviors and self-worth: it is not that one is a bad person, but that he is behaving in a way which is not helping himself or others.
7. Description and affirmation of productive behavior reinforces this behavior and makes reccurence more likely. Example: "Johnny, you participated in our class discussion for the first time today. I am pleased to hear you speak up and appreciate what you said."

Describing Your Feelings

A feeling is an inner signal of a need, or the satisfaction of a need. If I feel hungry, this tells me I need something to eat. When I feel full, this tells me I have eaten enough.

A strong case can be made for the theory that anything one does is in response to a personal need. So even action to help others arises from an inner need to help others.

If this is true, our feelings are very important factors in our behavior. Feelings signal us that we have needs and motivate us to take action to meet these needs. Other feelings indicate to us we have been successful in meeting these needs.

This is not to say that our behavior cannot be modified by thinking. A child may feel hungry and want to eat a cookie. But if mother has said no, the action prompted by the feeling can be restrained by thought and will. Of course, in this case other feelings come into the picture: fear of what will happen if mother is disobeyed, and some frustration and anger perhaps.

Training and conditioning helps us to control feelings which could be destructive if unleashed in our complex society. But this also can cause us to lose touch with our basic feelings. We then tend to respond automatically, like trained animals, rather than as thinking, feeling persons.

Also, feelings which are suppressed rather than communicated in some way tend to have an effect anyway. These feelings may affect a person physically with psychosomatic illness. And feelings may be expressed deviously. Person 1 says something and person 2 feels hurt by it. Person 2 does nothing at the time to communicate his feelings of hurt. But later when person 1 offers a suggestion in a meeting, person 2 blocks it and starts an argument. Or feelings may be misdirected. You may feel angry because the children have misbehaved in class, but express this feeling toward your spouse or children at home.

So feelings do affect us and the ways in which we relate to others. It is important to be able to communicate feelings clearly and appropriately. This is difficult to do. Often people tend to blame others, rationalize their actions, deny feelings, project their feelings to others, and do everything but clearly communicate what they are feeling. This leads to confusion and unresolved conflict between persons.

Feelings are communicated in many different ways: actions, words, tone of voice, bodily changes, and facial expressions. Sometimes these messages are difficult to decode. And even if you think you got the message, there is still a question about whether the sender knows what he is communicating, how the feeling is likely to affect his behavior, and how you are likely to respond.

One way to communicate more clearly is to *describe what you are feeling.* We usually try to convey our thoughts accurately. But description of feeling is frequently neglected. Often we talk about "feeling" something when what we really mean is that we "think" something. I may say, "I feel this lesson is too long." What I really mean is, "I feel bored. I think this lesson is too long."

In order to describe your feelings, you must be able to recognize what you are feeling. This in itself is often difficult. Your actions may be affected by feelings of which you are unaware. One way to get in touch with your feelings is to notice what is happening to you physiologically and interpret this in terms of feelings.

Here are some ways that feelings can be described to someone else:

1. Identify the feeling with words, "I feel annoyed." "I feel happy." At the end of this section is a sample list of words which may be used to describe feelings.
2. Use figures of speech. "I feel full of sunshine." "I feel as though a storm were raging inside me."
3. Tell what kind of action the feeling urges you to do. "I feel like walking out of the room." "I feel like staying here all day."
4. Tell what is happening to you physiologically. "My heart is pounding." "My palms are moist."

It is both possible and healthy to be able to identify and describe your feelings objectively. To do this you must be able to "own" your feelings. That is, you accept your feelings as being a part of you, rather than blaming yourself or someone else. Not—"You make me angry." But—"When you did that, I became angry." The first statement imputes blame to someone for making you angry. The second statement associates the feeling of anger with the action of another person, but does not necessarily blame the action of another person. It is an objective statement of fact: "You did that, I became angry." This leaves an opening to explore factors in both of us which may have caused the reaction, without imputing blame to anyone. To "own" your feelings means also that you accept it as OK to have and admit having any feeling. Otherwise, much denying of feeling is done. This serves only to submerge feelings, making their effects more devious and difficult to cope with.

The purpose in describing your feelings is to start a dialogue which can improve understanding. Unless you make your feelings known, another person cannot accurately consider them in his relationship to you. And unless you know what another person is feeling, you cannot accurately consider his feelings in your relationship to him.

Suppose you are having negative feelings toward someone. These are signals that the relationship between the two of you is not satisfactory. What will you do about these signals and the relationship? You may ignore the signals or deny them, but they are still there. Or you may assume that the other person is at fault and begin pinning blame on him. Or you may assume that you are at fault and begin kicking yourself for having such feelings.

Instead, by describing your feelings objectively you can avoid casting blame in either direction. His feedback to you may show you that your feelings resulted from a misinterpretation of him. In this case, your feelings would probably change because of new understanding. Also, your feedback to him may help him to see that his behavior is bringing responses from you of which he was not aware. He may recognize a behavior pattern which should be changed.

But description of feelings should not be used to coerce someone into changing to accommodate your feelings. It is a statement of fact, without judgments, about what you are feeling. It is the kind of information that must be communicated if two people are to understand each other and build a relationship.

WORDS TO DESCRIBE FEELINGS

POSITIVE		NEGATIVE	
happy	intelligent	hurt	dominated
pleased	clever	angry	manipulated
joyful	attractive	afraid	used
exuberant	beautiful	scared	controlled
exhilarated	well	insecure	shut-out
refreshed	bright	irritated	shut-in
stimulated	confident	annoyed	incompetent
invigorated	assured	put down	unworthy
enthused	certain	aggravated	confused
relaxed	cleansed	frustrated	mixed-up
affectionate	triumphant	disgusted	dull
loved	free	discouraged	bored
cared for	liberated	inadequate	uneasy
loving	comfortable	depressed	uncomfortable
secure	at ease	hopeless	lonely
safe	calm	hostile	rejected
accepted	rested	violent	sad
included	soothed	furious	grieved
united	relieved	hate	embarrassed
trusted	healed	guilty	ugly
trusting	open	hostile	misunderstood
appreciated	honest	jealous	foolish
respected	real	defensive	stupid
self-esteem	alert	defeated	bad
self-reliant	aware	excluded	lost
worthy	interested	powerless	undecided
reinforced	excited	sick	unsure
satisfied	exciting	impotent	tired
successful	potent	helpless	rushed
fulfilled	virile	weak	up tight
understood	pleasant	crushed	strung out
competent	self-controlled	exasperated	tense
together	whole	hysterical	hungry
strong	rewarded	uncontrolled	thirsty
rational	important	exhausted	dirty

The clearest communication occurs when the message is conveyed *congruently* (with all elements of communication in agreement). If I say I am angry, but am smiling, you have a difficult message to decode. You are getting a mixed signal. But if I say I am happy and am smiling, have a pleasant and enthusiastic voice, and perhaps some body and hand movement, you are getting multiple signals, all conveying the same message. This is easily understood and more believable. When I am angry, I need to communicate this with words, tone and volume of voice and body expressions which make the message clear to the receiver.

Examples of describing feelings	Examples of expressing feelings without describing them
"I feel embarrassed"	Blushing and saying nothing
"I feel pleased"	Blushing and smiling
"I feel annoyed"	Blushing and frowning
"I feel angry"	Arguing, talking loudly
"I'm feeling shut out"	Becoming silent in a group
"I'm worried about this"	Blaming, arguing, and frowning
"I feel hurt"	Making cutting remarks
"I enjoy her sense of humor"	"She's funny"
"I respect her ability"	"She's an able person"
"I like her"	"She's a wonderful person"
"I am getting bored"	"You are talking too much"
"I feel angry with myself"	"I always goof up"
"I am angry with you"	"You are acting foolishly"

A teacher's describing his own feelings in key situations can help in several ways to solve problems.

1. It identifies teacher as a real human being who has and is willing to admit having feelings. This tends to break through the stereotype "teacher" role and facilitates person-to-person classroom relationships.
2. It establishes a classroom norm in favor of accepting, rather than denying, feelings and in favor of describing feelings, rather than acting out feelings in disruptive behavior. It is acceptable to say, "I am angry with you," but not to hit.
3. It establishes a classroom norm in favor of owning, rather than projecting feelings. It is acceptable to say, "I am angry with you," but not to call someone a liar.
4. It gives pupils information on how their behavior adversely affects teacher. This breaks up the game of "let's drive teacher crazy" by exposing the game and insisting on an authentic rather than manipulative game-playing relationship. Example: "I am angry right now. Several of you are talking in the back of the room while I am giving instructions. If you need to speak, raise your hand. If not, be quiet while I am speaking."
5. It gives pupils information on how their behavior positively affects teacher. This reinforces problem-solving behavior as teacher expresses positive feelings about such behavior. Example: "I am so pleased with the work you have just done. It's a pleasure for me to try to help you learn when you respond like that."

6. Such a "feeling" statement can be more effective than an "evaluative" statement, either positive or negative. "I feel very annoyed when several of you are talking at the same time." NOT — "This is a thoughtless class. You constantly interrupt each other." "I feel pleased at the report you made." NOT — "You are a good student."

Of course, most pupils may appreciate a positive evaluation like, "You are a good student." But some will not find this believable because of low self-esteem. A "feeling" affirmation is more credible than the evaluation, especially if expressed with genuine feeling, a smile, and a pat on the shoulder.

THE PROBLEM SOLVING PROCESS

The communication skills which have been discussed can facilitate the process of solving problems.

Several steps in this process can be identified:

1. Statement of the problem.
2. Gathering data bearing on the problem.
3. Clarification of the problem.
4. Consideration of alternative solutions.
5. Commitment to try one or more alternatives.
6. Evaluation of attempted solutions.
7. Implementation of continued action.

The following example illustrates how the communication skills are used in the problem-solving process.

Mr. Tate teaches low-phase high school students. His course is Comparative Political Systems. He has had severe discipline problems and low achievement in past classes. This semester, after learning some new communication skills, he decides to try to apply them in classroom meetings as well as in person-to-person transactions.

Desks are arranged in a tight circle as class begins.

Mr. Tate: "I am concerned about what we are going to accomplish here this semester and how we will get along." (description of feelings, statement of the problem) "I want to know how you feel about being in this class and what you hope to get out of it." (request for data bearing on the problem)

Long silence. Further encouragement from teacher to speak up.

Mike: "I don't expect nothin' from this class except maybe a passing grade. It's a drag I've heard from other kids. But we're required to take it."

Mr. Tate: "You mean you don't expect to learn anything worth while in here, but you want to make a passing grade because it's required? (reflective listening feedback)

Mike: "Right. It's just something you have to put up with."

Joan: "I think there are helpful things in this course. I would like to learn more about politics and why different nations do the things they do."

Betty: "Yes. It's important to understand how governments work. That's the only way to change things."

Ben: "Baloney! You can't change anything. And all you'll get in here is a lot of propaganda."

Mr. Tate: "Ben, you think I'm here to give you propaganda?" (reflective listening)

Ben: "Yes. This course is just supposed to brainwash us to fit the system."

Jerry: "I don't agree with that. We can disagree with what's taught if we want to."

Ben: "Not if you want to make a grade."

Mr. Tate: "Let me check my understanding so far. Some of you are saying you see no value in the course, others that you do see value in learning what's going on in different governmental systems, and some concern about being given propaganda and forced to accept it. Right?" (summary of reflective listening, clarification of problem, and question for verification)

Some heads nod approval.

Mr. Tate: "OK, I want to deal with those concerns. I will try to help you learn about different political systems presently operating. There is factual information I will expect you to know, such as the way the government of the Soviet Union is organized. As to opinions of the way a system works, we will freely explore various opinions and the reasons for these opinions. You are welcome to your opinion. You will not be penalized for having opinions different from mine, so long as you know the facts." (consideration of alternative solutions)

Mike: "But if our opinions are different don't expect a good grade on a test."

Mr. Tate: "Mike, are you feeling doubtful about what I am saying?" (perception check, opening way to verify feelings expressed indirectly)

Mike: "Yeah, I doubt that I can make as good a grade by disagreeing with you as I can by agreeing."

Mr. Tate: "OK. If at any time anyone thinks he is being graded down for an opinion differing from mine, I want to know about it. I am willing to consider such a case with the whole class and to get help from the class in making an adjustment." (consideration of alternative solution)

At this point several persons begin speaking to each other while one person speaks out more loudly than they and to the teacher.

Mr. Tate: "Hold it! Several of you are talking and I am getting annoyed. I cannot hear more than one at a time. I want to hear what you have to say, so please speak one at a time." (description of behavior, description of feelings, description of alternative behavior)

Mr. Tate: "All right, now I want someone to repeat back to me what I have said about this course and let me know how you feel about it."

Jerry: "You have said we will study various governments. You expect us to know some facts about them. And we can have our own opinions, which we will not be graded down on."

Mr. Tate: "Right. Now, how do you feel about that?" (checking for commitment to solution)

Mike: "That sounds OK to me, if it really happens."

Mr. Tate: "You are still somewhat doubtful?" (perception check)

Mike: "Yeah, but I'm willing to go along."

Mr. Tate: "How about the rest of you?"

Most heads nod approval. (commitment to solution)

Mr. Tate: (Smiles and leans back more relaxed) "I'm feeling better already about working with you this semester. I really appreciate this discussion, and I hope we can be happy together." (description of feelings) "We will have discussions like this frequently to evaluate our progress and make adjustments." (provision for evaluation and further implementation)

Mr. Tate used reflective listening to demonstrate an openness which encouraged pupils to give him information. They soon sensed they would not get a defensive or punishing reaction to what they said. This maximized their input of data. Also, this technique enabled him to verify and clarify data received. And it enabled pupils to hear his interpretation of what they were saying and clarify and perhaps modify their own thinking! He set a norm for open, nonjudgmental listening which should greatly help the classroom climate. This listening model is a good one for pupils to emulate, and they should pick it up as the class progresses.

He checked his perception of feelings of others, thus verifying his perceptions and helping pupils to become aware of feelings they were expressing. This also communicated his willingness to accept feelings, even when hostile. And this helped him to come through as a sensitive, perceptive person. Such a person tends to receive respect because he gives respect to others.

He described his own feelings, both positive and negative, appropriately and congruently. This gave pupils data on how their behavior affected him, for better or worse. It helped establish person-to-person caring relationships, and helped eliminate possible manipulative game-playing in which feelings are hidden or projected through blaming tactics.

He described behavior and set limits on behavior which adversely affected the class task. He described alternate behavior and got commitment to try it. He demonstrated effective use of communication skills in a problem-solving process. The problem was identified. Data was gathered. The problem was clarified. Solutions were considered. Commitment was made to alternatives. And provision was made for evaluation and on-going action.

8

Communication

Communication is perhaps one of the most universal concepts of paramount importance in nursing practice. Communication pervades every phase of the nursing process. Essentially, everything one does involves communication— with clients, colleagues, and selves. Spoken or unspoken messages are the guides for accomplishment of each and every intent; communication involves "all."

Chapter 8 closely follows the material presented in the previous chapter on concepts of observation and listening. The specific focus of this chapter, however, is the communications of the nurse. Looking at the overall purpose, the chapter seeks to present a broad perspective on the communications concept, thereby providing a basis and rationale for an individual practitioner to develop a personal philosophy and conceptual framework for communicating that can be heightened further through experience.

The chapter basically responds to the following:

1. What is communication?
2. The model for communication.
3. Purpose for communication in nursing.
4. How does one communicate?
5. What does a nurse communicate?

WHAT IS COMMUNICATION?

In one sense, communication is everything, for no human being exists in an autonomous vacuum, going through life in an impermeable cell; being born, living, and dying in isolation from others; or reaching only to self to fulfill needs. Even though one would suspect from Slater's (1970) exposition of American culture, for example, that one positive goal of life is to be independent of and from others, this outcome is never purely achieved and is considered an aberration from the recognized fact that humans are social beings. Groups have developed languages by which to reach out to closely-related others, as well as dialects that are subsystems of the larger framework. Body language is often considered to be universally understood.

Shannon and Weaver (1949) provided an early definition of communication when they said that it encompasses all that occurs between two or more minds. They included written and spoken language, art, music, theater, and *all* of human behavior. It can be concisely stated that behavior is communication and all communication produces behavior. Gibran (1951) included in his discussion of talking a message that crystallized verbal speaking as a way of also communicating with self. Johnson (1972) defined the concept as a means for one person to relay a message to another with the goal of receiving a response. Although the others add to our view of the complexity of communication, it is this latter definition that most closely lends into formation of a theoretical model of communication.

Theoretical Model

Theorists have developed an almost universally accepted model for communication processes. Berlo (1960) and Miller (1966) made major contributions to Hein's (1973) presentation of the model in nursing. Hein describes six elements (Johnson [1972] closely parallels these steps in his portrayal of the model):

1. the reason for communicating or referent
2. the sender or source-encoder
3. a message that involves content
4. method(s) of communicating—channel(s): verbal and/or nonverbal
5. the receiver or decoder
6. feedback

Figure 8-1 portrays the model.

It is easy to see from the rather simplistic example in the figure that the model is dynamic; senders become receivers and vice versa, until the communication ceases. Even though patterns of communication are rarely as simple as denoted, the example is meant to illustrate the model. All communications can then be studied within this framework.

The feedback process is the same validational procedure described in Chapter 7. Berlo (1960) emphasizes the point that what and how one communicates relates to the attitudes, knowledge, and sociocultural system of the individual. Ergo, what is received relates to the same. Effective communication necessitates discovering a relatively positive related wavelength between senders and receivers; the goal is congruence between the message intended and that received.

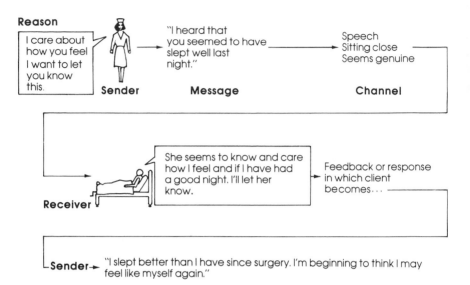

FIGURE 8-1
THEORETICAL MODEL: COMMUNICATION

PURPOSES FOR COMMUNICATING

The purpose for communicating with clients and colleagues specifically relates to one's definition of nursing and the reasons for care. As has been elucidated in earlier portions of this book, nursing involves facilitating clients' movement toward fulfillment of their health potential; when nurses intervene, it is toward this same goal. Specific assistance or interventions are required of the nurse to erase nursing diagnoses. It becomes necessary, therefore, to narrow communication in nursing practice and speak of therapeutic communication, a phrase mentioned by Hein (1973), effective communication (Johnson, 1972), or purposeful, effective communication in response to the client (this author). Communications with colleagues or health personnel should be directed toward the same purpose, with the client being of major concern.

Johnson, Dumas, and Johnson (1967) suggest that skillful nurse/client interactions are the essence of care. If one were to operate under the basic assumption (and this author does!) that all nurses care about their clients as do all health professionals, then it becomes necessary to explain why there is a growing body of literature pointing to consumers' perceived inhumane treatment by health care professionals. Nevertheless, it would be folly not to operate with the positive assumption. After all, if nurses do not care, what is there to prove? What is there to strive for and why bother? It becomes a death wish. You see, if the author believes nurses do not care, the author, being a nurse, is most specifically pointing at self. Responsibility for the profession rests within the individual first! Moving from this slight digression, the explanation for the consumers' perceived qualities of non-caring, inhumaneness, abruptness, or whatever must rest within the effective/ineffective communication process, for *communication is behavior,* and behavior is all that anyone can perceive. Furthermore, communication is defined only as what is perceived by others. If there is a discrepancy between one's attitudes of caring and one's perceived behaviors of caring, guilt must lie in communication. Conversely—and positively speaking—if a nurse's attitudes are consonant with caring, that is, desiring to help another grow and actualize self (Mayeroff, 1971), and the client so perceives this, it can be only a result of purposeful and effective communications. And so, the needs for effective communication become explicit. It is our only means for fulfilling our responsibilities, relating to either physical or emotional dimensions of care, guided by the desire to facilitate a positive experience for all members of the interaction. This relates to achievement of physically-oriented client goals as well as emotional ones.

Ponthieu (1977) elucidates some characteristics of an authentic communicator. Even though Ponthieu's perspective is from a manager's viewpoint, his thoughts nevertheless are deemed pertinent to discuss within a nursing framework. According to Ponthieu:

1. *Communication should not be determined by a role.* This involves genuineness on the part of the nurse rather than the mask of being "professional." It means meeting people on an adult-to-adult level (Berne, 1964), according to a transactional analysis model. Hierarchical placements have no reality base.
2. *The communicator must be aware of and in touch with his or her own attitudes (feelings, beliefs, and values).* Dissonance between a sender's attitudes and behaviors can be and usually is perceived by the receiver. If one's goal is to communicate clearly, it follows that one must be clear on what one wishes to communicate. Factual content and emotional overtones should correspond.
3. *Communicator must be self-confident and accepting.* Remembering that the nurse is a unique person first, it is vital to recognize that the nurse's feelings *are* valid; this facilitates acceptance of self. Since the nurse further desires to enable a client to accept self respective of givens in health and illness, the best way may be as a role model. This involves recognition of both one's strengths and weaknesses.

METHODS OF COMMUNICATION

Communication is bimodal: verbal and nonverbal. Within each category, it further may be one-way or two-way.

Verbal communication generally includes all that is spoken and written. Verbal interactions between the nurse/client, nurse/nurse, nurse/other health professional, and so forth, form the basis for this primary area. Secondary sources of verbal patterns include messages sent by people to others and may be directed toward a specific person or generally to parts of the system. These sources include nurse's notes, discharge summaries, memoranda from all sources, requests, and similar items.

Nonverbal communication involves all that is unsaid but implied by body language, which is also behavior. Included are gestures, eye contact, facial expressions, posture, and space variations between interactors. These generally amplify or detract from verbal statements but can stand alone in communicating meanings of silence. Very often, dissonance between attitudes and verbal behaviors are perceived through nonverbal messages. Table 8-1 portrays various nonverbal attending skills and ineffective/effective uses of each (Walters, 1975).

One-way communication involves no feedback; two-way uses feedback. Johnson (1972) continues this definition by saying that one-way communication is when the sender is unable to discover how the receiver is perceiving or decoding the message. Two-way communication is when the sender receives feedback or validation. Obviously both types of communication are used in health care, as in the following:

1. Sender gives message and does not provide avenue or time for feedback (one-way).
   Example: Physician writes stat order and leaves.
2. Sender gives message and provides avenue for feedback but receiver does not comply with request, at least verbally (one-way).
   Example:
   Nurse: "You look like you are hungry."
   Client: Silence
3. Sender gives written message and waits for or requests a reaction (two-way).
   Example: Head nurse in a written memo requesting reactions to the introduction of staff development programs on the unit and content of same. Space provided on memo to respond.
4. Sender gives verbal-message and waits for response; receiver replies to message (two-way).
   Example:
   Nurse: "Your record states that this is your third admission to this unit."
   Client: "Yes. . . .I was admitted two years ago with the same problem. I didn't know that is important right now."
   Nurse picks up message and goes on with conversation.

The literature is replete with broad and specific discussions of methods used during communication processes. For this reason, discussion has not been lengthy. Building from the information presented, it becomes important to look at what a nurse communicates.

TABLE 8-1
ATTENDING SKILLS

INEFFECTIVE USE	NONVERBAL MODES OF COMMUNICATION	EFFECTIVE USE
Doing any of these things will probably close off or slow down the conversation.		These behaviors encourage talk because they show acceptance and respect for the other person.
Distant; very close	Space	Approximate arms-length
Away	Movement	Toward
Slouching; rigid; seated leaning away	Posture	Relaxed, but attentive; seated leaning slightly toward
Absent; defiant; jittery	Eye contact	Regular
You continue with what you are doing before responding; in a hurry	Time	Respond at first opportunity; share time with them
Used to keep distance between the persons	Feet and legs (in sitting)	Unobtrusive
Used as a barrier	Furniture	Used to draw persons together
Does not match feelings; scowl; blank look	Facial expression	Matches your own or other's feelings; smile
Compete for attention with your words	Gestures	Highlight your words; unobtrusive; smooth
Obvious; distracting	Mannerisms	None, or unobtrusive
Very loud or very soft	Voice: volume	Clearly audible
Impatient or staccato; very slow or hesitant	Voice: rate	Average, or a bit slower
Apathetic; sleepy; jumpy; pushy	Energy level	Alert; stays alert throughout a long conversation

SOURCE: The amity book: Exercise in friendship and helping skills, p. 39. Copyright 1977 by Richard P. Walters. Reproduced by permission.

What a Nurse Communicates

In addition to the content involved in nurse/client and nurse/nurse inter-actions, there is a pattern of communication that is unique to the helper and should be reflective of counseling. Using this technique, interactions are based on a personal philosophy and conceptual framework. It should be noted that purposeful, effective communication is a nursing goal with and for the client. Counseling is an interchange of opinions, feelings, and the like with the planned purpose and design of assisting or facilitating others to help themselves. Communication in nursing often is counseling.

What a nurse does in communicating involves his or her practice according to one or more theories of counseling. The latter effect is called an eclectic approach. Whether or not this is used or one theory is applied, counseling should be based on an application of theory. The individuality of the helper remains whether the person bases counseling on one or more schools of thought (Arbuckle, 1974).

There are a number of counseling theories that pattern the process of communication for a helper. Arbuckle (1974) eloquently elaborates on several; his article is found in the suggested reading section of this chapter. The theory of Carl Rogers (1961, 1965) later researched and documented as effective by Carkhuff (1969) is discussed. The reader is referred to a broader presentation of this client-centered approach in Parts I and V of the book. Steps of the counseling process are the foci at this point.

Carkhuff (1969) delineated eight core conditions which the helper must facilitate in the communication process. These were previously explicated by Rogers (1961, 1965). They involve two phases: understanding and action. Aspects of these phases are listed.

Understanding Phase

1. Empathy—getting inside another's skin and understanding the world as the other perceives it to be.*
2. Respect—believing in another, respecting the other's world and rights as well as the validity of the other's unique feelings.
3. Warmth—involves caring; being concerned and loving.
4. Concreteness—the ability to be specific, succinct, and clear.
5. Genuineness—being a real human being; being honest and true.
6. Self-disclosure—being able to communicate one's own humanness; sharing feelings.

Action Phase

7. Confrontation—pointing out conflicts, discrepancies, or problems; saying what one observes constructively.
8. Immediacy—focusing on the here-and-now; looking at what seems to be happening between the helper and helpee.

Both Rogers (1961, 1965) and Carkhuff (1969) pointed out the need for both phases to occur within a relationship. If one goes to a helper because one is unable to meet the problems faced and one requires intervention, the helper becomes an expert—one that possesses the knowledge and experience needed to assist. The understanding phase is meant to build a relationship between nurse and client; the action phase is the content phase, possibly requiring changes in the client's habits, routines, and behavior patterns. The understanding phase precedes the action phase with empathy being the key ingredient (Carkhuff, 1969).

The following example is intended to clarify this process: Suppose you are a client, meeting a nurse for the first time in a clinic. You enter wearing green pants and an orange shirt. The first statement from Nurse Jean X is: "Green

*Descriptions are adapted from the work of Gazda, et al (1973), and Walters (1975).

and orange do not match; you would look much better if you wore complementary colors!"

What would your reaction be? Some of my feelings would be: "Who are you to tell me what to wear?" You see, the nurse has no information about the reasons you wore what you did. It may be that your clothes represented your best; or your mother's last gift to you was the blouse. Who knows except you? The tendency at this point is to discharge or block the nurse's statement plus have a negative reaction.

Now further suppose that you had been going to this nurse for six months; you trust her and know she is interested in all that is best for you; she cares about you. If she made the same statement as before, would you be likely to listen? Would you think she was trying to help? If your green pants were treasured by you, would you be likely to tell her?

In this situation, the trusting, cared for, understood person will have a greater probability for listening and maybe changing, if the change were appropriate and/or needed in the client's world.

Carrying this example into practice, much of nursing involves facilitating change within the client, teaching, and dealing with life styles and attitudes. (Remember that change is synonymous with learning.) It follows, therefore, that an understanding relationship must be developed prior to actions. Time in a relationship is a significant variable because one must meet demands and priorities reflected in nursing diagnoses and discussed in Chapter 3. The understanding phase can be compressed into a five-minute, meaningful interaction or lengthened over years; it corresponds to needs and the time available to meet them. In each phase, perceptions should be validated and messages should require feedback. This is all a part of communication.

SUMMARY

This chapter focused on communication, moving from a broad perspective to one that is pertinent in nursing practice. Communication was discussed and defined with a theoretical model illustrated. Purposes for communicating in nursing were followed by methods. Nonverbal and verbal patterns were presented and one-way/two-way processes exemplified. The chapter concluded with what a nurse communicates; this was built on the counseling theory of client-centered and humanistic therapy.

REFERENCES

Arbuckle, D. The practice of the theories of counseling. *Counseling Education and Supervision* 13:214–222, 1974.

Berlo, D. *The process of communication*. New York: Holt, Rinehart and Winston, 1960.

Berne, E. *Games people play*. New York: Grove Press, 1964.

Carkhuff, R. *Helping and human relations: A primer for lay and professional helpers*. Vols. 1 & 2. New York: Holt, Rinehart and Winston, 1969.

Gazda, G., Asbury, F., Balzer, F., Childers, W., Desselle, R., and Walters, R. *Human relations development: A manual for educators*. Boston: Allyn and Bacon, 1973.

Gibran, K. *The prophet*. New York: Alfred A. Knopf, 1951.

Hein, E. *Communication in nursing practice*. Boston: Little, Brown and Company, 1973.

Johnson, D. *Reaching out: Interpersonal effectiveness and self-actualization*. Englewood Cliffs, N.J.: Prentice-Hall, 1972.

Johnson, J., Dumas, R., and Johnson, B. Interpersonal relations: the essence of nursing care. *Nursing Forum* 6:324–334, 1967.

Mayeroff, M. *On caring*. New York: Harper and Row, 1971.

Miller, G. *Speech communication: A behavioral approach*. Indianapolis: Bobbs-Merrill, 1966.

Ponthieu, J. Open communication: The key to self-actualization and success. *Health Services Manager* 10:8–9, 1977.

Rogers, C. *On becoming a person*. Boston: Houghton-Mifflin, 1961.

Rogers, C. *Client-centered therapy*. Boston: Houghton-Mifflin, 1965.

Shannon, C., and Weaver, W. *The mathematical theory of communication*. Urbana, Illinois: University of Illinois Press, 1949.

Slater, P. *The pursuit of loneliness*. Boston: Beacon Press, 1970.

Walters, R. *The amity book: Exercises in friendship and helping skills*. 1975 (In G. Gazda, et al. Human relations development: A manual for educators. Boston: Allyn and Bacon, 1973.)

SELECTED READING

The suggested reading for this chapter is an article by Arbuckle (1974). This chapter built heavily on the need for nurses to have a theoretical basis for the communication (counseling) process. The client-centered approach was discussed as one framework. Arbuckle's article provides a synthesis of other counseling frameworks; one or more can be adopted as a basis for practice.

The Practice of the Theories of Counseling

Dugald S. Arbuckle

Some of the characteristics of the major theories of counseling and differences in practice among counselors of these theoretical orientations are discussed.

It is likely that most thinking, feeling, and questioning counselors have periodically wondered what kind of a counselor they are, if indeed, they could be described as a "kind" of a counselor. The most difficult kind of counselor to pin down, of course, is the fellow who calls himself eclectic, since this means that he can easily justify anything he does. I have a hunch, however, that most effective counselors who call themselves eclectic do have certain patterns of counseling behavior which are unique to them, so that one eclectic counselor could be distinguished from another eclectic counselor. The effective counselor, I would think, must show the uniqueness of his person in his counseling procedures with any client. He does not, in a sense, hold sacred any method or procedure, new or old. Just as the masters of yesterday and today developed their own ways, so he develops his. He is not a disciple. He does his own thing.

The purpose of this article is to attempt to spell out some of the functional characteristics of the major theories of counseling and to find out if what is actually done by counselors with different theoretical orientations does differ in a distinguishable fashion. In other words, does the gestalt therapist actually do certain things as part of the counseling process that are different from what is done by the existential therapist? I am concerned with what counselors actually do, not with what they say they believe about counseling and man and nature.

I will attempt to pull together what would appear to me to be acceptable descriptions of the counseling behaviors that characterize different theories of counseling. My sources for this task will be those individuals who are considered to be the developers or the most noted practitioners of the theory being discussed. There will be no specific references, but the basic sources will be listed in the bibliography at the end of this article.

CLIENT-CENTERED COUNSELING

Of all counseling theories, client-centered counseling is the one in which it is most difficult to determine what the counselor does. This is for the very

Reprinted with permission from *Counselor Education and Supervision*, vol. 13. Copyright 1974 by American Personnel and Guidance Association.

simple and obvious reason that in client-centered counseling the primary counselor function is to create an environment in which constructive personality change will take place. This, in turn, is directly related to the personal attitudes of the counselor. If effective counseling is to take place, the counselor must reflect genuineness and congruence, empathic understanding, and unconditional acceptance and positive regard. If these counselor conditions are present, if they are perceived by the client to at least some degree, and if the client has some level of anxiety and vulnerability, then positive change will take place.

The major technique of client-centered counseling continues to be reflection of feeling, which includes clarification, reformulation, and summarization. I would think that reflection of feeling must also include interpretation if, that is, we think of interpretation as meaning the counselor's perception of what the client is communicating to him in a feeling sense. That is, a client might say, "I love my mother very much..." and an accurate reflection of feeling (which to me would also be the counselor's interpretation) would be, "You feel angry, even though you say you love her...." It should be noted too that this reflection and/or interpretation is highly verbal, and the person of the counselor is relatively uninvolved and unexposed.

The only responsibility of the counselor is to create the right environment. If this is done, growth will take place, but the responsibility for growth rests solely in the hands of the client. The counseling is, literally, client-centered; it is the client who is in control; it is the client who determines what will happen and where he will go. Unconditional acceptance means that the counselor accepts the client as he is and has no preconceptions as to what the outcomes of the counseling should be.

Thus the client-centered counselor's primary technique is the verbal reflection and/or interpretation of feeling, including clarification, reformulation, and summarization. The client-centered counselor does not manipulate or direct since he has no goals for the client. For the same reason he would see no point in adivising the client nor would he be seen as a source of information as to how the client might better live his life. Nor does the counselor become involved with the client as a person in an emotional or physical sense. He is kind, and gentle, and caring, but he remains relatively aloof and does not share very much of himself.

EXISTENTIAL COUNSELING

Existential counseling is like client-centered counseling in that it has minimal concern with technique. Technique implies manipulation, and the existential counselor, like the client-centered counselor, views the client as a person. It is objects and things that are to be manipulated, not persons. The person of the counselor is even more important in existential counseling; it is, indeed, crucial since the heart of existential counseling is the human-with-human sharing between the counselor and the client. The counselor is not, as some critics have claimed, acting or playing a role. He is living with the client in an intimate human relationship. More than in any other kind of counseling the basic communication between the client and the counselor is nonverbal. It is a human sharing of two people with each other.

The counselor is interested in the client's past only in the sense of the degree to which it is part of the client's present. This means, of course, that the past often does become part of the immediate involvement between the client and his environment and the client and the counselor. But the client is experiencing now what the past may be doing to him. He is not analyzing the diagnostic meaning of the past.

Intimacy also implies that the counselor is experienced in life and living and is not just a personally removed student of life and living. There are confrontations in existential counseling—verbal, physical, personal. In a very literal sense, there will be a transference of feelings from the client to the counselor and from the counselor to the client. These feelings are part of the humanness of the counselor and the client and they are faced and shared. They are not analyzed to determine their real meaning by the personally aloof expert, as in more traditional psychoanalysis, nor are they considered to be a form of resistance which must be worked out.

The existential counselor would share with the client-centered counselor the feeling that the client must accept responsibility for his actions and that he must determine the goals of counseling. On the other hand, the human involvement of the existential counselor must inevitably mean that at least some of the responsibility for what happens must be shared by the counselor. For the same reason, too, there will be more counselor control and counselor direction. This is not done deliberately, but since the values of the counselor are exposed, this is obviously going to affect what the client does. It would seem almost inevitable that the existential counselor, more than any other kind of counselor, will serve as a human model for the client. This is a very grave responsibility, a responsibility which some existential counselors may refuse.

A client, for example, may be killing himself on drugs and he says to the counselor, "So, okay, I'll likely be dead in six months—what the hell difference does that make to you?" If an existential counselor is consistent with his philosophy, he is not going to reflect this feeling; he is not going to analyze the meaning of it; he is not going to discuss ways by which the client may feel more positive about himself. He is going to share his own feelings with the client, and he might say with emotion: "It makes a hell of a lot of difference to me—I care for you, you big lug, and I'd feel bad, real bad, if you keep right on and die in a gutter—but you've got to decide that—you can kill yourself if you want to. . . ."

BEHAVIORAL COUNSELING

The behavioral counselor does very little with the client, but does a great deal to him and, the counselor would doubtless feel, for him. The person of the counselor is of minimal importance as far as the client-counselor relationship is concerned. The counselor is the expert who provides effective experiences to modify client behavior in appropriate directions.

The behavioral counselor stresses the use of techniques and procedures determined by him, perhaps in collaboration with the client, to remedy the inappropriate behavior patterns of the client. Needless to say, this means that the counselor is very much in control of the counseling process. Behavioral counseling is, quite literally, counselor-centered. This being the case, it would seem obvious that manipulation of the client and/or the environment by the counselor would be a deliberately planned technique used by the counselor.

Since client choice is considered only as a fantasy, the client can hardly be expected to accept major responsibility for what happens in the counseling process. The counselor as the expert accepts responsibility for determining the behavior modifications to be used and the means by which their effect can be measured.

The counselor is an objective scientist, and his professional goal is the modification of inappropriate behavior to more appropriate behavior. He feels free to use any technique that works. Manipulation, interpretation, advising, reflection of feeling, questioning and probing, the use of information—all of these would be acceptable techniques. The only criterion measure would be "Do they work?" There would be little likelihood of transference or counter-transference because of the minimal personal involvement of the client and the counselor.

In stressing the what rather than the why, the behavioral counselor is putting emphasis on the immediate inappropriate behavior. This, in turn, means that primary attention is given to the symptom rather than the cause, the belief being that modification or removal of the symptom will in turn have a positive effect on the cause of the inappropriate behavior. The why also implies human values. These play little part in behavioral counseling since the client is viewed as a conditioned set of behaviors rather than as a human being too complex to be measured.

A final characteristic of the behavioral counselor is his certainty. He sets up the experiences which will develop more appropriate behaviors in the client and the effects of these experiences must be measurable if they are to be used. Behavioral therapy is effective with all kinds of neuroses, or at least so the behavioral conselor believes.

REALITY THERAPY

Reality therapy is very much akin to behavioral counseling, but it is mentioned here because of one major and very significant difference. As in behavior therapy, reality therapy is centered in learning theory. The patient is taught new ways of behavior and the new behavior in turn promotes further behavioral change. It is the initial change in behavior that starts the process; thus the attitude of the patient changes regardless of whether or not he understands his old ways. Insight is not viewed as an important or necessary ingredient for behavioral change.

Since it is believed that the reasons for the behavior do not make a difference in changing the behavior, the stress in reality therapy is on the what rather than the why. In these aspects reality therapy might be considered to be simply a somewhat restricted version of behavior therapy.

There is, however, one very crucial difference. The basic ingredients of reality therapy are that the patient is held responsible for his behavior and that he is helped to learn that his inappropriate behavior is irresponsible. Thus the message communicated to the patient is that he does have a choice either to move in the direction of more appropriate behavior and thus be more responsible or to remain with his current behavior and accept his irresponsibility.

At the same time, however, it is the therapist who determines to a great extent just what appropriate behavior might be. Patients are patients because they deny the reality of the world around them. They must learn to face this reality and at the same time learn how to satisfy their needs. Thus appropriate behavior, it would appear, is behavior in keeping with the demands of society, which is viewed as "reality." The reality therapist refers to facing the reality of the world around the patient, but the implication is that the therapist provides the patient with experiences so that he is more accepting of the reality of the therapist and of society in general. The young man who considers fleeing to Canada to avoid being drafted would probably be regarded as unrealistic and irresponsible—guilty of inappropriate behavior.

Thus there is a contradiction in reality therapy. The reality therapist stresses the obligation of the client to become more responsible by developing more appropriate behavior, but the meaning of "reality" and "appropriate" is determined by the therapist, not the patient. The reality therapist is unlike the behavioral therapist in that he does hold the patient responsible for his behavior, but he is like the behavioral therapist in that he is very much in control as to the determining of the future behavior of the patient.

GESTALT THERAPY

Like reality therapy, gestalt therapy would appear to be another somewhat restricted version (since certain techniques are not to be used) of behavioral therapy. The stress is on the here-and-now and the past or the future is viewed as a means of escaping from the reality of now. The patient is regarded as having the potential to function in a responsible manner, whereas it is the responsibility of the therapist to help the patient fulfill that potential.

Providing opportunities is considered to be more effective than verbal explanation; this means that a major tool of the therapist is manipulation of both the patient and the environment. The therapist deliberately manipulates circumstances so that the patient is forced to face the meaning of the affective relationship between the therapist and himself. This means that nonverbal communication is viewed as being more authentic than verbal communication; thus there is a good deal of stress on the immediate person-to-person relationship between the patient and therapist. Needless to say, there is no question as to who is in control since the act of manipulation obviously implies therapist direction and therapist control.

Interestingly enough, while the gestalt therapist views manipulation as a major technique, he is opposed to interpretation for a reason which I would think would also apply to manipulation. It is felt that interpretation implies that the therapist knows more about the patient than the patient knows about himself. Surely manipulation of the patient by the therapist implies the same thing!

PSYCHOANALYTIC THERAPY

While the psychoanalysis of today has changed somewhat from the psychoanalysis of Freud's day, it still retains the same basic characteristics and is still a pessimistic view of man. The two major differences are the current stress on the total developmental history of the patient rather than on the psychosexual and the greater involvement of the therapist as a person.

However, the therapist is still the expert and he operates in the same way as the medical doctor with a sick patient. The person coming to see the therapist is, indeed, viewed as a sick patient. The doctor is in control and the patient has little choice as to what is done to him and what happens to him. The personal relationship between the patient and the therapist is of minimal importance.

Through free association the therapist uncovers and interprets the unconscious repressed feelings which dominate and control the patient's life. The interpretation of the element of resistance, part of the transference relationship, is crucial in helping the patient achieve a higher level of self-understanding. In a broader sense, the patient is taught how to understand and control his instincts so that they will not destroy him.

More than any other current form of psychotherapy, psychoanalysis stresses the intellectual understanding of the past since the past is crucial for understanding the present.

RATIONAL-EMOTIVE PSYCHOTHERAPY

Although the term used is "rational-emotive," the therapy described here is overwhelmingly rational. The rational therapist believes that what we feel depends on what we think and that we are capable of thinking our way out of our negative and harmful feelings. The major function of the therapist is to teach in a dominant directive manner, using any kind of effective technique— challenging, confronting, prodding, manipulating. The patient is taught how to get rid of his anxiety as an irrational feeling for which he has little or no responsibility. The stress is on intellectual insight and understanding.

The rational therapist, like the behavioral therapist, sees himself as teaching the patient more appropriate modes of behavior. Unlike the behavioral therapist, however, he sees much of this behavior as being inborn. Thus irrational thinking and behavior is a natural human state. Since the patient is not to blame for his irrational behavior, he cannot be expected to accept responsibility for it. For this reason he cannot be considered to be irresonsible because of inappropriate behavior which may be damaging to himself or to others.

Needless to say, the dominating therapist is in control. The patient would appear to have as little say as to what happens and where he goes as would the sick patient of the medical doctor or the inappropriately behaving client of a behavioral therapist. In reality therapy it is the therapist who determines what is realistic and what is unrealistic. In behavioral therapy it is the therapist who determines what behavior is appropriate and what is inappropriate. In rational therapy it is the therapist who determines what is rational and what is irrational. These words—realistic, appropriate, rational—are synonymous and they all spell out therapist control, domination, and direction.

Rational therapy, like most modern therapies, stresses the present rather than the past. There is a difference, however, in that it is not so much the event or the behavior of the present that is stressed but the patient's perception of the event or the behavior. The perception, according to the rational therapist, is what causes the problem. Thus the pregnant teen-aged girl who is feeling guilty is taught that it is quite irrational to feel guilty. When she then comes to accept the irrationality of her feelings, she will be able to make some logical rational decisions as to what she is going to do about her pregnancy. It is not the event, but how we feel about the event that creates our neuroses. Since our feeling is due to either innate factors or environmental pressures over which we had no control, it is irrational for us to feel bad about ourselves.

With this stress on directive teaching and rationality, it is obvious that the person-to-person relationship between patient and therapist is of minimal importance. The relationship is that of student to teacher or patient to doctor. One person—the expert—knows what is wrong and what should be done about it. The other person feels that something is wrong but doesn't know what is wrong or what should be done about it.

SUMMATION

Are there really any differences in the practice of counselors of different theoretical orientations? The answer appears to be "Yes, some—but what is common is much more evident that what is different."

1. Counselor control and direction is stressed by the client-centered therapist, to some extent by existential and reality therapists, and very much so by the rest.
2. Stress on intellectual insight and verbal communication rather than affective client-counselor relationship occurs least with existential and gestalt therapists, somewhat with client-centered and reality therapists, and very much so with the rest.
3. The external reality of society is stressed least by existential and client-centered counselors, somewhat by psychoanalytic and rational-emotive therapists, and very much so by the rest.
4. The what of behavior is stressed least by the psychoanalytic therapist, somewhat by the client-centered and existential therapist, and very much so by the rest.

5. All practitioners, with the exception of the psychoanalytic, tend to stress the present rather than the past.
6. In terms of specific techniques, manipulation is stressed least by client-centered and existential therapists, used as the major technique by the gestalt therapist, and used by the rest whenever it is felt to be effective.
7. Interpretation is stressed least by the client-centered and gestalt therapist, but used by the others whenever it is felt to be effective.
8. Such techniques as advising, questioning, probing, and the use of information are used least by the client-centered counselor, but used by the others whenever they are felt to be effective.
9. Reflection of feeling is used as a major technique by client-centered counselors and used by all the others whenever it is felt to be effective.

BIBLIOGRAPHY

Arbuckle, D. S. *Counseling: Philosophy, theory and practice.* Boston: Allyn & Bacon, 1970.

Barclay, J. R. *Foundations of counseling strategies.* New York: Wiley, 1971.

Brill, A. A. *The basic writings of Sigmund Freud.* New York: Random house, 1927.

Carkhuff, R. R., & Berenson, B. G. *Beyond counseling and therapy.* New York: Holt, Rinehart & Winston, 1967.

Dreyfus, E. A. *Youth: Search for meaning.* Columbus, Ohio: Charles E. Merrill, 1972.

Ellis, A. Rational-emotive psychotherapy. In D. S. Arbuckle (Ed.), *Counseling and psychotherapy: An overview.* New York: McGraw-Hill, 1967. Pp. 78–99.

Ellis, A. *Reason and emotion in psychotherapy.* New York: Lyle Stuart, 1962.

Freud, S. *Beyond the pleasure principle.* London: Hogarth, 1924.

Freud, S. *The future of an illusion.* New York: International Psychoanalytic Library, 1943.

Glasser, W. *Reality therapy.* New York: Harper & Row, 1965.

Guntrip, H. J. S. *Psychoanalytic theory, therapy and the self.* New York: Basic Books, 1971.

Hart, J. T., & Tomlinson, T. M. *New directions in client-centered therapy.* Boston: Houghton Mifflin, 1970.

Hosford, R. E. Behavioral Counseling. *Counseling Psychologist,* 1969, *1,* 1–33.

Kemp, C. G. Existential counseling. *Counseling Psychologist,* 1971, *2,* 2–30.

Krumboltz, J. D., & Thoresen, C. E. *Behavioral counseling: Cases and techniques.* New York: Holt, Rinehart & Winston, 1969.

May, R. *Existential psychology*. New York: Random House, 1961.

Osipow, S. H., & Walsh, W. B. *Strategies in counseling for behavior change*. New York: Appleton-Century-Crofts, 1970.

Patterson, C. H. *Theories of counseling and psychotherapy*. New York: Harper & Row, 1966.

Perls, F. *Gestalt therapy*. Verbatim. Lafayette, Calif.: Real People Press, 1969.

Rogers, C. R. *Client-centered therapy*. Boston: Houghton Mifflin, 1951.

Skinner, B. F. Beyond freedom and dignity. *Psychology Today, 5*, 37–82, 1971.

Van Kaam, A. *The art of existential counseling*. Wilkes-Barre, Pa.: Dimension Books, 1966.

Wolpe, J., & Lazarus, A. A. *Behavior therapy techniques*. London: Pergamon Press, 1966.

Wolpe, J.; Salter, A.; & Reyna, L. J. *The conditioning therapies*. New York: Holt, Rinehart & Winston, 1964.

9

Interviewing

While useful in other phases of the nursing process, the interview is the primary procedure used in data collection. It is especially important in the gathering of information from the primary source—the client—but is also appropriate with secondary sources such as the family, social workers, friends, and others. Gathering of data related to the nursing history is by means of an interview; this skill, therefore, is often considered a technology in nursing. It is a skill built on other skills; some skills discussed in previous (and subsequent) chapters are important in carrying out an interview: observation, listening, and communication are particularly essential in interviewing.

WHAT IS AN INTERVIEW?

Bermosk (1966) denotes the interview as a special time when the nurse focuses particular attention on the client and/or the client's system with the purpose of understanding the client's world of experience, feelings, beliefs, attitudes, and behavior. Hein (1973) simply states that interviewing is a human interaction during which information is needed and/or shared. The eventual purpose of this process is observed by Keltner (1970) as determined by the interactors or people involved in the interview process. Bermosk and Mordan (1964) denoted the interpersonal nature of the interview but also starred it as a developmental procedure. Their rationale for this description was based on their view that the interview involves sequenced, directed, and progressive changes in all participants of the interview process—especially the nurse and client.

In many areas of the literature, the interview is recognized as a strategy. Kahn and Cannell (1964) conceived the interview as purposeful conversation; Schatzman and Strauss (1973) have agreed, even though their perspectives were as field researchers in the areas of sociology and anthropology.

Purposes of an Interview

Perhaps the primary purpose for an interview that relates to our definition of nursing has been explicated by Hein (1973, p. 27): "The interview in nursing is the deliberate use of verbal behaviors by the nurse to communicate with the patient in a manner directly concerned with the restoration of his health."* It is, therefore, a strategy for data collection to help the nurse discern the client's world, recognize areas requiring nursing assistance, and plan individualized care that is aimed toward alleviating nursing diagnoses and facilitating the client's movement to the fullest health potential.

It is evident that the interview must be specific to the client: the client's system and world. Categories of information that may be obtained during the interview process have been delineated by Hein (1973). These areas follow those of the PELLEM Pentagram (Chapter 20):

1. description of the happening
2. perceptions of client regarding the event
3. behaviors
4. attitudes and beliefs
5. feelings
6. values

Questions and statements by the nurse or interviewer should be purposeful toward generating information on the above categorical guidelines. They should describe and elaborate, clarify, validate, substantiate, interpret, and compare. In a sense, interviewer comments are levers by which the interviewee can find further self-expression.

Conditions and Principles of Interviewing

Kahn and Cannell (1964) view the interview as a lengthy conversation in which they denote three conditions for success: accessibility, cognition, and motivation. The first requires that the information received by the interviewer is in a conscious, clear, and relevant form. It must relate to the purposes of the interview for each unique client. Cognition requires that the person interviewed understand his role, the reasons for data collection, and the mode of informational transaction required. Finally, motivation or willingness to interact is the major requirement for a successful interview.

Since client motivation has been observed as a paramount and necessary condition, much research by social scientists has been devoted to the area. In one example, Kahn and Cannell (1964) postulate both instrumental and intrinsic factors in their motivational framework (Figure 9-1).

It is easy to observe that the interview can and should be regarded as a

*Reprinted with permission. Copyright 1973 by Little, Brown and Co., Inc.

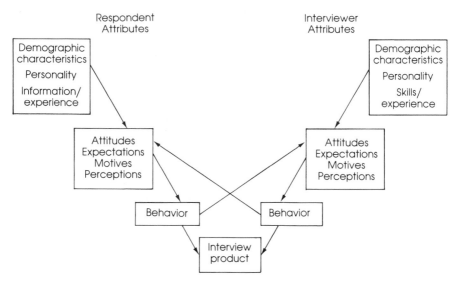

Respondent   Interviewer
Attributes   Attributes

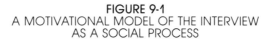

SOURCE: Kahn, R., and Cannell, C. The dynamics of interviewing. Copyright 1964. Reproduced by permission of John Wiley & Sons.

FIGURE 9-1
A MOTIVATIONAL MODEL OF THE INTERVIEW
AS A SOCIAL PROCESS

complex social phenomenon. *Instrumental factors* of motivation focus heavily on the interviewee's belief that the results of the interview will have some positive effect on what happens to him. The second type of motivation factors, *intrinsic* (Kahn and Cannell, 1964), reflect the qualities of the interviewer. Receptiveness, warmth, understanding, and interest are all seen as important. It is also pertinent to note that Carl Rogers' (1961) ingredients of a meaningful counseling relationship were noted by Kahn and Cannell (1964) as equally valid for a productive interview. This confirms the importance of effective communication skills in all that a nurse engages.

Certain principles for an effective interview must be integrated into the process. Hein (1973, p. 28) explicated the following essentials:

1. The freedom with which the patient expresses himself to the nurse is determined by the atmosphere the nurse creates in the presence of the patient.
2. An interview is effective to the degree that the nurse clearly establishes and understands the nursing goals in the interview.
3. An interview is effective to the degree that the nurse can relate to the patient without using value judgments.
4. An interview is effective to the degree that the nurse examines, encourages, and clarifies mutual thoughts and feelings that may affect nursing care.

5. An interview is effective to the degree the nurse consistently evaluates patient needs, nursing goals, and the behavioral responses of the patient to his nursing care.
6. An interview is effective to the degree that the nurse employs and encourages the use of feedback with patients in conveying, implementing, and evaluating nursing goals.*

In addition, Bermosk (1966, p. 207–210)† stated other requisites:

7. The climate the nurse creates within the patient-nurse interaction influences the substance of the interview.
8. Professional attitudes of warmth, acceptance, objectivity, and compassion are essential for effective interviewing.
9. The identification and clarification of conflicting thoughts and feelings of the patient and of the nurse lead toward a harmony of goals in the interview.

The social process involved in the interview can again be noticed by studying the principles; the interpersonal facet involves the nurse interviewer, the client, and the interaction of both.

DESIGNS AND CONTINGENCIES OF THE INTERVIEW

The interview can be structured or nonstructured. Structure implies that specific questions related to topic areas are posed by the interviewer; nonstructure relates to the fact that wording by the interviewer of questions relating to topics are not specified prior to the interview. Questions flow from the interview context, spontaneously. The purposes, however, are a constant in both.

Formal and informal are words used to further classify interviewing. Formality broadly represents the fact that time, place, and content are arranged prior to the interaction. It generally denotes a longer period for interviewing than the informal one. Informal interviewing can be anywhere from a five-minute, spontaneous interaction in which data are collected to a lengthy, unplanned talk.

Schatzman and Strauss (1973) have stated various contingencies that shape the interview's form and content:

1. Expected duration: How long is it expected to last? Will it be interrupted? Can it be extended or shortened as the process implies?
2. Single interview versus a series: Is this the only one? Is there a series? Where in the series does this one fall?

*Reprinted with permission. Copyright 1973 by Little, Brown and Co., Inc.
†Reprinted with permission from W. B. Saunders Co.

3. Setting: Is this a public or private place? What does the environment feel like? Is this feeling conducive to the interview's purpose? Is a specific conversational style more appropriate in the setting?
4. Identities: Is the interviewer an outsider or insider to the system? Can the interviewer and interviewee be seen as part of the same group?
5. Style of respondent.

In addition to these, this author includes the following:

6. Style of interviewer.
7. Harmony between respondent's style and that of the nurse.

SUMMARY

It becomes clear that interviewing is a complex social process involving the principal interactors, purposes guided by principles of interviewing, and extraneous variables that must be considered.

REFERENCES

Bermosk, L. Interviewing: A key to therapeutic communication in nursing practice. *Nursing Clinics of North America* 1:205–214, 1966.

Bermosk, L., and Mordan, M. *Interviewing in nursing.* New York: Macmillan, 1964.

Hein, E. *Communication in nursing practice.* Boston: Little, Brown and Company, 1973.

Kahn, R., and Cannell, C. *The dynamics of interviewing.* New York: John Wiley and Sons, 1964.

Keltner, J. *Interpersonal speech-communication: Elements and structures.* Belmont, Calif.: Wadsworth, 1970.

Rogers, C. *On becoming a person.* Boston: Houghton-Mifflin, 1961.

Schatzman, L., and Strauss, A. *Field research: Strategies for a natural sociology.* Englewood Cliffs, N.J.: Prentice-Hall, 1973.

SELECTED READING

Bermosk's (1966) classic article is included for further study of the interviewing process. She views interviewing as a key in therapeutic communication and comprehensively discusses five principles for interviewing in nursing practice.

Interviewing: A Key to Therapeutic Communication in Nursing Practice

Loretta Sue Bermosk, B.S., M. Litt.

Interviewing in nursing is a specific kind of communication which is in operation when the professional person (the nurse) focuses her attention on the patient (client, subject, group, family) and attends to the business of helping this person to better understand what is happening or what has happened to him at a particular moment in a particular situation. She encourages him to describe his actions and to express his thoughts and feelings so as to identify needs and to establish goals which will help him to regain, maintain, or improve his health status. With the acceptance of the interpersonal relationship as the context within which the actions of nursing are performed, and wherein the nurse functions as a counselor, teacher, technician, and socializing agent, it seems imperative that patient-centered, purposeful, and goal-directed communication be initiated and maintained by the nurse.

Principles of interviewing and supervised practice in applying these principles are currently seen as essential content in undergraduate and graduate nursing curricula. The specific content which provides the knowledge necessary for the implementation of the interviewing process has been derived from the theories and concepts of social psychology, personality, growth and development, normal and abnormal behavior, humanities, linguistics, and psychiatry. The supervised practice within the performance of nursing care in a variety of situations, with the intent of making the conversational aspect of the nurse-patient interaction purposeful and meaningful, allows nurse and supervisor and/or student and teacher to scrutinize both verbal and nonverbal responses and evaluate their effect on the patient. From this learning experience, the nurse is enabled to develop a nursing approach to each patient which incorporates an organization of verbal and nonverbal actions directed toward promoting a relationship with the patient in which the messages exchanged are patient-centered, clear, mutually understood, and goal-directed.

As she experiences working with patients who present deep-seated difficulties or are faced with overwhelming problems in adjusting to life or death situations, the nurse grows in her understanding of and ability to recognize patient needs, and develops increased skill in selecting those verbal and nonverbal responses that will be most helpful to the patient. Thus, she reaches a point in her administration of nursing care when the *communication*

Reprinted with permission from *Nursing Clinics of North America,* vol. 1, no. 2.

between professional person and patient is of a therapeutic nature and truly comprehensive in intent.

In this paper, the five principles of interviewing described by Bermosk and Mordan are presented as knowledge that becomes a key to open the door and bring the nurse to the threshold where she can communicate therapeutically as a psychiatric nurse practitioner. These principles guide the nurse's actions in relation to (1) the climate for the interview, (2) the nurse's attitudes and role, (3) and (4) the content of the interview, and (5) evaluation of the interview and the nurse-interviewer.

Although the psychiatric nurse has been chosen as the exemplar here, for the reason that the interview is a vital tool in her particular metier, the principles and the examples cited can all be applied to the broad field of general nursing care. In all verbal interchange with patients, nurses can find application of one or more of these principles.

PRINCIPLES OF INTERVIEWING IN NURSING

1. *The climate the nurse creates within the patient-nurse interaction influences the substance of the interview.*

Climate is composed of those immediate conditions, circumstances, and influences which surround and affect people interacting with each other. The physical, emotional, external, and internal factors are seen as dynamic forces which cause the climate within which the interview is conducted to change in relation to the specific areas or subjects being explored. The physical setting, the day's experiences, interactions with other patients and staff, and physical and emotional status affect the thoughts and feelings of patient and nurse. The expectations the patient has for himself and for the nurse, and the expectations the nurse has for herself and for the patient, are an influence on climate.

A graduate student, working with a woman patient who had many neurotic and psychophysiological complaints, expressed dissatisfaction, boredom, and loss of interest in this patient, because "nothing's happening. The patient says that everything's going great since she has this new boy friend. Neither her kids nor boss bother her anymore."

Instr.: You're bored with what she tells you?

G.S.: I think I should be spending my time with a patient who really needs me.

Instr.: You're saying this woman doesn't need your help.

G.S.: Not as much as some others.

Instr.: What would you like her to talk about in your sessions?

G.S.: Well, it would be nice if she thought she was getting some help from the clinic.

Instr.: From you?

G.S.: Well, yes. I have been seeing her for some time. I do want to help her, and I think I have, but she attributes any change in her mood to her boy friend.

Instr.: And now you find yourself losing interest in her because she isn't meeting your expectations of her.

G.S.: Seems that way. I'm not meeting my own expectations either with this lady—she jumps from one topic to another so quickly that I am unable to keep her focused on any subject long enough to identify what the problem really is. She makes me feel inadequate.

In exploring the situation, we find that the nurse's feeling of inadequacy in relation to her interviewing skills (not meeting expectations of self) was emphasized when she thought that the patient was saying that she (the patient) was being helped more by the boy friend than by the nurse (patient not meeting nurse's expectation that patient would recognize that nurse was helping her). This heightened feeling of inadequacy influenced the climate of the interview so much that the nurse was consciously aware of being bored, disinterested, and dissatisfied with the patient's responses. The patient may have kept the substance of the interview centered on her boy friend who wasn't bored, disinterested, and dissatisfied with her responses as a defense against the nonverbal communication of the nurse. Discovering the impact of her feelings of inadequacy on the climate of the interview and on the developing relationship between patient and nurse, the nurse can put more of her energies into developing her interviewing skills. Meanwhile, she goes into her next interview with her patient with a greater awareness, a little more objectivity, and a strengthened intention to focus on the patient.

How does the nurse create and maintain a climate which reflects her intention of helping the patient so that he will come to believe that she wants to help him, and will trust her and talk about those actions, thoughts, and feelings that concern him?

Knowledge of the concept of climate within the interview will increase the nurse's awareness of and sensitivity to those factors in the immediate surroundings that may enhance or interfere with the interaction between patient and nurse. Her intention must be sincere or the patient will sense the masquerade and avoid her.

In her initial contact, whether the patient is interested or not, actively verbal or passively nonverbal, the nurse approaches the patient in a relaxed, unhurried manner, introduces herself so that he knows who she is (name, discipline, and echelon)—so he can fit her into some frame of reference; tells him what she will be doing that concerns him (talking with him, going to activities, etc.); and arranges with him for a time to meet that will be mutually agreeable (hour, day, length of each conference, extent of total period of nursing therapy—if feasible at this time). She screens the bed unit, or seeks an alcove, a room, or an out of doors area for the conference where privacy, confidentiality, and relative freedom from noise and interruptions are possible. She provides comfortable chairs that can be arranged in such a way as to facilitate ease of listening and responding. She attends to both the verbal and non-verbal expressions of the patient, encourages him to tell her about his experiences and concerns, and helps the patient organize the telling by asking the who, where, what, and when of each incident. Thus, she demonstrates her interest and intent and the patient experiences an interaction wherein he is the center of attention and his concerns are listened to and responded to in an attempt to understand their import and meaning.

2. *Professional attitudes of warmth, acceptance, objectivity, and compassion are essential for effective interviewing.*

The development of these professional attitudes is dependent upon how well the nurse is able to work through her personal attitudes arising from her life experiences and sociocultural milieu. Identification of these attitudes and recognition of the strength of their influence on her behavior is an on-going process, and, when started early in the nursing curriculum through analysis of nurse-patient interactions in a variety of clinical settings, allows the nurse to experience her reactions to both subject matter and patient behavior. Comprehensive discussions of such subjects as pain, fear, sexual identification, masturbation, promiscuity, infidelity, birth control, abortion, unwed mothers, birth anomalies, race, religion, suicide, dying, and death, all of which relate to the nature of man and his adaptations to living and dying, are essential to achieving some degree of objectivity in relating to all patients. Identification and working with such personal feelings as shock, helplessness, inadequacy, heterosexual and homosexual attractions, anxiety, rejection, or dependency also become part of the learning experience. If the nurse is to communicate therapeutically with the psychiatric patient, she must be clear in her understanding of the dynamics of behavior so as to help the patient whose intrapsychic and social communications are distorted and impaired to arrive at some organization and clarity of ideas. Conscious awareness of her personal attitudes and how they have developed prepares her to respond to the patient's attitudes in terms of helping him to understand how his attitudes developed and how they influence his behavior.

How does the nurse demonstrate the professional attitudes of warmth, acceptance, objectivity, and compassion?

The nurse demonstrates *warmth* when she is kind, gentle, and thoughtful. She shows respect for the patient as a person by addressing him by name, and by remembering his personal preferences, idiosyncracies, and problems.

She demonstrates the attitude of *acceptance* when she views the patient's behavior as purposeful, meaningful, and a method arrived at for handling a stressful situation She attempts to learn to identify the need being expressed, and to take appropriate action. Behavior that is helpful and behavior that is harmful to the patient or to others are recognized in terms of the needs being expressed, and the nurse intervenes either to facilitate or to inhibit the action. If the patient says he is going to kill himself, she accepts this statement as an expression of a need, but in light of her responsibility to help the patient through this stress period, she institutes precautions to protect the patient from this action against himself.

Complete *objectivity* is an impossibility, but the nurse works at being relatively objective—relatively free from bias and prejudice—when she bases her assumptions on the collected data gathered in the reality of the situation—

that which is seen and heard—and attempts to validate her conclusions with the patient and with other professionals in the situation.

The nurse demonstrates *compassion* when she has reached the point where she is truly working with the patient within the sphere of his feelings and needs. She has learned to tolerate and harbor the impact of the emotion expressed by her patient with sufficient absorption that she can accept its meaning and enter into a feeling of fellowship with him. This implies that she has arrived at the point where she herself is comfortable with the feeling being expressed, and can move forward into translating the attitude of compassion into nursing action.

3. *Defined needs and goals (for the patient and for the nurse) determine the purpose of the interview.*

There is a time sequence involved in developing the ability to define needs and goals. Theory related to growth and development and the dynamics of human behavior orients the nurse to the existence of needs and to the physical, psychic, and social forces that generate these needs. Through the supervised practice of interacting with patients of all ages with varying degrees of illness, and the careful analysis of process recordings describing the words and actions of patient and nurse within these interactions, the nurse learns to recognize the overt and covert ways in which she and the patient express their needs. At the same time, she learns to recognize elements within each situation that threaten the security of patient and nurse, and works toward diminishing or removing the threatening element. She also experiences the sequence of phases found in the nurse-patient interaction—orientation, identification, exploitation, and resolution—and learns that her role in each phase will change as the patient becomes clear in his thinking and gains sufficient strength from the relationship to progress on his own.

4. *The identification and clarification of conflicting thoughts and feelings of the patient and of the nurse lead toward a harmony of goals in the interview.*

The patient will become clear in his thinking only as the nurse is able to become organized and clear in her thinking and can give direction to the communication that she shares with the patient. In her role of therapeutic agent, the nurse identifies the area in which the patient's conflict lies—in his thought processes, or at a deeper emotional level. She helps the patient describe events that happened to him and works toward a logical and sequential description of time, place, people, and event, so that the chaos of thoughts causing the patient's confusion have a time sequence, a beginning and an end, a cause and an effect, and can be looked at by patient and nurse as an experience that has meaning to the patient. She helps the patient to separate "this is what I was doing" from "this is what I was thinking" and from "this is what I was feeling," so that he can gain some perspective and objectivity in looking at his behavior during the particular event. He learns to distinguish between action, thought, and feeling along with discovering their relationship to each other. The conflict itself becomes less threatening as patient and nurse discuss it objectively. The conflict is visualized by both patient and nurse and the way is

clear for setting up a goal to deal with this conflict which is mutually understood and accepted by each.

The actions of the interview that help the nurse to define needs, to identify
and clarify thoughts and feelings, and to arrive at a harmony of goals with the
patient are observation, listening, verbal and nonverbal responses, interpretation of data, and recording of data.

Observation Observation that is planned, specific, and oriented in time,
place, people, and events and associated with a particular patient behavior
provides data about the patient which help the nurse learn the patient's reaction to stress, and to make assumptions about the degree of anxiety
experienced by the patient and his methods of handling it. As the nurse learns
the patient's habitual behavior patterns, she assesses the degree of organization
and/or disorganization, his awareness or unawareness of others around him,
his appearance, dress, stature, and walk, and carefully notes when a change
appears and looks further to note what in the situation may account for the
change. She also notes her own behavior and assesses its influence on the
patient.

Listening Listening accompanies observation, and adds words and greater
meaning to the observed actions. It adds another dimension in learning about
the patient—the pitch, tone, harshness or softness of his voice, his vocabulary
and choice of words, his hesitancy or intensity in speaking. The nurse listens to
the patient's words and attempts to identify those themes that are stressed and
those that are vaguely hinted at; those that indicate healthy aspects of the
patient's personality, and those that indicate the areas where he experiences
the most conflict and disturbance.

Nonverbal responses Nonverbal responses include all the methods by which
one communicates other than by the spoken word, e.g., gestures, body
movements, sweaty palms, limp handshake, pushing away from a persona or
moving closer, physical appearance, and choice of make-up and clothing.
Silence may be an indication of many emotions or complete apathy, the exact
meaning of which must be explored with the patient.

Verbal responses Verbal responses include questions, statements, and those
words that indicate that one is listening, such as "yes," "go on," "uh huh."
Questions and statements that contain a single idea will elicit the clearest
responses. The "what," "where," "when," and "who" open-ended questions
related to a specific topic introduced by the patient aid in helping the patient
get the specific event organized so that he and the nurse are able to explore it
together. Learning to focus on an event so as to see the relationship to the
patient's thoughts and feelings becomes the intent and purpose of the nurse for
communicating with the patient. She helps the patient look more closely at his
strengths in particular situations and, in looking at his failures, provides him
with information to consider in handling the situation differently the next
time. For the most part, she encourages the patient to organize his thoughts,

reconstruct situations, take a look at what really did happen and what the patient thought happened.

In working with psychiatric patients, the nurse learns to become aggressive in intervening in the stream of words issuing from the patient in an effort to break into the stereotyped thinking, the rigid, the biased, the prejudiced, the judgmental, the self-effacing, and to introduce new ideas to increase or decrease the amount of reflected light on the subject, to separate the real from the fantasy, to clear up the dark areas—the unknown, the frightening, the prohibited, the unexplored—to help the patient obtain a different, new, or altered perspective of himself and the "others" in his world.

Interpretation of data Interpretation of data within the interview is an on-going intellectual function of the nurse. She listens and observes and from her knowledge of behavior relates principles and facts to her collected data. She interprets the meaning of the patient's behavior to herself and makes certain assumptions about his needs. She then can do one of three things: she can respond to the data and test her assumption, she can ignore the data and change the subject, or she can physically retreat from the situation. Her decision directs her action. Whatever her action, her recognition of the selected action and its influence on the nurse-patient relationship will dictate her next approach.

In learning to interpret behavior and to respond appropriately (constructively), the nurse learns to test her assumptions and the validity of her interpretations. She may err. Her intention of helping the patient is not lost; this gets communicated nonverbally. Aware of her error, she reviews and evaluates the process of thinking that led to the incorrect assumption. This too is learning. To err is human, and for the nurse to discuss her error with the patient sometimes paves the way for the patient to talk more freely with her about his inadequacies and/or failures. In the role of professional practitioner, the nurse assumes the responsibility for the results of her nursing actions whether she attempts to meet the patient's needs or to ignore them.

Recording of data Recording of data follows two patterns, each with a specific purpose: (1) the recording of the raw data—the content of the interview—so as to study the behavior of patient and nurse, to obtain a record of patient progress and learning, and to assess the skill of the nurse as an interviewer and psychiatric nurse practitioner; and (2) the recording of certain aspects of her interaction with the patient for other team members through written nurses' notes and verbal conferences to contribute toward continuity of patient care.

In recording the actual interview, nurses are becoming adept in using a notebook and pencil and/or a tape recorder. The most accurate reproduction of verbal content will be gained by using the recorder. However, the nurse also needs to note and remember the nonverbal responses. With the notebook and pencil, the nurse develops a code for herself so she can keep pace with the patient and herself, as well as noting silent periods and other nonverbal responses. Recording the action of the interview after one leaves the patient allows memory loss and distortion to enter the record, and if this method is used, the recording should be done as soon after the event as possible.

One great advantage of recording by tape or writing during the interaction is the opportunity to review content with the patient. The nurse may play back certain sections of the tape to help the patient hear the anger in his voice when talking about a particular person or situation, or hear the words he used in describing a person or place. With the notebook, she can refer accurately to some of the patient's statements in an attempt to help him clarify meaning or sequence of time and events.

5. *Continuous and terminal evaluations of the interview are made in terms of behavior changes in the patient and in the nurse related to the defined needs and goals.*

In the activity of the interview, in concentrating upon the patient's behavior, each observation and response of the patient is attended to by the nurse. She is continuously trying to ascertain whether or not the words used are conveying the meaning each intends, to search for meaning in each exchange, to assess level of anxiety, to keep the focus on a particular subject matter until it is explored and understood, and to make associations betwen events the patient chooses to introduce. She is continuously in the process of evaluating, making a quick judgment, and then selecting her own response to the patient based on this judgment. Sometimes her responses bring her and the patient closer to their goal and sometimes they do not. Often, she may be able to reword, rephrase, or retract her response on the spot if she is immediately aware of the situation. Other times, it is only in retrospect as she reviews her recording of the interchange that she becomes aware that she and the patient were miles apart. Then she attempts to reconstruct the sequence of exchanges within the interaction to pinpoint the ideas, feelings, or behavior which interfered or interrupted the patient and the nurse in working toward their defined goal. She reviews data from other interactions with this patient to support or negate her assumptions about patterns of behavior which indicate her own difficulties in handling certain behavior or situations. She confers with her professional colleagues both to gain other points of view and to be as objective as possible in reading her data. She peruses the literature to add to her knowledge of behavior and psychiatric nursing.

Learning to communicate with the psychiatric patient in a therapeutic manner evolves from the application of interviewing principles and psychiatric nursing principles practiced within the context of the nurse-patient relationship. When the principles of interviewing and guided experiences are introduced early in the nurse's education, and she is both encouraged and expected to expand her interviewing knowledge and to develop her interviewing skills in each clinical situation as she progresses from relatively simple to more complex health problems, she possesses a key to open the door to therapeutic communication in her nursing practice.

REFERENCES

1. Bermosk, Loretta Sue, and Mordan, Mary Jane. *Interviewing in nursing.* New York: Macmillan, 1964.

2. Peplau, Hildegarde. *Basic principles of patient counseling.* 2nd ed. Philadelphia: Smith, Kline & French Laboratories, 1964.

3. Reusch, Jurgen. *Therapeutic communication.* New York: Norton, 1961.

4. Spiegel. Specific problems of communication in psychiatric conditions. In Arieti, S., Ed.: *American handbook of psychiatry.* New York: Basic Books, 1959, Chap. 46.

10

Decision-Making

Decision-making is a vital skill throughout the nursing process. This chapter begins by examining the nature of the decision-making process and its pertinence in nursing practice. Steps of decision-making are delineated, following a problem-solving model, and the leadership skills necessary to put the process into operation are described. The chapter concludes by discussing factors that can facilitate or hinder effective decisions made by groups.

NATURE OF DECISION-MAKING

As an essential aspect of modern management, decision-making is a basic function of managers (Finch, Jones, and Litterer, 1976) and leaders. By recognizing the nurse's role in managing client care and providing leadership to the client so that the client may achieve maximum health, one can easily see the necessity for decision-making in nursing as well. Basically speaking, Radford (1975) defines decision-making in its simplest form: making a choice between two or more feasible options following evaluation of each as it reflects progress toward fulfillment of a goal or objective.

Ackoff (1971) and Ackoff and Emery (1972) view decision-making as an essential characteristic of all systems that move toward goals or objectives. They term this type of system as *purposeful*. Radford (1975) describes a system as a set of interrelated elements and considers the human being an open system. The environmental variables plus ever-changing stimuli bombard and affect the individual. This point of view further substantiates the conceptual framework of the nursing process discussed in Chapter 5.

Extensive research shows that work teams, who have successfully achieved their goals over time, have a theoretical rationale and method for making decisions. Eminent authors in this field, such as Churchman (1961), Cyert and March (1963), Eilon (1969), Raiffa (1968), Simon (1959, 1965), and

Simon and Newell (1971), have all documented that effective decision-making *is* the road to successful goal accomplishment.

Decision-Making in Nursing Care

Recognition that professional nurses need to become effective leaders has pervaded the writings of nursing theorists and practitioners over the years (Beyer and Phillips, 1971; Douglass and Bevis, 1974; Eckelberry, 1971; Kron, 1971). Most writings have discussed decision-making as a function of nurses who are leading other health workers in delivering nursing and/or health care. The importance for *all* professional nurses to possess effective decision-making skills has been underemphasized. This may be because of previous narrow definitions of the leader concept.

This book's definition of leadership takes in a broad area. Any time a person is a recognized authority, whether this be by position or personal traits, and has followers who count on this person's expertise to carry out their objectives, *the person is a leader.* Furthermore, anyone who is responsible for giving assistance to others is also a leader. It becomes apparent that with this definition, every nurse is a leader.

The nurse who is responsible for the care of one or more persons is the leader and is recognized as the authority by the client(s). Within the nursing care team, even though the nurse may or may not be a leader by designated position, *the nurse is an expert* in all matters regarding the care of client(s). Consultation with others on the team is often indicated and decisions are made based on all input that is received. Table 10-1 shows various situations in which nurses can be recognized as leaders.

It should be obvious that the organizational framework of a hospital is also a clue to who is a leader as well as to whom the leader leads. Figure 10-1 presents a hypothetical organizational chart.

TABLE 10-1
SITUATIONS IN WHICH NURSES ARE LEADERS

LEADERS	SITUATIONS
1. Student Nurse Staff Nurse Primary Nurse	Caring for one or more clients in direct service Recognized as an authority by clients and families Presenting client in a team conference Consulting informally with associates regarding client care
2. Team Leaders Head Nurse	Delegating and/or participating in the care of client(s) with followers, associates and/or superiors
3. Supervisors Directors	Delegating care of clients to followers

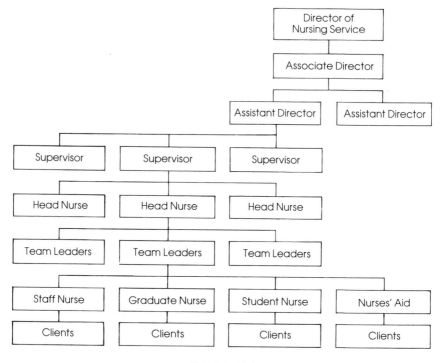

FIGURE 10-1
HYPOTHETICAL ORGANIZATIONAL CHART

In Figure 10-1, moving from the bottom of the chart upward, the staff, graduate, and student nurses, as well as the nurse's aide in some respects, are leaders in the care of the client. Team leaders are responsible by position for all people beneath them; head nurses, supervisors, and directors follow the same pattern. It does not matter whether people are in top, middle, or lower management positions; if someone relies on them, they are leaders.

Moving back to decision-making as a function in successful leadership, it is clear that knowledge and experience in this concept is necessary for all professionals. Writings in this area have consistently documented the importance for decision-making to be grounded in theory.

STEPS IN THE DECISION-MAKING PROCESS

The steps of the decision-making process have been postulated by a number of authors, most notably Tannenbaum (1950–51), and generally follow a scientific problem-solving method. With the goal or objective in mind, the decision process consists of the following steps:

1. Defining the problem
2. Collecting information
3. Identifying alternative solutions
4. Testing or weighing of alternatives
5. Determining the best alternative/action and who does what
6. Acting.

It is usually the function of the leader initially to define the problem and collect all the information relating to it. Group involvement usually becomes prominent in steps 3, 4, and 5. The amount of group involvement is designated by the decision-making style of the leader, in response to the nature of the situational variables. These styles have been eloquently described by Vroom (1973) and are:

1. The leader makes the decision based on available information—*authoritarian style.*
2. Followers provide necessary information and then a decision is made by the leader—*authoritarian style.* (Followers may not be aware of the problem.)
3. Problem is individually shared with followers who offer ideas and suggestions; decision is made by the leader and it may or may not reflect the suggestions of the followers—*consultative style.*
4. Problem is shared and discussed with the collective group; decision is made by the leader—*consultative style.*
5. With the group of involved people, the problem is shared, discussed, and agreement is reached by the constituents—*democratic style.*

A sixth style described by Vroom and Yetton (1973) is delegation.

6. Problem is given by the leader to the followers for complete analysis— *delegative style.*

A complete discussion of these aforementioned decision-making styles can be found in the selected reading at the end of this chapter (La Monica and Finch, 1977).

Application of Steps in Decision-Making

In carrying out the steps of the decision-making process using appropriate styles, the leader must use specific skills effectively. Generally speaking, these skills are listening, observing, communicating, and the use of facilitative group or interpersonal processes. Application of the steps of the decision-making process are described in detail as follows:*

---

*The skills are derived from materials compiled by an anonymous source.

1. Stating the problem:
   In terms the group understands
   Includes necessary information
   Clear definition
   No slanting
   Importance
   Relationship to the group's broader purposes
2. Clarifying the problem:
   Restating
   Asking for missing information
   Asking for specific meanings
   Asking for statement of responsibility, boundaries, deadlines, use of solution, etc.
3. Developing alternatives:
   State, consider, and amend possibilities
   Relate alternatives to a statement of the problem
4. Keeping discussion on the beam:
   Knowing when it is off
   Giving individuals a chance to relate their comments to the issue
   Restating contributions which tend to invite digression
   Inviting exploration of questions not yet considered
5. Summarizing:
   Timing
   Sensitivity to place where the group has given the consideration probably required
   Choosing significant data for restatement
   Rejecting data according to consensus already achieved
6. Testing consequences of the group's tentative choice, questioning concerning the emerging decision:
   What it means
   How it relates to other tasks
   Is it possible
   Where such things as cost, time, facilities are considered
   What are the effects
7. Testing understanding of member commitment:
   Making sure of the willingness and availability of those responsible
   Repeating above if necessary
8. Decision-making:
   Consideration as to whether all are involved
   Sensitivity to agreement*
   Use of firm statement of agreement
   Recording and reporting

*There is a difference between agreement and consensus. Agreement requires unanimity of thought, whereas consensus requires unanimity of thoughts and feelings.

FACTORS WHICH FACILITATE OR BLOCK
GOOD DECISIONS

To understand further the nature of decision-making and strive to upgrade its quality, it becomes necessary to understand the nature of the factors that facilitate or block such choices.

Factors that facilitate good decision-making are:

1. Willingness to work with the real problem.
2. A clear definition of the problem about which a decision is to be made.
3. Placing the responsibility for decision-making at that level where most appropriate data are available and relevant.
4. Effective communication among the group that is to make the decision, so that the maximum number of effective solutions are brought out for consideration.
5. Some mechanism for building a commitment to action. This means that action steps should be specified, clearly understood, and delegated to appropriate persons.

Factors that block good decisions are:

1. Avoidance of real problem.
2. Lack of problem clarity.
3. Failure to pin down responsibility for making the decision to a clearly defined group of people.
4. Looking at the first few alternatives that appear as the only alternatives.
5. Haste in making decisions before they are appropriately tested.
6. Asking a group to make a decision without data.
7. Failure to build in an action commitment.
8. Placing responsibility for decision-making too high in the organization. People who are involved in taking action should be involved in making decisions.
9. Having the status figure or chairman state attitudes too early in the decision-making process.
10. Failure to make an experimental, provisional attitude toward action programs. This produces fear of failure.
11. Mixing the idea-getting function with the testing function. Idea producing should be divorced from evaluation during the "bright idea" stages. Many good ideas die before they are born because of self-censure.
12. Inappropriate size in group for decision-making. Groups that are too large produce threats that decrease creativity. Groups that are too small do not guarantee a broad experience base for decision-making.

SUMMARY

The nature of decision-making began the discussion in Chapter 10. Decision-making was described as making a choice between options for the purpose of meeting an objective. Application in nursing practice followed with the recognition that all nurses are leaders. The steps of a problem-solving model were portrayed as the components of the decision-making process and leader styles for involvement of the group discussed. Skills and factors that can impede or facilitate good decisions concluded the chapter.

REFERENCES

Ackoff, R. Toward a system of system concepts. *Management Science* 17:661–671, 1971.

Ackoff, R., and Emery, F. *On purposeful systems.* Chicago: Aldine-Atherton, 1972.

Beyers, M., and Phillips, C. *Nursing management for patient care.* Boston: Little, Brown and Company, 1971.

Churchman, C. *Prediction and optimal decision.* Englewood Cliffs, N.J.: Prentice-Hall, 1961.

Cyert, R., and March, J. *A behavioral theory of the firm.* Englewood Cliffs, N.J.: Prentice-Hall, 1963.

Douglas, L., and Bevis, E. *Nursing leadership in action.* St. Louis: C. V. Mosby, 1974.

Eckelberry, G. *Administration of comprehensive nursing care.* New York: Appleton-Century-Crofts, 1971.

Eilon, S. What is a decision. *Management Science* 16:172–189, 1969.

Finch, F., Jones, H., and Litterer, J. *Managing for organizational effectiveness.* New York: McGraw-Hill Books, Inc., 1976.

Kron, T. *The management of patient care.* Philadelphia: W. B. Saunders, 1971.

La Monica, E., and Finch, F. Managerial decision-making. *Journal of Nursing Administration* 7:20–28, 1977.

Radford, K. *Managerial decision making.* Reston, Va.: Reston Publishing Company, 1975.

Raiffa, H. *Decision analysis: Introductory lectures on choices under uncertainty.* Reading, Mass.: Addison-Wesley, 1968.

Simon, H. Theories of decision-making in economics and behavioral science. *American Economic Review*, 1959.

Simon, H. *Administrative behavior.* New York: Free Press, 1965.

Simon, H., and Newell, A. Human problem solving: The state of the theory in 1970. *American Psychologist* 26:145–159, 1971.

Tannenbaum, R. Managerial decision-making. *Journal of Business* 23:22–39, 1950.

Vroom, V. A new look at managerial decision making. *Organizational Dynamics* 1:67, 1973.

Vroom, V., and Yetton, P. *Leadership and decision making.* Pittsburgh: University of Pittsburgh Press, 1973.

SELECTED READING

The selected reading concluding this chapter is an article by this author and a colleague in business education. It discusses the rationale for selecting decision-making styles given certain variables that must be considered if effectiveness is valued. Application is made in nursing situations.

Managerial Decision-Making

Elaine La Monica
Frederic E. Finch

A decision-making and problem-solving tool which provides alternative processes is presented. It includes a method for diagnosing different situations and selecting appropriate techniques. Case examples and teaching outlines for classroom and inservice comprise the experiential exercise that brings the theory to life.

DECISION-MAKING STYLES

The ways that problems are solved and decisions made in organizations have been conceptualized in many different ways[1-4]. Most theories are based on value preferences rather than on research. For example, one of the prevailing biases in academic circles is a strong preference for democratic, participative problem-solving and decision-making processes. This has resulted in a generalized prescription that managers should always involve others. This generalization carries a strong evaluative component in the sense that managers who do use these participative processes are "good" and those who do not are "bad."

Another strong value bias comes largely from practicing managers who believe that since they are held responsible for decisions, they are going to make them. There are a host of other assumptions imbedded in such a stance, such as a lack of trust in the capacity of subordinates or a fear of "losing control" if decisions are delegated.

Research in the behavioral sciences is demonstrating that neither extreme position is tenable. The problem-solving and decision-making process used in a particular situation depends on *that* situation's nature. A general guide for managers can be depicted by the following equation:

$$\text{Effective Decisions} = f\ (\text{Quality} \times \text{Acceptance})$$

Thus, if the problem to be solved has a high quality characteristic (quality being critical) and does not require acceptance or commitment from others to implement it, then seek someone with the relevant expertise. For example, to obtain funding for a new hospital wing, it makes little sense to involve the nursing staff.

If the decision has a high acceptance component and a low quality requirement (scheduling coffee and lunch breaks on a unit yet maintaining adequate coverage), then the nursing staff can be profitably involved. Their involvement facilitates communication, brings relevant information to bear on

Reprinted with permission from the *Journal of Nursing Administration,* vol. VII, no. 5.

the problem, and increases motivation and commitment to the implementation of the decision.

If the problem has both quality and acceptance characteristics, then appropriate experts have to be brought together with those who are responsible for implementing the decision (if they are different).

This basic insight into the styles of problem solving and decision making is useful, although highly simplistic. Most of the literature dealing with the involvement of subordinates proposes group decision making as the most appropriate, or only, participative technique; but consultation and delegation are others. Although the literature deals with situations in which individuals are more effective than groups, it rarely details what situational variables should be examined in order to select the most effective decision process[5]. Recently a powerful model was developed by Vroom and Yetton which not only uses a range of processes, but provides a means to diagnose situations to determine the most appropriate technique for different classes of situations[6].

THE VROOM AND YETTON MANAGERIAL DECISION-MAKING MODEL

In order to examine how this model[7, 8, 9] works we would like you to go through part of the method we have used in teaching the theory to students and practicing managers. Table 1 identifies five different managerial decision

TABLE 1
TYPES OF MANAGEMENT DECISION STYLES

AI	You solve the problem or make the decision yourself, using information available to you at that time.
AII	You obtain the necessary information from your subordinate(s), then decide on the solution to the problem yourself. You may or may not tell your subordinates what the problem is in getting the information from them. The role played by your subordinates in making the decision is clearly one of providing the necessary information to you, rather than generating or evaluating alternative solutions.
CI	You share the problem with relevant subordinates individually, getting their ideas and suggestions without bringing them together as a group. Then you make the decision that may or may not reflect your subordinates' influence.
CII	You share the problem with your subordinates as a group, collectively obtaining their ideas and suggestions. Then you make the decision that may or may not reflect your subordinates' influence.
GII	You share a problem with your subordinates as a group. Together you generate and evaluate alternatives and attempt to reach agreement (consensus) on a solution. Your role is much like that of chairman. You do not try to influence the group to adopt "your" solution and you are willing to accept and implement any solution that has the support of the entire group.

styles. Read each and then study the four cases. Select the decision-making style *you* would use if you were the manager described in the case. Later, you will have an opportunity to compare your selections with those chosen by the model.

Case #1

You are an assistant director of nursing in a large city hospital. The management has recently put into effect, at your request and consultation, the unit manager system on two floors. This was expected to relieve the nurses of administrative responsibility, increase their abilities to provide quality care to clients, insure that health assessments and care plans could be accomplished for every client and lower the nursing budget. Quality health care and nursing care plans reflected the suggestions made by the hospital accreditors. To the surprise of everyone, yourself included, little of the above has been realized. In fact, nurses are sitting in the conference room more, quality has maintained a status quo, and employees and patients are complaining more than ever.

You do not believe that there is anything wrong with the new system. You have had reports from other hospitals using it and they confirm this opinion. You have also had representatives from institutions using the system talk with your nursing personnel, and they report that your nurses have full knowledge of the system and their altered responsibilities.

You suspect that a few people may be responsible for the situation, but this view is not widely shared among your two supervisors and four head nurses. The failure has been variously attributed to poor training of the unit managers, lack of financial incentives, and poor morale. Clearly, this is an issue about which there is considerable depth of feeling within individuals and potential disagreement among your subordinates.

This morning you received a phone call from the nursing director. She had just talked with the hospital administrator and was calling to express her deep concern. She indicated that the problem was yours to solve in any way you think best, but she would like to know within a week what steps you plan to take.

You share your director's concern and know that the personnel involved are equally concerned. The problem is to decide what steps to take to rectify the situation.

1. Decision style you would use:_____.

Case #2

You are the head nurse of a 50-bed orthopedic unit that is the first group to move to a new wing in one week. You must estimate the supplies and medications necessary to stock on the new floor so that nursing care can be maintained smoothly and without interruption.

Since you have been head nurse for ten years on this unit, you have the knowledge and experience necessary to evaluate approximately what you will need. It is important that nothing be forgotten since surgery will be uninterrupted and fresh postoperative patients will be arriving from surgery as well as preoperative patients needing preparation. Absent supplies may result in delayed surgery, confusion, frustrated personnel and poor nursing care. It is your practice to meet regularly with your managerial subordinates to discuss the problems of running the floor. These meetings have resulted in the creation and development of a very effective team.

2. Decision style you would use:_____.

Case #3

You are the nursing supervisor of 12 registered nurses in an intensive care unit. Their formal education, responsibilities and experience are very similar, providing for an extremely close-knit group who share responsibilities. Yesterday, your director of nurses informed you that she would supply funds for four of your nurses to attend the National Critical Care Nursing Association Convention for five days in San Francisco.

It is your perception that all of your nurses would very much like to attend and from the standpoint of staffing, there is no particular reason why any one should attend over any other. The problem is somewhat complicated by the fact that all of the nurses are active officers and members of the local organization.

3. Decision style you would use:_____.

Case #4

You are the executive director of a small but growing midwestern Visiting Nurse's Association. The rural location and consumer needs are factors which contribute to the emphasis on expanded roles in nursing practice at all levels.

When you took the position five years ago, the nursing care was poor and finances were slim. Under your leadership, much progress has been made. You obtained state and federal monies and personally educated your nursing resources. This progress has been achieved while the economy has moved into a mild recession, and, as a result, your prestige among your colleagues and staff is very high. Your success, which you are inclined to attribute principally to good luck and to a few timely decisions on your part, has, in your judgment, one unfortunate by-product. It has caused your staff to look to you for leadership and guidance in decision making beyond what you consider necessary. You have no doubts about their capabilities but wish they were not quite so willing to accede to your judgment.

You have recently acquired a grant to permit opening a satellite branch. Your problem is to decide on the best location. You believe that there is no formula in this selection process; it will be made by assessment of community needs, lack of available resources and "what feels right." You have asked your staff to assess their districts since their knowledge about the community in which they practice should be extremely useful in making a wise choice.

Their support is essential because the success of the satellite will be highly dependent on their willingness to initially staff and then educate and assist new nurses during its early days. Currently, your staff is small enough for everyone to feel and function as a team; you want this to continue.

The success of the satellite will benefit everybody. Directly, they will benefit from the expansion, and, indirectly, they will reap the personal and professional advantages of being involved in the building and expansion of nursing services.

4. Decision style you would use:_____.*

Obviously a variety of decision-making processes are possible. Note that a major style—delegation—is not included (later we will discuss how this can be incorporated into the model). The five styles can be considered as a continuum. AI and AII at one end, represent styles which do not (or minimally) involve subordinates, but are usually quicker processes than the others. CI and CII are consultative; they extend the degree of subordinate involvement. GII, the group style, permits greater subordinate involvement and is probably the slowest process. Delegation would be at the opposite end of the continuum from AI, representing the greatest amount of subordinate involvement. The time factor would depend on whether delegation was to an individual (the time would be the same as AI) or to a group (the time factor would duplicate GII).

Given these five decision styles, Vroom and Yetton identify seven central variables which theory and research suggest are critical in diagnosing situations and determining appropriate decision styles. These situational variables (which Vroom and Yetton call "problem attributes") are: 1) those which specify the importance of quality and acceptance for a particular situation (A and D in Table 2); and 2) those which have a high probability of moderating the effects of participation on quality and acceptance (all others in Table 2). These seven problem attributes are restated in question form for diagnostic purposes, and will be used in this form later in the diagnostic model.

Consistent with research findings, Vroom and Yetton developed a set of rules for choosing among the alternative decision-making styles. Rules 1, 2, and 3 were designed to protect decision quality; rules 4, 5, 6 and 7 to protect decision acceptance.

Finally, Vroom and Yetton took one important, further step to facilitate the use of the rules and attributes, making this model valuable to the practi-

*The first three nursing situations were adapted from business examples. The original material is presented in Vroom, V. H. A new look at managerial decision making. *Organization Dynamics*, Vol. 1, No. 9, Spring, 1973, pp. 72-73. The fourth adaptation is originally found in Vroom, V. H., and Jago, A. G. Decision making as a social process. *Decision Sciences*, Vol. 5, No. 4, October, 1974, p. 750.

TABLE 2
PROBLEM ATTRIBUTES USED IN THE MODEL

PROBLEM ATTRIBUTES	DIAGNOSTIC QUESTIONS
A. The importance of the quality of the decision.	Is there a quality requirement such that one solution is likely to be more rational than another?
B. The extent to which the leader possesses sufficient information/ expertise to make a high-quality decision by himself.	Do I have sufficient information to make a high-quality decision?
C. The extent to which the problem is structured.	Is the problem structured?
D. The extent to which acceptance or commitment on the part of subordinates is critical to the effective implementation of the decision.	Is acceptance of decision by subordinates critical to effective implementation?
E. The prior probability that the leader's autocratic decision will receive acceptance by subordinates.	If you were to make the decision by yourself, is it reasonably certain that it would be accepted by your subordinates?
F. The extent to which subordinates are motivated to attain the organizational goals as represented in the objectives explicit in the statement of the problem.	Do subordinates share the organizational goals to be obtained in solving this problem?
G. The extent to which subordinates are likely to be in conflict over preferred solutions.	Is conflict among subordinates likely in preferred solutions?

Reprinted by permission of the publisher: Victor Vroom. A new look at managerial decision making. Organizational Dynamics, Vol. 1, No. 4, Spring, 1973, p. 69. Copyright 1973 by AMACOM, a division of American Management Associations.

tioner. A decision model was constructed (Figure 1) with the problem attributes, in question form, arranged across the top. The rules are applied when one answers the diagnostic questions with respect to a particular situation. For example, if you had a specific situation in mind and answered "No" to the first question (A), you would follow the "No" branch to the next node (intersection), answer the question associated with that node (D), and continue in like manner until an end point (terminal node) is reached. At that point the decision style for a situation, as selected by the theory, is noted.

Alternatively, if you responded "Yes" to the first question (A), you would proceed along the "Yes" branch to the first intersection, answer the question associated with that node (B), and continue in a similar way until an end point is reached.

In using this model we discerned two major problems. First, people have trouble understanding the initial diagnostic question (A). Another explanation would be to indicate that if they can think of a number of possible solutions and if some alternatives clearly result in better outcomes than others, a quality requirement exists for that situation. For example, in Case 1 there are a number of possible solutions, some producing preferred outcome. In Case 3,

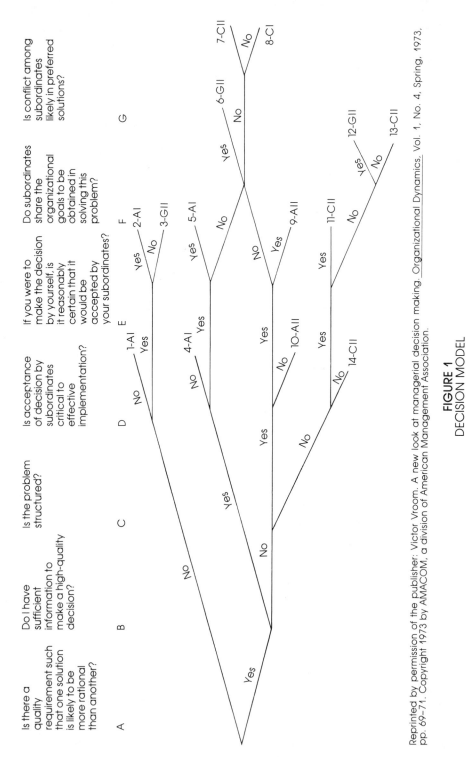

FIGURE 1
DECISION MODEL

Reprinted by permission of the publisher: Victor Vroom. A new look at managerial decision making. Organizational Dynamics. Vol. 1, No. 4, Spring, 1973, pp. 69–71. Copyright 1973 by AMACOM, a division of American Management Association.

however, all the nurses are equally qualified and, from the perspective of the manager, any of them could go. There is no quality requirement here. There are numerous situations which have low quality but high acceptance requirements. Maier indicates that many of these situations have "fairness" as a key variable (such as scheduling work, overtime, unpleasant tasks, coffee breaks)[10].

The other troublesome area is the third question (C)—is the problem structured? Even though the problem is clear, the variety of data required to solve the issue and steps toward problem alleviation remain undetermined and mandate further exploration. In rule 3 an unstructured problem is defined as one in which you neither know what information is needed nor where it is located. Case 1 is an example of an unstructured problem.

Finally, note in Figure 1 that there are 14 terminal nodes or "problem types." Each represents a particular type of problem or class of situation. Type 1 (terminal node 1) represents situations in which neither quality nor acceptance are important. Although each node is designated by one decision style, it is possible to use more than one style for many problem types. The styles were chosen for the 14 nodes by applying a third criteria not included in the preceding equation—time. Thus, that equation can be modified as follows:

$$\text{Effective Decisions} = f \text{ (Quality} \times \text{Acceptance} \times \text{Time)}$$

Therefore, the styles noted for each node were selected by applying the time criteria—they represent the quickest decision process for the particular problem type. As indicated previously, the various styles can represent a time continuum, with "A" usually being the quickest and the group style the slowest. Table 3 lists the 14 problem types and the associated feasible styles.

Thus, for problem type 1 all five styles would be appropriate for that class of situations. None of the styles violates any of the rules. AI would be used if time were a critical consideration. If the manager had other needs to be satisfied (such as providing subordinates with an opportunity to experience group problem-solving skills), the GII style could be used. For other problem types, such as 6 in Table 3, only one decision style is appropriate.

The core of the model developed by Vroom and Yetton is now complete and can be used for diagnostic purposes. We suggest that you use the decision model to diagnose the four cases you responded to earlier before reading the solutions and rationales.

Decision Rules

1. *The Information Rule.* If the quality of the decision is important and if the leader does not possess enough information or expertise to solve the problem by himself, AI is eliminated from the feasible set. (Its use risks a low-quality decision.)

2. *The Goal Congruence Rule.* If the quality of the decision is important and if the subordinates do not share the organizational goals to be obtained in solving the problem, GII is eliminated from the feasible set. (Alternatives that eliminate the leader's final control over the decision reached may jeopardize the quality of the decision.)

TABLE 3
PROBLEM TYPES AND THE FEASIBLE SET OF
DECISION PROCESS

PROBLEM TYPE	ACCEPTABLE METHODS
1.	AI, AII, CI, CII, GII
2.	AI, AII, CI, CII, GII
3.	GII
4.	AI, AII, CI, CII, GII*
5.	AI, AII, CI, CII, GII*
6.	GII
7.	CII
8.	CI, CII
9.	AII, CI, CII, GII*
10.	AII, CI, CII, GII*
11.	CII, GII*
12.	GII
13.	CII
14.	CI, GII*

*Within the feasible set only when the answer to question F is Yes.

Reprinted by permission of the publisher: Victor Vroom. A new look at managerial decision making. Organizational Dynamics, Vol. 1, No. 4, Spring, 1973, p. 71. Copyright 1973 by AMACOM, a division of American Management Associations.

3. *The Unstructured Problem Rule.* In decisions in which the quality of the decision is important, if the leader lacks the necessary information or expertise to solve the problem by himself, and if the problem is unstructured, i.e., he does not know exactly what information is needed and where it is located, the method used must provide not only for him to collect the information but to do so in an efficient and effective manner. Methods that involve interaction among all subordinates with full knowledge of the problem are likely to be both more efficient and more likely to generate a high-quality solution to the problem. Under these conditions, AI, AII, and CI are eliminated from the feasible set. (AI does not provide for him to collect the necessary information, and AII and CI represent more cumbersome, less effective, and less efficient means of bringing the necessary information to bear on the solution of the problem than methods that do permit those with the necessary information to interact.)

4. *The Acceptance Rule.* If the acceptance of the decision by subordinates is critical to effective implementation, and if it is not certain that an autocratic decision made by the leader would receive that acceptance, AI and AII are eliminated from the feasible set. (Neither provides an opportunity for subordinates to participate in the decision and both risk the necessary acceptance.)

5. *The Conflict Rule.* If the acceptance of the decision is critical, and an autocratic decision is not certain to be accepted, and subor-

dinates are likely to be in conflict or disagreement over the appropriate solution, AI, AII, and CI are eliminated from the feasible set. (The method used in solving the problem should enable those in disagreement to resolve their differences with full knowledge of the problem. Accordingly, under these conditions, AI, AII, and CI, which involve no interaction or only "one-to-one" relationships and therefore provide no opportunity for those in conflict to resolve their differences, are eliminated from the feasible set. Their use runs the risk of leaving some of the subordinates with less than the necessary commitment to the final decision.)

6. *The Fairness Rule.* If the quality of decision is unimportant and if acceptance is critical and not certain to result from an autocratic decision, AI, AII, CI and CII, are eliminated from the feasible set. (The method used should maximize the probability of acceptance as this is the only relevant consideration in determining the effectiveness of the decision. Under these circumstances, AI, AII, CI, and CII, are eliminated from the feasible set. To use them is to run the risk of getting less than the needed acceptance of the decision.)

7. *The Acceptance Priority Rule.* If acceptance is critical, not assured by an autocratic decision, and if subordinates can be trusted, AI, AII, CI, and CII are eliminated from the feasible set. (Methods that provide equal partnership in the decision-making process can provide greater acceptance without risking decision quality. Use of any method other than GII results in an unnecessary risk that the decision will not be fully accepted or receive the necessary commitment on the part of subordinates.)*

Case 1
Questions:

A. Quality	Yes
B. Manager's information	No
C. Structure	No
D. Acceptance	Yes
E. Prior probability of acceptance	No
F. Goal congruence	Yes
Problem type:	12
Minimum time decision style:	GII

Rule violations:
AI violates rules 1, 3, 4, 5, 7
AII violates rules 3, 4, 5, 7
CI violates rules 3, 5, 7
CII violates rule 7

Rationale: In this case there is a quality requirement. There are a number of possible solutions to the problem, some apt to be better than others. The

*Reprinted by permission of the publisher: Victor Vroom. A new look at managerial decision making. *Organization Dynamics.* Vol. 1, No. 4, Spring, 1973, pp. 69-71. Copyright 1973 by AMACOM, a division of American Management Association.

assistant director does not have the expertise to solve the problem by herself. She lacks sufficient, relevant information and does not know where it is located. Acceptance will be critical to the effective implementation of any decision. In fact, one cause for the system's failure might well be not involving personnel during the initial planning. It is unlikely that an autocratic decision would be tolerated and implemented. Finally, the question of goal congruence is a difficult one. The first sentence of the last paragraph states that those involved are also concerned—this could be indicative of goal congruence. However, this point is debatable. A "Yes" answer produces GII; a "No" answer, CII. In this situation, we would select GII, get the two supervisors and four head nurses together, make it clear that a group problem-solving process is to be used, and proceed in that manner.

Case 2
Questions:
A. Quality	Yes
B. Manager's information	Yes
C. Acceptance	No
Problem type:	4
Feasible sets:	AI, AII, CI, CII, GII
Minimum time decision style:	AI
Rule violations:	None

Rationale: There is a quality requirement, the head nurse has the requisite information, and the nurses are only concerned that the supplies be available. In this case any of the styles could be used. If the head nurse wanted to develop subordinates' problem-solving skills, this situation could be serviceable.

Case 3
Questions:
A. Quality	No
B. Acceptance	Yes
C. Prior probability of acceptance	No
Problem type:	3
Feasible set:	GII
Minimum time decision style:	GII

Rule violations:
AI and AII violate rules 4, 5, 6
CI violates rules 5 and 6
CII violates rule 6

Rationale: This situation is distressing for many managers. They would not trust nurses to make the decision by themselves, feeling they lack the ability to resolve the issue fairly if unaided. CI is often suggested as an alternative. It offers rapid communication among members and the development of individual reasons, for each person's selection, but it can induce suspicions of favoritism if the head nurse makes the decision. If the group members are competent, responsible individuals, they can work out a solution they can live with, perceiving aspects unknown to the head nurse. The head nurse might also indicate that if the group could not make the decision, she would use AI as a backup. Probably the head nurse would attend and lead the discussion, but refuse to become involved in the problem's substance. In this way information would be accessible if the group could not decide or chose to let her do so.

Case 4
Questions:

A. Quality	Yes
B. Manager's information	No
C. Structure	No
D. Acceptance	Yes
E. Prior probability of acceptance	Yes
Problem type:	II
Feasible set:	CII, GII
Minimum time decision style:	CII

Rule violations:
  AI violates rules 1 and 3
  AII and CI violates rule 3

Rationale: This is a fairly straightforward case. The only issue is whether to use GII or CII. If the nurses lack confidence in their own ability, the CII style provides an opportunity for the director to involve them as a group in the problem-solving process while retaining the ultimate decision. It is also an excellent chance to use the GII style if the director knows their capabilities and also possesses effective group management skills.

Issues Raised by the Model

There are some paramount issues to be considered in using this model. First, it does not provide hard and fast answers and should not be used rigidly. All of its aspects are open to a variety of interpretations. In teaching the model to students or in using it with practicing managers, it becomes apparent that each situation can be interpreted in a variety of ways and that even the diagnostic questions can be construed differently by individuals. Thus, the tremendous power of the model lies in its ability to stimulate people to think differently about problem solving and decision making, to increase their flexibility, to consider their own behavior, to provide a vehicle for contemplating behavior changes.

Secondly, a critical limitation of the model is that it does not include delegation as a decision style. (Vroom and Yetton attempted this in another model which focused on the two-person superior/subordinate relationship[11].) It is possible, however, to delegate to a group as well as to an individual. One way to incorporate this element in the model presented here is to consider those problem types where GII is a possible style. In these situations the extent to which the manager trusts the capacity of subordinates to resolve issues by themselves and has no reason to be involved in the process, delegation could be used.

A third concern is the skill needed by the manager to use the various styles satisfactorily. Managers ordinarily have the ability to exercise the authoritarian styles (AI, AII), consultative styles (CI, CII), or delegation. Authoritarian and consultative styles are widely used; people have numerous opportunities to observe and practice them. There is little skill necessary to use delegation, although it is not widely employed. Most managers, however, do not have the expertise to manage a group problem-solving and decision-making process effectively, but this can be acquired[12, 13].

Finally, it is important that managers explain lucidly what style they are using in a particular situation, sharing theory with subordinates and involving them when a situation concerns them. Frequently, subordinates are invited to participate in a group meeting and believe they are going to make significant contributions to the process. When the manager uses the meeting as a forum for her own ideas, or presents a solution and ignores suggested alternatives, or behaves in any way which signals that subordinates are not going to have a voice, then they feel manipulated. Trust diminishes rapidly, and the problem-solving process becomes a waste of time. Apprising personnel of the nature of their involvement beforehand can eliminate such dysfunctional outcomes.

Teaching Methodology

Our initial experiences in teaching this model by traditional methods were largely negative, resulting in confusion, misunderstanding, frustration, resistance and rejection on the part of learners. We felt that our lack of success was due to the method, not the theory. As a consequence, we designed and extensively utilized an alternative technique, modifying it as we moved from teaching in the classroom and in inservice to consulting with ongoing organizational units. The basic process is described in the classroom design with extensions for inservice and ongoing units.

TEACHING DESIGN FOR THE CLASSROOM

Materials: Duplicated copies of: Tables 1, 2, and 3; the four cases; the decision rules; and Figure 1.

Step 1. Hand out the four cases and Table 1. Read the five decision styles to the class and tell them that they are to read the four cases and select the decision style they (as individuals) would use if they were the manager in each situation.

Step 2. After everyone has completed Step 1, divide the class into groups of five or six people each (no larger than six so everyone has a chance to be heard). The task is for each individual to share her choice of decision style with her group and the reasons for the particular selection. Caution the groups against consensus on the "best" style, or they will waste time and experience frustration. Even when told simply to share selections and reasons for individual choices heated discussion usually occurs. We allow this, but put a time limit on the total discussion time to complete the four cases (40-45 minutes).

We also urge students to note the two or three major reasons for their style selections for each case. This expresses their own implicit theory about effective decision processes.

Step 3. Following the group discussion, hand out Tables 2 and 3, the decision rules, and Figure 1. Give a mini-lecture about the theory, starting with the "effective decision" equation, the identification of the seven problem attributes, and the seven decision rules. We usually read through the attributes and rules, discussing their implications with the class. Then note that the decision model is a reformulation of the rules that makes their application feasible and describe how the decision tree functions.

Step 4. Instruct each group, as a group, to diagnose the four cases using the decision model.

Step 5. Collect the styles selected individually by participants and then those arrived at collectively by each group and post these results on the board. Hold an open class discussion case by case for each of the four examples. Table 4 is one way such information can be displayed.

General Comments: You will find a wide range of interpretation and results. We encourage such diversity, noting the difficulty of interpretation of the problem attributes and that reasonable people can differ on their views of a particular situation. We encourage experienced students to select a particular work situation and run it through the model. We also use the general class discussion to explore any patterns students observed in their own individual choices and their reasons for them. Some people will tend to choose authoritarian and consultative styles, excluding the group style; others will use the group and consultative, avoiding the authoritarian. These patterns can provide a basis for interesting analysis.

Time: Approximately two hours.

TABLE 4
DECISION-MAKING STYLES

CASES	INDIVIDUAL CHOICES*					GROUP CHOICES**			
	AI	AII	CI	CII	GII	1	2	3	4
I									
II									
III									
IV									

*For posting of individual choices have students who choose AI for Case I raise their hands, count them and post in the AI, Case I space. Repeat for each decision style until the whole class has registered their choices for Case I.

**Do the same for Cases II, III, and IV. Then collect the styles arrived at by each group for each case using the decision model.

TEACHING DESIGN FOR INSERVICE

The situational decision model is a potent tool for inservice management development. For example, head or supervisory nurses can be encouraged to examine the way they function as managers and to reflect on changing the way they function.

Step 1. Begin with Steps 1 through 5 of the classroom design above.

Step 2. After the general discussion, each individual thinks of two recent major decisions she has made and the style used. Then each uses the model to diagnose the two situations to determine the appropriate, recommended decision style.

Step 3. Form the participants into groups of three to share and discuss situations, style used and style suggested by the model (we strongly urge use of triads; dyads can limit the range of experience and discussion, and larger groups often do not provide enough air time for each participant).

Step 4. Initiate a general discussion to share insights and learnings generated.

Step 5. Ask each person to think of two recent major decisions by their superior and the decision style used. As in Step 2, use the decision model for diagnosis. Repeat Step 3, then move on to Step 6.

Step 6. In a general discussion, focus on any discrepancies between how they see themselves as managers and how they see their superiors. Another point should emerge with respect to how their subordinates would perceive the two situations each participant discussed in Step 2.

Time: Four to five hours.

TEACHING DESIGN FOR ONGOING UNITS

The most exciting use of this model is with ongoing organizational units. The manager and subordinates should be involved equally in each step of the model. The model provides an excellent opportunity for structured feedback to the manager on how subordinates view her decisions. How decisions are made has a tremendous impact, not only on the quality and acceptance of the decision, but also on how people feel about their work and their organization. Thus, it is important what decision styles are used and how subordinates react to them.

Step 1. Begin with 1 through 5 of the classroom design.

Step 2. Ask the group to list major decisions made in the past three or four months. When eight to ten items have been generated, let them select three or four to work on.

Step 3. After the situations have been selected, each individual notes the decision styles used.

Step 4. Ask the individuals to share their perceptions of the style used. After a discussion, there is usually substantial agreement, although subordinates often view the manager's techniques differently.

Step 5. After the discussion, the group then analyzes the situations using the decision model to determine what the theory suggests as an appropriate style. They evaluate both the actual and the recommended.

Step 6. Conduct a general discussion of the model and its implications. Usually, the manager and the subordinates are surprised by the assumptions each made about the other. In some areas the manager thought subordinates wanted to be involved, but they often preferred that the manager use less involving styles or make the decision unilaterally. In other areas they wanted to be more involved. The process of clarifying such preferences, and negotiating decision styles on this basis is one of the positive outcomes of such an experience.

Step 7. Have the group identify major decisions to be made in the next three to four months and replicate the rest of Step 2 and Steps 3 through 6 above. This step allows participants to express their preferences.

General Comments: In using this design it is critical that the manager be fully aware of the model and its implications and that she volunteer for such training. Usually, more effective managers who are fairly secure in their ability are able to risk involvement with subordinates in a discussion such as this design generates.

Time: Six to seven hours (a full day workshop).

CONCLUSIONS

Central to the task of a nursing leader and to the functioning of health organizations is the development of effective processes for solving problems and making decisions. The qualitative growth and development of leaders embraces these essential components. It is difficult to conceive of any meaningful process of either personal or professional growth and development that does not comprise problem solving and decision making. Moreover, it is equally difficult to conceive of a process of learning *how* to solve problems and make decisions which does not include tangible practice by direct involvement. The growth and development of effective managers, and of all people in organizations, depends upon the depth of their participation in these processes and in learning the associated skills. Sadly, many managers feel they only have two choices—make the decision or delegate it to subordinates. There are a range of alternatives between these extremes.

Additionally, many leaders fail to use sufficiently the human resources available to them. In many cases (and numerous observers would say "most cases") the manager does the bulk of the problem solving and decision making. From some perspectives, (his own growth and development), the authoritarian style is satisfactory, but often an overload hinders devoting adequate time to any one area, and acquiring ample knowledge to formulate sound decisions. Thus the quality of decision declines. In addition, subordinates are denied practice in solving problems and making decisions; their growth and development is retarded.

Finally, research links involvement in problem solving and decision making with the implementation of decisions. Most decisions are implemented by employees whose understanding and motivation are improved when they have a voice in the process.

Thus, there are authoritative reasons for involvement of those who have a stake in the problem or are responsible for implementing it. Unfortunately, participation has been treated as an "ought" in much of the nursing literature, so that many managers find themselves feeling guilty for not involving followers. The use of a particular decision-making process, however, is a situational matter. In some instances followers should not be (and often do not want to be) involved; in other situations, they should (and want to be) involved. The question then becomes "how and how much."

By delineating the situational factors which may be encountered while providing quality nursing care, the Vroom and Yetton model increases the probability that decisions will reflect an awareness of the variables that interplay in a system. These include the leader, followers, clients, environment, goals, time and urgency. The tool and experiential model have been successfully utilized in educational settings as well as in staff development programs. The results have been consistently positive, and follow-up studies have further documented its usefulness in practice.

The range of decision process alternatives, then, can be depicted analytically with substantial, concomitant benefits to administrators, personnel, and, ultimately, our patients.

REFERENCES

1. March, J. G., and Simon, H. A. *Organizations.* New York: Wiley, 1958.

2. Tannenbaum, R., and Schmidt, W. How to choose a leadership pattern. *Harvard Business Review,* Vol. 36, No. 2, 1958, pp. 95–101.

3. Maier, N. R. F. *Problem Solving and Creativity in Individuals and Groups.* Belmont, California: Brooks-Cole, 1970.

4. Vroom, V. H., and Yetton, P. W. *Leadership and Decision Making.* Pittsburgh: University of Pittsburgh Press, 1973.

5. Maier, N. R. F. 1970.

6. Vroom, V. H., and Yetton, P. W. 1973.

7. Vroom, V. H. A new look at managerial decision making. *Organizational Dynamics,* Vol. 1, No. 4, 1973, pp. 66–80.

8. Vroom, V. H., and Yetton, P. W. 1973.

9. Vroom, V. H., and Jago, A. G. Decision making as a social process. *Decision Sciences,* Vol. 5, No. 4, 1974, pp. 743–769.

10. Maier, N. R. F. *Problem Solving Discussions and Conferences.* New York: McGraw-Hill, 1963.

11. Vroom, V. H., and Yetton, P. W. 1973.

12. Maier, N. R. F. 1963.

13. Finch, F. E., et al. *Managing for Organizational Effectiveness.* New York: McGraw-Hill, 1976.

11

Teaching-Learning

The focus of this chapter is on the teaching-learning process. Discussion revolves around diagnosing the learning needs of care-givers and -receivers in order to carry out the nursing process methods to their fullest potential. Learning principles and teaching strategies are discussed and form the foundation for teaching and learning in nursing practice.

TEACHING–LEARNING AND THE NURSING PROCESS

Teaching involves a behavioral method for facilitating another person's learning. Learning is an internal experience for the receiver. It denotes an integration of thoughts, ideas, theory, and experience—past and present. The areas of self included in the PELLEM Pentagram (Chapter 20) are guides through which one can understand the integration of teaching behaviors into a person's cognitive, affective, and psychomotor processes, resulting in learning. Further, learning is change since new matter added within a system (specifically a person) produces an added mind-dimension that makes a person different than before the process began.

Keeping the focus of teaching and learning in mind while using the nursing process and interacting with a client and the client's system, two functions are involved. First, the nurse assesses the learning needs of the client; these become the teaching responsibilities of the nurse. Second, to carry out teaching responsibilities, the nurse must assess learning needs of self relative to teaching the client—does the nurse have the background to know what should be taught and the best method for doing so? The teaching-learning process can therefore be conceptualized as a two-way interaction between learner and teacher, each dimension being dependent on the other with both parties learning.

It follows that the nurse becomes involved in two diagnostic steps:

1. Assessing the learning needs of the client—nursing diagnoses; and,
2. Assessing the nurse's own learning needs to carry out teaching responsibilities—self-diagnosis.

It is deemed essential that the professional nurse consider both steps to provide comprehensive nursing care. The experience of the author has found that learning needs infinitely exist. This open-end must be clothed with the variables of priority, time, and space, reflective of a given purpose. Further, the author admonishes continual consideration of these steps so as not to close doors before realizing what is being shut-out. With this rhetoric, learning needs should be considered in light of past and present educational theory.

LEARNING THEORY PRINCIPLES

Conley (1973, pp. 212–214) explicates eight generalizations from the literature on learning theories. She has synthesized a wealth of theory and research. Each principle is discussed separately and applied into the framework of the chapter:

1. *"Learning requires perceiving* (Conley)." Many years ago Dewey (1938, 1961) interpreted learning as a sociologic phenomenon between an organism and the organism's environment. It is important that learners perceive a situation or subject matter as something that is important for themselves and is relevant and/or needed. Bruner (1977) calls this learning readiness.
2. *"Unique characteristics of the learner govern the extent of what is integrated* (Conley)." Differences between learners have been noted by many theorists in education. Piaget underscored intellectual variations based on the developmental maturation of a human being (Ginsburg and Opper, 1969; Wadsworth, 1971). Thorndike noted individual differences while developing "connectism" as a theory (Hilgard, 1956) and Wertheimer (1945), a Gestalt psychologist, earmarked the importance of past experience in learning. Research has consistently proven that learning differences exist between individuals and the disparity can be attributed to a variety of factors.
3. *"The degree of learning is influenced by one's environment* (Conley)." Again coming from a sociological framework, behaviorists such as Watson (1916, 1928), Dewey (Hilgard, 1956) in his functionalist perspective, and von Bertalanffy (1968) in systems theory have shown that the environment is an important learning variable.
4. *"Learning is dependent upon the activity of the learner* (Conley)." This principle involves problem solving and behavior toward goal accomplishment by the learner. Hull (1942) discussed this in terms of his drive reduc-

tion theory. When one has a need or drive to learn, problem-solve, or accomplish, one is so motivated to satisfy this need.

5. *"Motivation of the learner influences what is learned* (Conley)." Internal motives such as achievement, esteem, and self-actualization (Maslow, 1954), as well as external drives and incentives must be considered. Both play a key role in determining what one learns.

6. *"Reinforcement of desired behavior increases the probability that the behavior will reoccur in another situation* (Conley)." Behaviorist theories have long documented this principle; positive reinforcement of those behaviors that one desires is effective.

7. *"Transfer of learning occurs when similar conditions are present in old and new situations* (Conley)." Thorndike (Hilgard, 1956) was very early in documenting this principle. Guthrie (1952) later reaffirmed that a stimulus pattern that produces a certain response will tend to replicate the response if it or a similar pattern is repeated. Bruner (1977) underscored the importance of transfer in learning through this principle.

8. *"Practice determines the effectiveness and efficiency in learning* (Conley)." Repetition is of primary importance in learning but the learner must possess knowledge of practice at each point. Thorndike (Hilgard, 1956) was early in noting this effect. Research has found that time between practice periods and evaluation between intervals facilitates learning.

Understanding and use of general principles developed by learning theorists must ground a nurse's teaching processes. Within this framework, there are a variety of instructional modes and media that the nurse can employ to meet the learning needs of client and self.

TEACHING STRATEGIES

The use of teaching strategies must be based on principles of learning, as well as dimensions of the learner and the teacher. The term strategy implies a means or method for achievement of a goal. It is not the aim of teaching but rather the vehicle through which teaching occurs. This vehicle should reflect the best way to accomplish teaching objectives synchronized with the perceived best means by which the learner will integrate new knowledge and the experience and ability of the teacher in using the strategy.

There are no absolutes in choosing a teaching strategy and the instructor is limited only by personal ingenuity and creativity in composing a variety of modes and media around teaching objectives and what is known about the client and self. It is with this background that this portion of the chapter broadly discusses teaching strategies—modes and media—as they apply in nursing practice. They can be considered as a resource pool from which a nurse can draw but not be limited.

Conley (1973) distinguishes modes from media by designating *modes* as types of conversations between teacher and learner; *media* are devices or props used in instruction to extend what is discussed. Conley provides the types of modes and media; the author amplifies each in nursing practice, when appropriate.

Modes

1. *Lecture.* This is the most widely used mode in education systems and consists mainly of one-way communication—teacher-to-learner. In one to one teaching situations, this framework has little application. It is useful, however, in reaching large groups of clients who share a particular learning need and remains best when followed by group discussion, thus reinforcing the intended learning.
2. *Group Discussion.* This is a group learning format that facilitates integration of new material by enabling two-way conversation between teacher-learners and learner-learners. It is one of the best means for development and discussion of ideas, feelings, beliefs, and experiences around a particular content area. In this mode, the teacher is often seen as a facilitator of learning with expertise in the topic. This has been found as most beneficial when learners shared a particular problem or disability and support can be given and shared. It tends to destroy the myth of being alone and can build bonds of assistance between clients, staff, and colleagues.
3. *Panel discussion.* Again, this a more formal method and can be used in teaching client groups as can the lecture. An interplay or mini-group discussion can occur between panel members on a topic with the audience being listeners and occasionally raisers of questions addressed to members of the presenting panel.
4. *Seminar.* Respecting nursing practice, the seminar is most useful for self-learning situations in groups of peers. The typical format involves one or two members presenting an idea, problem, or issue, with everyone then discussing it. The team conference, as discussed in Chapter 6, can be equated with this mode.
5. *Demonstration.* The demonstration involves use of media by the teacher to personify what is intended for learning by the audience. This can occur with any number of participants from large groups. An example is a nurse demonstrating the act of giving insulin, using the necessary equipment, plus an orange, doll, or self. Steps and procedures of the task are the foci and learners may then be given the opportunity to practice also. This latter aspect is reflective of the next mode.
6. *Laboratory instruction.* Instruction in a laboratory is usually used in formal student learning where self-discovery is the primary basis for learning. Simulations may be involved and didactic presentation may precede or

follow the event. In nursing practice, laboratory instruction may follow teacher demonstration, thereby providing the opportunity for "trying on" the new behaviors in a safe environment with assistance if this is required.

7. *Team teaching.* Team teaching occurs when two or more professionals carry the responsibility for fulfilling specific teaching objectives with a client or group. In reality, this is most often the case in nursing practice situations, especially with a team nursing model of delivery. Communication between teachers on the team is underscored as essential and the learner has the opportunity to experience several perspectives in a given area. Learning can be enhanced if the team concept is put into operation but two separate people doing the same thing can be oppressive; team teaching mandates coordination and integration of all efforts.

Media

Media are devices chosen and used to amplify the aforementioned modes of teaching.

1. *Programmed instruction and computer-assisted instruction.* Both media comprise teaching machines or books that carry a learner step by step through content. They offer immediate feedback to the learner in terms of correct responses to questions that usually follow theory. Two-way communication indirectly occurs between the author of the material and the learner. This method has benefit as an augmentor of learning in nursing practice environments. It is best when preceded and followed by group discussion or one-to-one talks with the teacher.

2. *Television.* Closed circuit and public television is becoming increasingly popular in education. Closed-circuit television can employ videotapes prepared by teachers on a given content area for teaching a specified audience. It is commonly found in medical and dental offices for use by clients in learning. Public television involves many areas; some are specific in content and others provide vicarious experience of direct health education. Hospital situation dramas are a prime example of the latter; television specials addressing such topics as life after death or rape, for instance, are examples of the former.

3. *Motion pictures.* These can be useful in learning when they are specific to the content requiring teaching. Conley (1973) describes motion pictures as similar to demonstration when the films amplify content.

4. *Simulations.* This is primarily involved with laboratory learning and demonstration. Everything that must be achieved is presented in a hypothetical situation, with low-risk and a safe environment provided by the teacher. Cognitive, affective, and psychomotor aspects of learning are all amplified and group or one-to-one discussion usually precedes and follows

the simulation. Further, these simulations can be videotaped and used as media in future endeavors. The humanistic exercises in this book are examples of simulations.

5. *Pictorial presentations and printed language.* These forms of media are most often employed by nurses. Pictures and figures with adjacent explanations are helpful in reinforcing learning that has occurred via a specific mode. They should be used to augment learning. Filmstrips and slides are other examples of this teaching mode.

6. *Tape and disc recordings.* These can be helpful in self-learning, group discussions, and seminars when what is recorded focuses on a situation or presentation that talks to the topic in focus. Often, tape or disc recordings provide narration or an explanation of slides.

7. *Models.* These are usually representations of objects needed in demonstration. A model may be a female pelvis that can be taken apart in order to portray childbirth. Again, as with other media, models illustrate what one wishes to teach.

It should be recognized that whatever mode or method is chosen for teaching objectives, personality aspects of both the learner and teacher should be considered. If the client is observed as shy and uncomfortable with groups, that mode is contraindicated. Moreover, if the nurse is inexperienced or nervous demonstrating with groups, another mode is indicated. The decision of using modes and media must portray the best possible learning environment for all the interacters in the situation.

SUMMARY

Discussion of teaching-learning began with its pertinence in nursing practice. Principles gleaned from learning theory were presented followed by specific teaching strategies. Within teaching strategies, a variety of modes and media were presented.

REFERENCES

Bruner, J. *The process of education.* Cambridge, Mass.: Harvard University Press, 1977.

Conley, V. *Curriculum and instruction in nursing.* Boston: Little, Brown and Company, 1973.

Dewey, J. *Experience and education.* New York: Macmillan, 1938.

Dewey, J. *Democracy and education.* New York: Macmillan, 1961.

Ginsburg, H., and Opper, S. *Piaget's theory of intellectual development*. Englewood Cliffs, N. J.: Prentice-Hall, 1969.

Guthrie, E. *The psychology of learning*. New York: Harper and Row, 1952.

Hilgard, E. *Theories of learning*. New York: Appleton-Century-Crofts, 1956.

Hull, C. Conditioning: Outline of a systematic theory of learning. In *The psychology of learning*. Forty-first Yearbook of the National Society for the Study of Education, Part II. Chicago: University of Chicago Press, 1942.

Maslow, A. *Motivation and personality*. New York: Harper and Row, 1954.

von Bertalanffy, L. *General system theory*. New York: George Braziller Company, 1968.

Wadsworth, B. *Piaget's theory of intellectual development*. New York: David McKay Company, 1971.

Watson, J. The place of the conditioned reflex in psychology. *Psychological Review* 23: 89, 1916.

Watson, J. *Psychological care of infant and child*. New York: W. W. Norton, 1928.

Wertheimer, M. *Productive thinking*. New York: Harper and Brothers, 1945.

SELECTED READING

The following article by O'Connor (1978) describes the process of assessing learning needs of self. O'Connor provides a means for studying one's own needs for continued education; this process can stand alone in its purpose. It can also be applied, however, in similar situations involving the assessment of learning needs.

Diagnosing Your Needs for Continuing Education

Andrea B. O'Connor

The increased interest in continuing education has resulted in a proliferation of formal continuing education programs, self-study devices, as well as inservice education offerings to provide learning resources for nurses. The learning needs of nurses as a whole have been surveyed, but little is available to help the individual practitioner design a continuing education program to meet personally determined needs.

Too often, nurses who recognize continuing education as necessary enroll in programs simply because they "seem interesting" or "are available" or "offer CEUs." Most of us would agree that selection from the learning resources available should be based on an assessment of learning needs that will provide a basis for improving skills and adding knowledge for use in present or future practice. To do this one must know how to diagnose one's own learning needs.

There are three areas nurses can examine in their self-diagnostic process: the present level of their practice competence; their future professional goals; and their professional awareness, which includes issues and trends in the health care field in general and in nursing in particular. By assessing individual learning needs in each area, the nurse should be able to determine those needs and develop an education program that can be revised and expanded as old needs are satisfied and new ones emerge.

In his book *Self-Directed Learning,* Malcolm Knowles[1] provides an approach to self-assessment of learning needs that is applicable in these three areas. This involves

1. Developing a model of required competencies;
2. Assessing one's practice in relation to the model;
3. Identifying the gaps between one's own knowledge and skills and those required by the model.

There are numerous models that can be used to assess one's present level of practice.

Such formal criteria of competence as the American Nurses' Association's Standards of Nursing Practice give a broad picture of the knowledge, skills, and behaviors which constitute competent professional practice. These standards include those for nurse practitioners and standards formulated by the divisions of Community Health Nursing, Gerontological Nursing,

Reprinted with permission from *American Journal of Nursing,* Vol. 78, No. 3. Copyright 1978 by the American Journal of Nursing Company.

Maternal and Child Health Nursing, Medical/Surgical Nursing, and Psychiatric and Mental Health Nursing. Specialty nursing organizations have also developed other statements or standards either for nurses now practicing or those entering a specialty.

Nursing journals frequently publish articles on "ideal" nursing practice in particular care situations, and these constitute an additional model source.

Self-administered tests, such as "Test Yourself," which appears monthly in the *American Journal of Nursing*, the nursing examination review books published by the Medical Examination Publishing Co.,[2] and "Nursing Decisions," published by Docent Corp.,[3] provide a model of competence in terms of a knowledge base required in specific practice settings.

Peers or coworkers offer an at-hand source of model identification that can be used in two ways to identify an "ideal" practitioner whom one might wish to emulate, or, in group meetings with peers, to identify a model of practice that might serve as an "ideal" in a particular setting.

The model against which a nurse can assess her present practice may be one or a combination of these models, depending on the practice situation. For example, a nurse working in an acute neurosurgical setting may select aspects of models identified in the American Nurses' Association standards, in literature, and in and by peers and coworkers to construct a picture of competent nursing practice in a neurosurgical setting.

Diagnosing one's own level of practice is a difficult aspect of self-directed learning. Traditional educational experiences provided a built-in assessment in the form of grading: one knew where one was and took little formal responsibility for determining competence. Objective examination of one's weaknesses and strengths in practice is a skill that takes time to develop.

A beginning approach to self-assessment most obviously occurs in the course of practice. During one week, a nurse might focus on her professional competencies by jotting down questions that come to mind while giving nursing care. Perhaps it is a new drug whose actions are unknown to her, or the realization that she is uncertain about the normal values of test results to be interpreted. I'm sure we have all thought to ourselves, "I'll have to look that up later," but never do. By making notes of such questions as they come up, a nurse can begin to formulate a list of knowledges valuable to her in the clinical setting.

Also important in assessing one's practice is an awareness of those nursing activities one tends to avoid or that make one uncomfortable. Later examination of these situations can provide clues regarding areas of deficiency.

Another obvious basis for assessment is identification of skills one wishes to improve or knowledges that seem superficial.

In the course of self-diagnosis one must be careful to take note of those aspects of practice which represent competence and skill; that is, both positive and negative practices should be recognized, assessed and recorded.

The opinions of others also can be helpful. These may be presented in formal performance ratings by superiors or be elicited from peers or superiors.

Once a model of practice has been identified and one has completed a self-assessment of present practice competence, the two should be compared. Knowles suggests listing those "performance elements" (knowledges, skills, and behaviors) identified in the model and then rating oneself on a scale of 1 to 10 (low to high) for each of the identified elements. Such a rating would reveal areas that need work and form the basis for planning continuing learning projects.

A similar approach to that outlined above can be used in assessing learning needs for future practice. A first step would be the nurse's identification of what expanded or extended roles might be pursued for the future. For example, a nurse in an acute medical setting may decide she would like to become a respiratory care nurse specialist in the future; a nurse working in a delivery room may be attracted to midwifery; or a nurse in a clinic setting or a doctor's office may identify a family nurse practitioner role as a possible future career.

Having decided on one or more goals or possible areas for extended or expanded practice, the nurse should locate models to determine the competencies and educational criteria for these roles. Such models may exist, again, in formal standards or nursing literature and certainly can be found in nurse specialists who are practicing in these areas.

The nurse's self-assessment in relation to such models should extend to the practical aspects of pursuing an educational program to attain such goals. For example, a clinical specialty role may require a master's degree. The nurse must determine whether pursuit of such a degree is feasible. Or, an intensive continuing education program may be requisite for entry into an extended role. Will time and finances or personal considerations permit attendance at such a program?

The area of "professional awareness," encompassing issues and trends in the health care field and in nursing, and including legislative and legal problems, is a more nebulous area for needs assessment in terms of continued learning. The nurse who is satisfied with her present level of practice competence or is pursuing a continuing program of learning to maintain or update practice skills may still feel some deficiencies in terms of involvement with or understanding of issues and trends affecting professional nursing practice.

Here, one can turn to journals and publications of nursing associations for news of the profession or health care in general. Attendance at meetings of professional groups, such as district or state nurses associations, the local chapter of the National League for Nursing, or a local group of specialty practitioners can provide information on emerging issues and trends important to the profession.

With "professional awareness" thus enhanced, the nurse can now go on to develop a list of knowledges required to actively pursue a solution to a problem or to broaden understanding and awareness of a trend. Pursuit of a learning program to achieve such knowledges coupled with active engagement in programs to solve problems in the profession will serve to further broaden the nurse's "professional awareness" and provide yet another program for continued learning.

REFERENCES

1. Knowles, Malcolm. *On self-directed learning.* New York: Association Press, 1975.
2. Medical Examination Publishing Co. 65-36 Fresh Meadow Lane, Flushing, N.Y. 11365.
3. Docent Corp. 430 Manville Rd., Pleasantville, N.Y. 10570.

12

Group Processes

Group processes involve the study and analysis of how people communicate with each other. Chapter 8 emphasized the importance of effective communication skills in nursing and all helping professions. The study of group processes provides a means to analyze communications of groups with the goal of rendering them more effective.

Chapter 12 begins with a discussion of rationale for looking at a group's behavior followed by its importance in nursing practice and education. Common group tasks follow with role functions exhibited by members concluding the chapter.

RATIONALE FOR STUDYING GROUP BEHAVIOR

Group process is one of the most important facets of organizational work, especially when human beings are the focus of the system. Further, when several people must pool their knowledge, experience, and skill in carrying out goals of helping, the need for effective group functioning must be underscored. It must be noted that "group process" and "individualized care" are not contradictory terms. The former helps to accomplish the latter when more than one individual must be involved in whatever process is in focus. (For example, developing nursing care plans involves all care-givers plus the client's system.) Group process is a means for accomplishing individualized care.

According to system theory (described in Chapter 19), a system (or group) is more than a sum of its parts (von Bertalanffy, 1968); the outcome of group functioning is a combination of what each member contributes plus the interactive effects that occur between members. It can be concluded, therefore, that when people are working toward a common goal, in addition to the task other things are happening. Theorists in group behavior name these dimensions content and process variables.

Content variables are simply concerned with the task(s) of the group. They involve what the group is talking about, what it needs to accomplish, and/or its goals and objectives. The foremost sub-tasks of a group are usually to make decisions, problem-solve, and draw conclusions regarding group content. Practically speaking, if a group of nurses meet in a team conference to pool knowledge that each individual has regarding a client—with the goal of developing a care plan and determining the best nursing orders that would have the highest probability for alleviating the nursing diagnosis—all knowledge and discussion would be considered content variables of the group's work.

The second classification of variables are *process dimensions* and generally involve the communication patterns of the group members, climate of the environment in which tasks are carried out, group conflict, decision-making procedures, and members' commitment to objectives.

Content and process variables both play an equally important role in the success of a group's work. Unfortunately, it is the latter variable that is often overlooked and rarely observed. Perhaps this may be due to a lack of knowledge on the procedures for studying process dimensions or little awareness of its importance; both are emphasized in this chapter.

THE IMPORTANCE OF EFFECTIVE
GROUP PROCESSES IN NURSING

As described throughout this book, nursing is a human service—it is a dynamic, open system. "Dynamic" means that it is ever-changing and growing/learning, and "open" refers to the fact that people and environmental factors move in and out in response to the system's goals. It can be logically deduced that the nursing care system is never totally independent or in isolation of others. The author wishes to clarify the difference between autonomous and independent. Autonomous refers to a particular nurse or nursing practice which governs its own actions; independence, interdependence, and dependence refer to the type of action that the nurse uses to fulfill the purposes. Independent actions are actions which rely on and are controlled by the individual nurse; interdependent actions rely on and are controlled by the nurse and other systems. Dependent actions rely on and are controlled by persons or situations other than the nurse. A nurse uses all of these roles, respective of the situation, but the nurse's purpose is always shared with others.

The literature continues to expand on the importance of group processes in nursing as well as health practices (Maloney, 1967; Marram, 1973; Sampson and Marthas, 1977). Marram (1973) states the scope of group work can include psychotherapy groups, therapeutic groups (such as those with a homogeneous factor such as aging), self-help groups, and growth or self-actualization groups. Sampson and Marthas (1977) more specifically delineate target groups for health professionals and their function:

Target Group	Functions
1. Patient care	a. Human growth and development
	b. Maintenance of health*
	c. Restoration to fullest health potential*
2. Patient and self-help groups	Health promotion and maintenance
3. Other health professionals/team practice	a. Behavior change
	b. Behavior maintenance
	c. Education*
4. Families	a. Behavior change
	b. Behavior maintenance
	c. Education*
5. Community groups/informal groups in institutions	a. Organizing ⎫ Toward
	b. Leading ⎬ Goal
	c. Managing ⎭ Attainment*
6. Persons undergoing training and supervision	a. Client and family support and education
	b. Learning in formal educative systems*

The reader is advised to comb the literature should more documentation of the indices for group work be required. There are very few instances in the day of a nursing professional when two or more people are not involved with a task. For this very important reason, effective group processes must be facilitated and studied. Moreover, the skills and systems addressed in this book all involve group work—from leadership activities, collaborating with associates or listening, to observing and developing care plans with and for clients.

Common Group Tasks

The various groups in which nurses are involved have been discussed in the previous portion of this chapter. Even though only examples are provided, it has been shown that the bulk of nursing practice and education involves working with and through a group. Common tasks of each group can be circumscribed with the goal of rendering group function more effective; subgoals are to increase the awareness of self, and foster inquiry, risk-taking, and

*The author's additions.

learning of each member. Common group tasks involve what participants must do to study content and process variables. They are outlined as follows:

Content
Accomplish a task
  Identify issues
  Discuss alternatives
  Make decisions
Information-sharing
Learning new material
  Cognitive
  Affective
  Psychomotor

Process
Study communication patterns between members
Discuss group climate
Identify points of conflict between members
Look at the manner in which decisions are made
Share individual's commitment to the group's goal(s)

Looking at the outline of content and process variables descriptions, these areas need to be applied specifically. Working first with content, accomplishing a task follows a problem-solving method. Whether the task is to develop a nursing care plan or decide on the protocol for a nursing procedure, gathering relevant expertise for input into the eventual outcome is viewed as necessary to insure the highest quality possible in the results. Further, acceptance of the results is also shared when members have had input in the outcome. Both of these facets, however, are qualified on the effectiveness of the group's process. If, for example, two divergent schools of thought emerge in the alternatives with no resolution and just a majority ruling, the members supporting the losing thoughts may not feel comfortable with a part of the decision, may not accept it, and may not fully implement it. This points out the interdependence of content and process.

Information-sharing may be a team leader's report regarding assignments. Two-way communication (Chapter 8) is essential in group work since the term "group" denotes more than two participants. Information-sharing emphasizes collaborative or consultative qualities rather than just authoritative decision-making. The author wishes to emphasize that a team leader's individual report, for example, may be indeed indicated; but call it as it is—one-way communication. If the group is or should be involved by design in the decision, then two-way channels of communication must be maintained.

Learning new materials, whether in formal or informal educational modalities (Chapter 11), must be presented accurately in terms of group involvement. If a mode or medium is used that limits or forbids two-way communication processes, then present it as such. If group learning is the intent, the same protocol as discussed in this section remains intact and indicated. Remember that affective and psychomotor learning is best facilitated when two-way processes are open. Another point is that leader clarity and honesty in intent is a positive group builder. There is nothing wrong with a leader just giving information or imparting knowledge; there is a potential problem when a leader says the group will be involved in solving a problem but then presents information that denotes the leader's decision has been made and will be followed.

Process variables encompass certain dimensions, according to the aforementioned outline, and generally have the effect of strengthening group relationships and achieving quality outcomes if they are facilitated and studied properly. The reader is directed to Benne and Sheats (1948) and Sampson and Marthas (1977) for congruent and in-depth discussions of the process variables synthesized by the author.

Communication Patterns   Communication patterns involve the social organization of the group. Who is talking to whom, informal leadership, word selection, nonverbal behavior, and many other nuances can be indicators of messages which may or may not be related to the group task. The purpose of studying social organization is to draw out member issues and focus in on task issues effectively.

Climate of the Group   The climate has to do with the overall tone of the group. Is it competitive? Tense? Polite? Friendly? Flat and lifeless? Energized? Enthusiastic? All these and many more adjectives give indication of how the group members feel about the task; all must be studied. If a group's climate is positive, it might be helpful in the future to be aware of why the group was so inclined. Future endeavors could be modeled after a positive group experience. Also, sharing enthusiasm can create positive experiences; enthusiasm is catching. The task, therefore, will be carried out with zest. Conversely, should a group engender a negative climate, this could (and usually will) affect the outcome and feelings of the members regarding working with that specific group and/or others, as well as the task at hand. This too has a ladder effect — only downward.

Points of Conflict   Conflict in the group must be identified and worked out before effective problem-solving can take place and before information can be received to its fullest potential. Conflict tends to dissipate energy away from the goals and directs it toward the point of conflict. It is difficult to quietly handle two items simultaneously.

If conflict is an issue and blocks goal accomplishment, it is necessary to set aside the task and work on alleviating the disagreement. The most effective avenue for identifying conflict is by allowing time for processing the group's work. This also tends to dampen the intensity of a conflict because it can open potential areas for concern before they grow out of proportion.

Manner of Making Decisions   The manner in which decisions are made by a group bears study. Schein (1969) discusses six ways in which this task can be accomplished:

1. *Decision by lack of response* ("plop"). This is seen as the least visible method and involves several members consecutively suggesting decisions without due discussion of any. The group in essence bypasses ideas and then decides immediately on one. There may be a hidden agenda operating and the suggesters may feel that the decisions they individually support remain not supported by fellow members. This engenders feelings of not being heard, having nothing to say worthy of listening to, and many other negative feelings.
2. *Decision by authority rule*. Involved in this process is power, and use of position power is fine if this intent is clear. Should a leader say that he or she will make the decision but desires consultation, then this method is positive. Conversely, if a leader proposes group decision-making and then ends discussion with his or her own conclusion, members may feel angry and rightfully so.
3. *Decision by minority*. This is a result of one, two, or three people employing pressure tactics to railroad a decision. The balance of the membership are usually left feeling helpless and impotent.
4. *Decision by majority rule: voting and/or polling*. By far the most familiar method for making decisions is to ask formally (voting) or informally (polling) for the members' position on the issue: for it, against it, or abstention. This is most positive following discussion of an issue and if members agree that this will be the decision-making style. Should implementation of a decision be fulfilled by the voting membership, it may be more effective to decide by consensus. This statement is based on the fact that one may not be committed to the decision unless one so believes in it.
5. *Decision by consensus*. Schein (1969) calls this a psychologic state whereby all members see rationale in the decision and agree to support it. This operates even though some members may be in the minority vote.
6. *Decision by unanimous consent*. This method is logically perfect but rarely attained. There may be instances when unanimous decisions should be made (crime conviction, for example) but usually consensus is sufficient in our operations.

Commitment   The last process variable is the individual's sharing commitment and interest in the group's goal. This factor can have an impressive effect on the quality of the outcome and the time it takes to reach the goal. It is mentioned last but should be considered equally.

Process variables must be studied throughout group work. An easy design is to set aside approximately ten minutes of the agenda time to look at these variables. It is a good investment!

Feedback   Study of process variables usually involves feedback. The purpose of giving feedback to group members or individuals is to increase shared understanding about behavior, feelings, and motivations; to help in developing a growth relationship—building trust and openness between members; and giving information to a person or group on how the person or group affects others. Napier and Gershenfeld (1973) suggest criteria for feedback, based on their belief that it should be done in a manner that creates minimal defenses and maximum acceptance.

1. The information about the group should be descriptive and not colored by value-laden adjectives of a good/bad nature.
2. The examples of group behavior being discussed should be specific and clarified through examples.
3. Whenever possible, the information should be given sooner rather than later. The longer the time between the behavior and its discussion, the less value it has for the listener.
4. The information must be confined to matters which are within the power of the group.
5. The group must seek the feedback. If it is not solicited, it will be met with resistance and probably have little positive impact.
6. A person and a group can only internalize a certain amount of information about itself at any one point in time. It is important not to overload the system with more than it can handle.
7. If a person presents a perception of how the group behaved in a certain instance, it is important to discover whether or not others share this view. This increases the reliability of the observation.

Role Functions of Group Members

Understanding of group process involves another dimension, that of studying the roles that group members assume in their group work. Roles are helpful to the group's learning regardless of its own structure, that is, communication and power; equally important is awareness by the members on how they perceive their own functioning, juxtaposed or harmonious with how others see them. All involve consciousness-raising toward the goals of increasing effectiveness in group endeavors. Benne and Sheats (1948) identified

three major categories through which group roles can be studied: task, maintenance, and personal. They further delineated each and noted that members
may assume one or more roles in group work.* Processing and using feedback
on perceptions of people in these roles is an important means to identify,
discuss, and increase awareness of group issues and problems.

Task functions   These relate to the task with which the group is involved:

1. *Initiator*—Introduces new ideas or procedures; tries to establish movement
   towards the goal.
2. *Information seeker*—Tries to obtain needed information or opinions; points
   out gaps in information; asks for opinions; responds to suggestions.
3. *Evaluator*—Tries to determine where the group stands on an issue; tests for
   consensus; evaluates progress.
4. *Coordinator*—Points out relationships among ideas or procedures; pulls
   ideas together and builds on the contributions of others; takes things one
   step further.
5. *Procedural technician*—Expedites group work by performing routine tasks,
   distributing material, etc.
6. *Recorder*—Writes down ideas, decisions, and recommendations; keeps
   minutes.

Maintenance Functions   These are oriented toward the functioning of the
group as a whole unit, building group centered attitudes, and strengthening its
productivity:

1. *Encourager*—Offers warmth and support to another's contribution; accepts
   what each member says.
2. *Harmonizer*—Mediates the differences between members; attempts to
   reconcile disagreements.
3. *Compromiser*—Seeks a middle position between opposing viewpoints.
4. *Standard setter*—Tries to bring to awareness the norms and standards of
   the group.
5. *Gatekeeper*—Keeps communication channels open; facilitates participation
   of all members; keeps track of time.

Self-oriented Roles   These roles involve attempts by members to satisfy their
own needs through the group and are usually not directed toward effective
group work. Self-oriented roles are often seen as dysfunctional.

1. *Aggressor*—Deflates the status of others; attacks the group, its individual
   members, or the task; displays envy towards the contributions by taking
   credit for them.

*The author presents a partial list of roles; please refer to the original source for a complete discussion.

2. *Blocker*—Negative, stubborn opposer who reintroduces issues that have been previously decided upon.
3. *Recognition-seeker*—Works in a myriad of ways to call attention to self; boastful and self-centered.
4. *Playboy*—Displays lack of interest by being cynical or humorous on heavy issues.
5. *Dominator*—Asserts authority or superiority over others by manipulating the group—flatters, interrupts, or gives authoritative directions.
6. *Help-seeker*—Calls attention to self and seeks a sympathetic response from the group.

SUMMARY

The importance of being aware of the part group processes play in goal accomplishment as well as factors that must be considered in analyzing group work were identified. Content and process variables were discussed.

REFERENCES

Benne, K., and Sheats, P. Functional roles of group members. *Journal of Social Issues* 4:41–49, 1948.

Maloney, E. Concepts basic to psychotherapeutic use of group process. In B. Bergersen, E. Anderson, M. Duffey, M. Lohr, and M. Rose. *Current concepts in clinical nursing*, Chapter 14. St. Louis: C. V. Mosby, 1967.

Marram, G. *The group approach in nursing practice.* St. Louis: C. V. Mosby, 1973.

Napier, R., and Gershenfeld, M. *Groups: Theory and experience.* Boston: Houghton-Mifflin, 1973.

Sampson, E., and Marthas, M. *Group process for the health professions.* New York: John Wiley and Sons, 1977.

Schein, E. *Process consultation: Its role in organization development.* Reading, Mass.: Addison-Wesley, 1969.

von Bertalanffy, L. *General system theory.* New York: George Braziller Company, 1968.

SELECTED READING

The selected reading for this chapter is by Elizabeth M. Maloney. Chapter 12 discussed the need for nurses to have knowledge of group process and function effectively in groups; these are requisite in planning individualized care for clients in our present health care system. Taking a different perspective on the need for nurses to know group process, Maloney looks at the expanding arena of therapy groups that she predicts will become widespread methods of health care delivery in our immediate future. Maloney's perspective on groups is different from this author's; however, knowledge of both is important for the practicing nurse.

A Perspective on Groups in the Health Field in the 1980s

Elizabeth M. Maloney

There are literally hundreds of sources where information about groups, group process, analysis of groups and their functioning, research studies on groups for professionals, and a multitude of other facets of the subject can be obtained. Just to give a cross section of nursing publications in the field a few follow: Clark (1), Marrem (2), Pearlmutter (3), and Ramshorn (4). The various kinds of groups deemed worthy of inclusion in the literature approximate several dozen. There are lay groups; professional groups operating along different dimensions; social aggregations; and those falling under the rubric of therapy along another axis. That some overlap exists is a given, since therapy groups for example can also become social groups even if in a sub-rosa fashion.

If one poses the question as to where a professional in the health field encounters groups in the execution of healing work, then again a sizeable list could be presented, this one being more focused. It is in the psychiatric field that the neophyte physician or nurse expects to locate the therapeutic group. Training for group psychotherapy is clearly a specialty within the specialization but it also cross cuts several disciplines such as social work, clinical psychology, nursing, and medicine. If the foregoing seems paradoxical, it is not.

In one university, there are bound to be at least four programs dealing in some curricular fashion with groups. Each one is usually focused on its own frequently repetitive, but closely patterned version of how that specific generic professional group should be educated in dealing with groups. There are then subcultures within each of the health professions whose practitioners are prepared to work out of several disciplines in one form of group work or another. They are most frequently found in psychiatry.

The number of groups, multiplying daily with almost mathematical precision in this country, is surprising in that there is such a climate of acceptance for so many kinds of organizations. Reusch and Bateson (5) pointed out many years ago that groups have always flourished in American soil and link this observation to our national history. Forced to depend upon each other sometimes for life itself in the earlier emigration-pioneer style of existence that prevailed in this country, groups became the sine qua non of existence. There are probably many other compelling reasons, not the least being that from birth onward we are, without having much choice in the matter, in the company of others.

Where then can one limit this vast field of group possibilities in considering available materials so that some direction for nursing practitioners can be mapped? It is probable that the most productive avenue is to lay out two or three directions which might be more future oriented than only related to current practice. These lines are: The need to develop facility in moving from the one-to-one model that is still the ideal of clinician and educator to a more flexible structure. That structure would allow new freedom for the health professional to use the classic one-to-one as the desirable base line and proceed to group processes as a preferred means to individualized care within a therapy group mode. Beginning consideration of this area will be attempted, with an eye to where other modes might be equally acceptable to the client system. A second consideration will be the use of the self-help groups and their relationship to the world of the professional. This phenomenon has many cultural and time bound roots which bear close scrutiny by those who professionally manage the world of the sick. Although nurses deal with such community groups all of the time, only a few have written about it. Bumbalo (6) for example, did a review of self-help groups including criteria for effectiveness and the same year a section on self-help groups was incorporated in a work on groups (7). Emotionally, most nurses are exposed to one or more visits to self-help groups (addiction groups such as Alcoholic Anonymous or various groups of ex-addicts). Whether or not the dynamics of groups such as this are considered theoretically in depth in most educational programs is uncertain.

ONE-TO-ONE: THE IMPOSSIBLE DREAM?

Private entrepeneurs are a vanishing breed in the western world, or nearly so. Most people—most professionals—work and practice in bureaucracies: scientists, social workers, nurses, teachers in public schools, and others all work within a bureaucratic structure. There are private practitioners in every field but becoming more and more common is group practice, certainly in medicine. To the extent that private practice is engaged in among nursing specialists, logistics lead some to form dyadic arrangements (8). Geiger, discussing the change from small medical partnerships to group arrangements, comments on the patients' movement from the "solo practice" (9) to a group practice. He sees it as part of the move towards a pre-paid, contractual arrangement which covers not only sickness but health. The patient, in the context of group practice, learns to accept more than one person as purveyor of care or the "plural provider image in the mind of the patient." (10) The parts may be said to be interchangeable when a person belonging to a group has a health problem over a weekend, for example.

The one to one has been said by Howard (11) to "be useful in studying health care relationships, but it has its limits." Continuing along these lines, one cannot but agree again with Howard that this is an idealized version of practice (12). Looked at critically (seldom done in nursing), it has some identifiable flaws. It follows then that at least an initial critique must be undertaken as to the origin and value attached to what has been called over the years "the one to one."

The likelihood is that this almost mandatory public pairing of nurse and patient in the nursing literature has its genesis in the same tradition as the development of the largely sacrosanct doctor/patient relationship. It is probably necessary to take this ancient partnership as a given, to acknowledge its historical origins in the "art" phase of nursing, and to move to the era of nursing technology. It would be sufficient to note that many of the nursing texts of the last four decades have the word "art" in their title; courses taught were labeled "Nursing Arts"; and in general, this term was one implicitly understood by several generations of nursing. It can be argued that an increasing need to be scientifically technologic shunted the "art" off into a side stream—it has since emerged again in the concept of "humanistic nursing." Probably the last truly possible artistic practice of nursing was in the highest form of private duty (circa 1920) (13). This was the classic one to one.

In this same vein, one source notes that the literature in nursing is "saturated" with isolated factors related to the nurse/patient relationship (14), and goes on to make the point that there are two missing factors in any analysis of relationships between clients and nurses. First is what the reader judges to be optimal conditions for this relationship to proceed therapeutically, and second are the lack of instruments to measure the quality and effectiveness of this event. There is little doubt that a great many of the conceptual schemes in nursing have been set up along the psychoanalytic model lines or at the least, assume continuing and highly individualized nurse/patient contacts. Then, it is important enough to the argument that the "one to one" has assumed unreal significance in the theories of nursing practice, that comment must be made on what appears to be its psychoanalytic origins. A brief analysis therefore of some of the published impact on the folkways in the field yield a diverse array of psychiatric and psychologic sources. As an illustration, the earlier texts suggested that the nurse attend to the physical, emotional, and spiritual needs of patients. (The term *folkways* is used to indicate a discursive level of advice—"shoulds" and "musts" which characterized one era of text writing in American nursing.) Many of the other subsequent sources have an understandably heavy base of behavioral content.

It is now time to regard the nurse/patient duo. There is no question that both nursing and medical intervention are theoretically geared towards the idealized uniqueness of the individual presenting himself for treatment. Equally, there is no question that the orientation of the professional is inevitably in the direction of typification. Can it be otherwise, considering the education of professionals? The vast amount of information inherent in learning any field is geared towards classifying and sorting to a particularized end or "case," from a prior set of laws, rules, principles, hypotheses, and generalizations. In our pursuit of applying theory and science into the art of nursing, we have inadvertently pushed out the facets of care that personify human service. We have not integrated art and science but rather have exchanged science for art. It is a cliche to top all cliches to cite the hospital use of the depersonalizing disease or condition accompanied by a number—"gallbladder or knee in 106." Yet we must look at the persistence of the phenomenon, for it is the kind of behavior that has disenchanted public and practitioner alike.

It is possible the crux of the dilemma can (partially at least) be stated as follows:

1. What to a given individual is a unique health concern of major or minor proportions, is to the professional one of many such encountered conditions.
2. As the encounter passes from the unique (patient) to the common (practitioner), then the question of how much emotional coin can be paid out in tribute to *each* unique event has been, becomes, and will be the crux of the professional dilemma in any service organization.

Many of the concepts and supervised clinical experiences do not give the operational sustenance (real) to carry out the ultimate humanized, aware (ideal) practice. In any event, the precision of such a balancing operation is finely tuned. It is, as Bellin (15) said, also the end product of an educational system which, despite Herculean struggles, remains in the health field at least, in itself, dehumanized. It is yet again the product of focused introspection, considerable capacity for personal growth, and a context in which such practice is given value. This preparation is, among other things, very expensive and the climate of many modern hospitals does not place a high premium on those who would stop and ruminate. It is, however, as Howard (16) said, the best we have. Still, its rigid ideologic base as taught in some educational settings, makes for conflict in neophyte practitioners, for without flexibility, it is an impossible dream. It *is* also hard to posit a more fertile field for disillusionment than to produce practitioners who have this modus operandi as a central value.

PHENOMENA OF THE SELF-HELP GROUP

Health professionals can provide one sort of service for people presenting specific problems, but in the last two decades the rise of numerous self-help or nonprofessional groups has been nothing short of phenomenal. Frequently these groups are auxiliary or adjunctive to professional care, the acute dilemma being dealt with by the professional and the later period, commonly called rehabilitation, becoming the domain of the seasoned self-help group members.

Speculation as to why these groups arose in the first instance ranges across a wide area. It is certain that unsettled conditions in the 1960s exacerbated tendencies such as distrust of authority; an expanded demand for helping services arise and a militant consumer constituency developed. All in all, this perhaps constitutes what one source has characterized as a deprofessionalization (17) trend or movement in Western society. Added to this is the lack of former family unity, with an accompanying decline of the central roles of such institutions as the church and schools. This lack of a social glue common to the neighborhoods of yesterday has contributed heavily to alternate ways of securing support. Thus an expansion of groups which common usage has begun to call self-help groups (18) (19) (20) is a characteristic of urban society.

Nature and Structure of the Self-Help Groups

Who are the self-help groups and what is their structure? As noted earlier, Americans are a group-minded people and there is no question that the proliferation of the groups under discussion fills a vacuum or serves common need. It should also be noted that there are at least two related themes or occurrences which, while not under consideration, are probably part of the same phenomena. These two factors are self-care and self-improvement. The first, self-care, is exemplified by a recent publication by Levin et al (21). Second, there are also literally dozens of self-improving volumes as possibilities for the eager reader. Generally they deal in terms of gaining control of life, out-foxing or one-upping the other fellow through various stratagems, asserting oneself by diverse means, and the like. The only interesting question that might be raised in regard to the latter trend is how many of these books (if any) are read before seeking professional help?

As yet unstudied in any great degree is the process of self-diagnosis and subsequent selection of available treatment modalities. There are probably large numbers of persons who are self-referred to self-help groups, and who find them entirely appropriate in the solution of their specific problem. Subsequently, such individuals may never appear in the statistics of health and illness at all. To carry the point a step further, it can be said that almost always, other routes are tried before approaching the professional, whether the problem is legal, medical, or other. Bloom (22) develops this point in a recent publication.

It would be useful to explore this, since it is so common to find people first exhausting the nonprofessional means at hand in an effort to solve their pressing problems. The first resource at hand is of course the self. People try to deal with the difficulty alone before turning to family, people at work, or (as every physician and nurse has experienced) informal advice from professional friends. Only if no lasting or workable solution emerges, do we call for professional assistance. These days, there are quite a few persons also who unhesitatingly engage in selection of specialists directly. If, for example, they diagnose a sinus difficulty, they tap their informational network and make an appointment with an otolaryngologist. They do not wait for a generalist to refer them to a specialist. As has been pointed out elsewhere,

> The foregoing comments could be summarized operationally as follows: (1) A situation exists where individuals encounter a problem or difficulty in daily living; (2) They make abortive attempts to solve problems on their own; (3) They find that they do not have the necessary knowledge or skill for a solution; (4) Therefore they turn to one

designated by society as an expert in the specific class of difficulty; (5) By so doing, they have instituted a specialized helping process. These steps are the usual preliminaries to the initiation of any professional process. (23)

It is important to add that the selection of one of the self help groupsfollows the same process. An illustration follows: A person suffering from alcoholism can respond to a bus or subway placard with a telephone number to contact a local group, or can secure the same information from television "spots," or can call on the next door neighbor—who has a cousin known to benefited from Alcoholics Anonymous. The steps remain constant: self-diagnosis, self-referral, and avoidance of the professional mainstream when dealing with a health problem. The same process can be followed through with weight loss and smoking, two health problems not necessarily as immediately detrimental as the alcoholic one. (However, according to all current findings, the long term results may equally affect longevity.) Thus, as Levin et al point out, "a second central characteristic of the human services is the major extent to which the consumer serves himself or herself." (24)

Since the self-help group is playing a more prominent part than some health workers are little more than tangentially aware, it is logical to next examine the working structure of these groups, their clientele, and something of how they are perceived or used by professionals.

A partial listing of self-help groups quickly gives an overview of the range and kind available for selected use, and the clientele served usually appears in the title, for example, Gamblers Anonymous. There are groups for medical-surgical patients (ostomy) groups, groups for the aged (Gray Panthers), for the obese (T.O.P.s), for dwarfs (The Little People of America), for persons with Cancer (Cancer Anonymous), for released criminals (Fortune Society), and for drug addiction (Synanon). This is a very truncated list since these groups arise rapidly. New ones are added to the total every year.

Alcoholics Anonymous is frequently cited as a model for a great many of the other groups and is viewed both in medical and nursing texts in the following representative ways in its relationship to the care-cure system.

> Because Alcoholics Anonymous (AA) is the prime resource for the rehabilitation of most alcoholics, all individuals in the community mental health system should understand how AA works. It is a group process. . . .AA is the original self-help group. (25)

> Because AA is the prime resource for the rehabilitation of most alcoholics, all nurses should understand how it works. (26)

> The success of Alcoholics Anonymous in keeping members "dry" is well known and respected by many health professionals. The success of these groups over other orthodox therapies lies largely in the attributes of the groups themselves. (27)

In the above examples from nursing texts, these statements follow nursing care for (usually) the acute phase. It would appear then, that this particular self-help group is frequently viewed (or referrals made to) in terms of a rehabilitative function; in short as a backup to professional treatment. As was seen earlier it is a self-referral organization as well.

What makes these groups work, when they work? It must be noted that they work well for some but by no means for all. Professional care also works well for some but fails for some others. It is in part professional failure which makes some of these groups flourish.

Essentially such groups appear to break through an individual's sense of being alone with a dreadful problem, shared by no one else. Simply finding others who are so burdened relieves a sense of self-defeat and fosters, in some instances, an immediate identification with the people at least, if not the ideology of the particular group.

Available also are models of success; veterans who have gone the same way (someone who has lost 50 lbs in one of the weight reducing organizations, for example) and are available to describe how it was, how it came about, the way it is now, and steps to maintain the new way of life. To some degree, each of these organizations offers or requires changes in life style. Essentially, it is the influence and powers of the group with whom the seeker of help identifies that appears to be the crucial factor in effecting change and in the maintainance of it.

Areas of Overlap between Self-Help Groups and Professionals

Health professionals are more concerned with those persons who, after engaging in abortive attempts to deal with problems, cross over an ill-defined line and become a patient, or who sometimes arrive at hospitals via legal channels, due to an overdose of drugs, acute alcoholism, or severe onset of schizophrenia. Needless to say, these are not popular admissions for several reasons. Some of the reasons are rational, such as lack of suitable space and the like. Some are prejudicial to the individual in terms of embodying a stigmatic or stereotypical class of deviate. So it is with a sense of relief that when the acute phase is finished, referrals can be made to self-help groups. There is relief because there is genuine powerlessness many times as to suitable procedures following the acute phases in addictive and psychologically based "illnesses."

Referral is the concept which sets in motion the operations that go on between a professional and a potential member of self-help groups. There is this viable link, the referral process, from the care system to the self-help system. Many times, this relieves some serious rehabilitative problems for the client and generally solves a very tough problem for the professional group. It should be pointed out that there is often a return referral system from the self-help groups. Should a member fail, the veteran core or old guard of Emphysema Anonymous, for example, know where to direct a member, should the condition become worse and the member be without professional counsel, or there are physicians who deal specifically with addiction problems, known to the group. Each has its available rank of experts.

As pointed out in one excellent work on self-help groups by Gardner and Reissman (28), some diametrically opposed views may emerge when professionals and self-help veterans collide ideologically but the realization that each has a particular function has reduced some of the initial suspicion. It is outside of the scope of this presentation to discuss at any length the particular subculture which encompasses professionals as members of any of these self-help groups. Doctors and nurses are generally a population at risk when it comes to addiction to various drugs. For example, Bissell (29) has studied both doctors and nurses in relation to alcoholism and remission patterns.

CHRONIC AND LONG TERM ILLNESS

One of the most promising places to adapt the skills of group work is in the area of chronic illness. A longer life span has the effect of producing first, more illness, and then sometimes, the requirement for group, residential living. Most nurses are employed in hospitals dealing with short term, acute illnesses. The question as to whether that state of affairs can continue or not, revolves about the definition of illness in this culture as well as what the meaning of clinical practice is to the majority of nurses.

It would be worthwhile to examine some groups which any nurse would agree qualified for the term ill. The psychiatric patient, ill in sufficient numbers to be called the number one health problem; nursing home residents; and rehabilitation center patients are groups of patients in areas in which practicing nurses are conspicuous by their absence. It is probable that if the health needs of our country are to be met, one of two things has to happen. A large number of people entering the professional arenas of the health field have to learn to deal with large groups of people who are defined as ill that they are not now dealing with or the kinds of people who are entering the field will have to change so that care of the future is seen in terms of long-term care and deferred satisfaction for professional nurses. It is this latter area which appears problematic—the lack of quick results. Additionally, in many of the foregoing areas there are large areas of ambiguity to deal with as to probable cause and outcome. These patient cores, plus an increased acceptance of the old in our society, will have to receive additional curricular attention.

Chronic, long-term patients live where they are ill in the instances cited above. Since many are more often ambulatory than not, then facilities for group living must be built into these institutions. The day room is a ubiquitous part of such a setting, for example. Also included are swimming pools, playing fields, and organized game schedules, to name a few of the other accommodations where groups are expected to congregate. it is here that group skills would be very useful to make life more livable in nursing homes and long stay rehabilitation centers.

SUMMARY

An attempt has been initiated to make a case for the classic nurse/patient (now nurse/client relationship) as a desirable ideal; the goals of this ideal can be reached in the future by other forms of group work. An effort was made to call attention to the real need to accept limitations on the heretofore magical aspects of our present health care delivery systems. A renewed attention to groups outside of the psychiatric settings will partially serve this purpose. There are already in the community treatment facilities that are being staffed by professionals, apparently accepting the premise that several people will relate to one client. The interdisciplinary work with families is an excellent example, as was earlier work in the various therapeutic communities in which the total situation acted as "doctor" (26).

NOTES AND REFERENCES

1. Clark, Carolyn. *The Nurse as Group Leader.* New York: Springer Co., 1977.

2. Marrem, Gwen. *The Group Approach in Nursing Practice.* St. Louis: The C. V. Mosby Co., 1973. (See especially Chapter 3 Self-Help Groups.)

3. Pearlmutter, Deanna. Section 3, Working with Groups. In Lucille Joel and Doris Collins (eds.), *Concepts of Psychiatric Nursing.* New York: McGraw-Hill Book Co., 1978.

4. Ramshorn, Mary. The Group as a Therapeutic Tool. *Perspectives in Psychiatric Care,* Vol. 8, No. 5 (1970), 104–105.

5. Reusch, Jengen, and Bateson, Gregory. *Communication.* New York: W. W. Norton and Co., 1951, pp. 109–110.

6. Bumbalo, Judith. The Self Help Phenomenon. *American Journal of Nursing,* Vol. 9 (September, 1977), 1588–1591.

7. Marram, Gwen D. *The Group Approach.* St. Louis: The C. V. Mosby Co., 1973, pp. 39–54 (Chapter 3).

8. Kohnke, Mary, et al. *Independent Nurse Practitioner.* Garden Grove, Calif.: Trainex, 1974.

9. Geiger, Jack. The Causes of Dehumanization in Health Care and Prospects for Humanization. In Jan Howard, and Anslem Strauss, (eds.), *Humanizing Health Care.* New York: John Wiley and Sons, pp. 11–36.

10. Howard, Jan, and Strauss, Anslem, eds. *Humanizing Health Care* (Chapter 4), *Humanization and Dehumanization of Health Care.* New York: John Wiley and Sons, p. 71.

12. Ibid., pp. 70–71.

13. Maloney, Elizabeth. Philosophy in Nursing: Ideal and Real. (Notes from an unpublished paper), Conference on the Nursing and the Humanities: A Public Dialogue, Farmington, Conn., November 11, 1977.

14. Pluckman, Margaret. *Human Communication.* New York: McGraw-Hill Books, Inc., 1978, p. 153.

15. Bellin, Nowell. How Medical Practitioners Get the Scars that Distort Their Human Values. *Professionalism and Human Values.* In Seminar Report, Program of General Education in the Humanities, Columbia University, Vol. 3 (Fall, 1975).

16. Howard, Jan, op cit.

17. Haug, Marie. In Paul Halmos (ed.). *Professionalism and Social Change.* Keele, Staffordshire: The University of Keele, Sociological Review, Monograph No. 20, pp. 195–211.

18. Bumbalo, Judith, op cit., pp. 1588–1591.

19. Marram, Gwen, op. cit., pp. 39–54 (Chapter 3).

20. Gartner, Alan, and Riessman, Frank. *Self Help in the Human Services.* San Francisco: Jossey-Bass Publishers, 1977, p. 13.

21. Levin, Lowell S., Katz, Alfred H., and Holst, Erik. *Self-Care* (Lay initiatives in Health). Prodist, New York, 1976 (Proceedings on the Role of the Individual in Primary Health Care—Joint Center for Studies of Health Programs, Copenhagen, 1975).

22. Bloom, Martin. *The Paradox of Helping.* New York: John Wiley and Sons, 1975, pp. 100–113.

23. Maloney, Elizabeth. The Nursing Process. In Judith Haber (ed.) *Comprehensive Psychiatric Nursing.* New York: McGraw-Hill Book Co., p. 102 (Chapter 7).

24. Levin, Lowell, and Katz, Alfred, op cit., p. 40.

25. Burgess, Ann W., and Lazare, Aaron. *Community Mental Health Problems.* Englewood Cliffs, N. J.: Prentice-Hall, Inc., p. 127.

26. Burgess, Ann W. *Psychiatric Nursing in the Hospital and the Community.* 2nd ed. Englewood Cliffs, N. J.: Prentice-Hall, Inc., 1976, p. 458.

27. Pearlmutter, Deanna. Classifying Psychotherapy Groups. In Lucille Joel and Doris Collins (eds.), *Psychiatric Nursing: Theory and Application.* New York: McGraw-Hill Books, Inc., 1978, pp. 231–237 (Chapter 17, Section 3).

28. Gartner, Alan, and Reissman, Frank, op cit., Chapter 1–3.

29. Bissell, LeClair, Chief Physician, Alcoholism Unit, Roosevelt Hospital (and Smithers Rehabilitation Unit), New York City. Unpublished study presented under auspices of St. Vincent's Hospital, New York City, Spring, 1978.

30. Rapaport, Robert. *Community as Doctor.* London: Tavistock Publications, 1960.

HUMANISTIC EXERCISES

PART II
SKILLS AND COMPETENCIES

EXERCISE 1
Observation

PURPOSES

1. To observe another individual intently to sharpen one's observational skills.
2. To empathize with another.

FACILITY

A classroom large enough to accommodate participants.

MATERIALS

None.

TIME REQUIRED

Twenty minutes.

GROUP SIZE

Unlimited pairs.

DESIGN

1. Members should form pairs.
2. Pairs should sit facing one another for two minutes, each person observing everything about their partner. If necessary, it can be suggested that items be noted, such as: posture, eye contact, placement of hands and feet, facial expressions, dress, jewelry, and so forth.
3. Then members of each pair should turn back-to-back with the agreed-upon partner changing five things about herself or himself.
4. When changes have been accomplished, members should once again face each other. The observing partner attempts to verbalize the noticed changes.
5. Roles are reversed.
6. Discuss the experience.

VARIATIONS

The exercise can be lengthened by using the same pairs and requesting members to change five more things about themselves. This occasionally poses a problem and people often do not know what to change further. During discussion ask participants if they thought of asking for help from another close member of a pair who was also searching for changes. If they did, how did they feel about needing help on a seemingly simple task? If they did not request assistance, why not?

EXERCISE 2
Observation of Body Talk

PURPOSES

1. To become aware of how different emotions can be expressed nonverbally.
2. To validate one's perception of nonverbally expressed emotions.

FACILITY

Large enough room to accommodate participants sitting around tables or on the floor in a circle.

MATERIALS

Small pieces of paper and two hats or baskets.

TIME REQUIRED

Thirty minutes or more, depending on group size.

GROUP SIZE

12 to 15 is ideal; two or more groups may be formed if group is large.

DESIGN

1. In a large group, ask participants to verbalize emotions/feelings. Write one each on a slip of paper; fold and place in a hat.
2. Repeat #1, except this time ask that participants verbalize parts of the body which can be used to express emotions/feelings.
3. A person from the group should then distribute or have participants pick a slip of paper from each hat.
4. Request each participant who has picked an emotion and body part to role-play the emotion nonverbally primarily using the designated body part.
5. Group participants should then try to guess what feeling is being expressed.
6. Discussion follows.
7. Role-players should place papers back in each respective hat and steps #3 through #6 should be repeated. This should be done so that all members have a chance to role-play.

VARIATIONS

If two or more groups of twelve are possible, equalize the number of emotions and body parts for both groups and time how long it takes for groups to carry out the task. Then have groups work against one another; all role-plays should result in the group accurately diagnosing the emotion and body part used in expression. Only then may they proceed to the next role-play. The group finishing first has the sharpest observational skills, given those present.

EXERCISE 3
Perception

PURPOSES
1. To increase awareness of the variety of perceptions which can be elicited from a given situation.
2. To raise self-awareness regarding individual perceptual fields.

FACILITY
Room to accommodate the class size in groups of six.

MATERIALS
Paper and pencils.

TIME REQUIRED
One hour.

GROUP SIZE
Unlimited groups of six.

SCENARIO 1
It is 11:15 a.m. Ms. Blue, a supervisor, is making rounds on a surgical unit. She observes a patient with traction of the right leg, a basin of water on the bedside table, the bed stripped, a gown placed over patient's chest, and the patient, Ms. Green, reading a book. As the supervisor enters the room, the patient explains that the student nurse assigned to assist her with a bath had struck his head against the crossbar of the traction frame at 10:30 a.m. The nursing instructor had taken him to the emergency room. On the way to the nurse's station, the supervisor notices several nursing personnel, including the head nurse, drinking coffee in the utility room. As she begins calling the Nursing School office to report that a nursing student and instructor had left a patient unattended, the head nurse comes in to tell her about the accident.

SCENARIO 2*
The setting is a general hospital unit in an urban city. Three people are involved: Ms. King, the new head nurse of the medical unit; Ms. James, the Director of Nursing Services; and Ms. Carmichael, the Day Supervisor of the building. Ms. King gives the Kardex a last minute check to be sure all patients' activities, treatments, medications, etc., are taken care of or are in process. Then she checks the patients, going from room to room. "It's going pretty well" she thinks—she is

---

*This situation was received by this author at the University of Florida, College of Nursing, 1966. Author is unknown.

particularly satisfied with the way Ms. X is responding to the care plan now. She has spent a great deal of time working with Ms. X. Certainly, Ms. King thinks, Ms. James can find nothing wrong here; the patients are all receiving excellent care. Ms. King has heard a lot about these "spontaneous rounds" by Ms. James. Shortly thereafter, Ms. James and Ms. Carmichael arrive on the unit by the backstairs, so it is some time before Ms. King even knows they are there.

During the "rounds," with Ms. James and Ms. Carmichael, Ms. King makes several attempts to comment on certain patients, their progress, etc. Ms. James ignores the attempts and starts to jot down notes on her clip board. Ms. James and Ms. Carmichael maintain a general conversation about the unit while they finish "rounds." No attempt is made to draw Ms. King into the conversation. After rounds are completed on the unit, Ms. King asks if there is any additional information they need. Ms. James says, "No, however there are a few small items I would like to call to your attention, Ms. King. The shelves in the medicine cupboard are rather dusty, and the utility room is very cluttered. Will you please see that these things are taken care of?" With that Ms. James and Ms. Carmichael leave the unit.

On the way to the next unit Ms. James remarks to Ms. Carmichael, "On the whole, I think Ms. King is doing a good job with her unit. She should make a fine head nurse."

DESIGN

1. Have participants individually read Scenario 1 and write down their perceptions and reactions concerning what happened, their feelings in the situation, and what conclusions they would reach.
2. Ask that participants share these notations with their small group.
3. Observe and discuss perceptual differences, possible reasons for such, and rationale for conclusions. Dichotomous differences between members should be studied more fully.
4. Repeat the design with Scenario 2.

EXERCISE 4
Communication in Counseling

PURPOSES

1. To focus on the verbal and nonverbal cues which may be emitted in a counseling situation.
2. To validate perceptions with intent.
3. To become aware of one's own communications against perceptions by others.

FACILITY

Large enough room to accommodate participants seated around tables or in a circle on the floor.

MATERIALS

None.

TIME REQUIRED

One hour +, depending on group size and number of volunteers.

GROUP SIZE

Unlimited groups of twelve.

DESIGN

1. Paired volunteers should be given a couple of minutes to develop a hypothetical counseling situation. They should decide which of them is to be the counselor and the counselee. (A hypothetical counseling situation is a made-up story in which the counselee is seeking help/advice from the counselor. These should not be personal.)
2. The pair should then role-play the counseling situation with instruction being given to the counselor that he or she should decide whether he or she was to be effective or ineffective. Only the counselor should know what is decided.
3. Following the role-play, group members should give feedback on their reactions and perceptions of what was nonverbally and verbally communicated during the scenario. The players' intent should be backdropped against perceptions.
4. Discuss the experience.

VARIATION

The instructor can prepare the scenes prior to class. Situations from Carkhuff's Index of Communication, Helping and Human Relations, Vol. I, 1969, pp. 95–99, may be used.

EXERCISE 5
Communication: Process Recordings

PURPOSES
1. To raise self-awareness on communicative inter-actions with peers and clients.
2. To validate perceptions with peers and instructors.
3. To validate one's effective use of communication skills with peers and instructors.

FACILITY
Access to interactions with clients and peers in any setting.

MATERIALS
Process Recording Sheets; pen or pencil.

TIME REQUIRED
Variable.

GROUP SIZE
Dyads composed of instructor and learner or two peers.

DESIGN
1. Using the Process Recording Sheet (Worksheet A), have participants engage in an interaction with a chosen and agreeable peer. Notes can be taken during the talk or immediately following it.
2. Process recordings can then be discussed with another peer or a teacher. Rationale for perceptions, thoughts and feelings of the student during the interaction, and communication skills should be in focus. Alternatives in communicating may be suggested by both parties.
3. Repeat design using clients.

VARIATIONS
This exercise can be done with clients. The nursing history interview can also be done and studied using this format.

EXERCISE 5
WORKSHEET A

PROCESS RECORDING SHEET

What the client/peer communicates (verbal and nonverbal):	What the nurse communicates (verbal and nonverbal):	Perceptions of or about client/peer	Thoughts and/or feelings about these perceptions

EXERCISE 6
Decision-Making

PURPOSES

1. To gain experience in diagnosing situations in order to determine the most appropriate decision-making technique for different scenarios.
2. To gain knowledge of the problem-solving and decision-making styles.
3. To appropriately apply decision-making styles to diagnosed situations.

FACILITY

Large room with tables that will accommodate participants in groups of six.

MATERIALS

None (except Tables included in exercise).

TIME REQUIRED

Approximately two hours.

GROUP SIZE

Five to six.

DESIGN

Note: For the design of this exercise, please refer to the selected reading of Chapter 10, pp. 244–261, in which the complete version of this exercise can be found.

From: La Monica, E., Finch, F. Managerial decision-making, Journal of Nursing Administration 7:20–28.

EXERCISE 7
Teaching

PURPOSES
1. To gain experience in using different instructional modes and media to teach a content area.
2. To experience a variety of teaching strategies.

FACILITY
Large room to accommodate class.

MATERIALS
Specified by the students in their teaching module.

TIME REQUIRED
Ten minutes per member.

GROUP SIZE
Under 25.

DESIGN
1. As a homework assignment, ask students to think of anything (skill, philosophy, belief, etc.) that they know or do well.
2. Then have them prepare a 5–7 minute teaching module on the area chosen. The module should include objectives and teaching modes and media.
3. Request that preparation be made for a class presentation.
4. At a subsequent class, have students teach the module to their peers.
5. Encourage group discussion of the experience, focusing on the teacher's experience as well as that of the learner.

VARIATIONS
Nursing skills or competencies as well as theory can be substituted for the content in the original design.

EXERCISE 8
Teaching

PURPOSES

1. To broaden experience in diagnosing the teaching needs of clients and colleagues in a health environment.
2. To increase awareness of the teaching diagnoses which others perceive in the same situation.
3. To identify appropriate objectives and the most effective teaching strategies to accomplish same.

FACILITY

Large room to accommodate participants seated in groups of six.

MATERIALS

Paper and pencils.

TIME REQUIRED

One to two hours.

GROUP SIZE

Unlimited groups of six.

SCENARIOS*

1. Three times in the past two days you've found that elderly patients who have been gotten up out of bed rather early in the morning have stayed up sitting in chairs for the rest of the morning. In each case when you noted this the patients' respirations were either labored or rapid. The pulse was rapid, and the patients appeared and said they were tired.
2. A patient on your unit has been on a Stryker frame for two weeks. You have been told that tomorrow a newly employed graduate nurse and two senior nursing students will be with your team for the first time.
3. A patient on your unit has been on a Stryker frame for two weeks. Today when you go in to turn her, two beginning sophomore students ask you if they may come with you to see what you are doing.
4. During afternoon conference, a patient was mentioned who had just returned from the operating room following "repair of a fractured hip." A nurse said, "We'll have to be careful of his back since he'll have to stay on it for some time."
5. When making rounds on your unit after lunch, you notice that although many patients are in their beds, most of the beds are elevated and in many cases the linen is rumpled. A TV set is audible through most of the area, and three of your staff members are talking rather loudly in the corridor.

*Scenarios were received by this author at the University of Florida, College of Nursing, 1966. Author is unknown.

6. On Monday Mr. Smith tells you that his doctor told him he might be going home in a couple of days. Mr. Smith has congestive heart failure, has been on digitalis and a diuretic, still has some peripheral edema, and is on a low sodium diet.

7. Ms. Jones has asked for and received a prescribed narcotic for pain for several days prior to and following her surgery. The nurse assigned to give medications and the one assigned to care for her yesterday both questioned "if she really needed it." The doctor was told of this and gave permission for a prn placebo. Today it is discussed by others on the team. Ms. Jones responded well the first time the placebo was given but then seemed to "want the other medicine" (she recognized that a different injection had been given). The medicine nurse today said she felt Ms. Jones had no real need for the narcotic, but another nurse said he thought Ms. Jones acted as if she really had pain.

8. When an aide attempting to change a patient's position was experiencing evident difficulty, a graduate nurse came over to the aide, assisted, and then explained the procedure to the aide and patient.

9. You observe a patient walking down the corridor in a coat and hat, carrying a suitcase—an aide is walking beside the patient. A graduate nurse leaves the nurse's station, greets the patient, takes the suitcase, and hands it to the aide. The nurse discusses the patient's plans for discharge as they walk down the hall. The situation was discussed with the aide after the aide returned from taking the patient to the hospital lobby.

10. Team leader asked an aide to do a sugar and acetone test for a patient and reminded the aide not to obtain the urine for testing from the patient's tube (indwelling Foley catheter). The aide took a sample from the drainage bottle and reported the test to team leader who then recorded the results.

11. A patient is shaking side rails and stating in a loud voice that he wants to go to the lavatory. The aide and practical nurse remove side rails, explaining to patient why side rails are necessary. (He had slipped getting out of bed yesterday.) Practical nurse escorts patient to bathroom and waits to escort him back to bed.

12. A graduate nurse wheels a patient into the solarium, places the wheelchair close to another patient, and introduces them to each other. The nurse then asks each patient to demonstrate active and passive exercises of their arms. As the nurse leaves the room, patients continue exercises and discuss each other's progress.

DESIGN

1. Using all or any combination of the scenarios, ask participants to individually respond to the following (Worksheet A may be used):
   a. In the situation, is there a teaching need?
   b. If there is, to whom? What needs to be taught? Why and how?

c. Identify most appropriate teaching mode and any
　　　　 media which may be used.
　　2. In small groups of six, participants should share their
　　　 responses.
　　3. Different perceptions between students on all
　　　 questions should be discussed.

VARIATIONS　　　Step 1 may be done as a homework assignment.

TEACHING

Scenario Number	Is there a teaching need and for whom?	What needs to be taught and why?	What teaching strategy would be best? (mode and media)
1.			
2.			
3.			
4.			
5.			
6.			
7.			
8.			
9.			
10.			
11.			
12.			

EXERCISE 9
Group Process Observation Sheets

PURPOSES
1. To gain experience in studying small group processes.
2. To gain experience in communicating with group members on process observations (giving and receiving feedback).
3. To provide feedback on a group functioning in relation to the accomplishment of the task.

FACILITY
The same place where group experience occurred.

MATERIALS
Worksheets.

TIME REQUIRED
Ten to thirty minutes.

GROUP SIZE
The same as in the group experience.

DESIGN
These worksheets are to be used in any group experience in which the members of the group wish to study their group process in relation to accomplishment of their group task.
1. At the conclusion of group work, reserve fifteen minutes or more for group processing. Request members to individually respond to the items in Worksheet A or B.
2. Instruct the total group to share their responses with one another, amplifying their rationale for choices. Differences in point allocation should be discussed since they point out various group members' perceptions.

EVALUATION OF GROUP EFFECTIVENESS*

Rate the group on each statement below with 4 representing your highest agreement and 1 representing your lowest agreement with the statement. Circle the number that best approximates your rating of the behavior exhibited by the group.

1. Group members understood the problem under discussion.   1 2 3 4

2. Group members stayed on the topic.   1 2 3 4

3. Group members avoided premature closure on discussion.   1 2 3 4

4. Group members contributed equally to the discussion.   1 2 3 4

5. Group members agreed with group consensus and/or decisions.   1 2 3 4

6. Group members discussed their opinions openly without hiding personal feelings.   1 2 3 4

7. Group members were able to resolve conflict or discontent.   1 2 3 4

8. Group members displayed commitment to the group tasks.   1 2 3 4

9. Group members indicated satisfaction with the group process.   1 2 3 4

10. Group members indicated satisfaction with the group outcomes.   1 2 3 4

*This instrument was obtained by this author at the University of Massachusetts, School of Education, 1974. Author is unknown.

EVALUATION OF WORK GROUP EFFECTIVENESS*

The following five items: Commitment to Objectives; Communications; Decision-Making; Conflict; and Climate will be used to critique work group activity.

1. **Individual evaluation of work group.** Each person will distribute 100 points among the alternatives for **each item** as the person evaluates the activity of the work group.
2. **Work group evaluation.** The group will discuss the point allocation for every item to reach by consensus a **single** distribution that represents member understanding of how work group activity took place. Any approach that assures that the thinking of each member of each item is heard and considered may be used. Averaging of individual answers to get a single work group rating is to be avoided. The purpose is to probe for differences in points of view.

Climate

1. _____ Competitive, tense, win-lose conflict; one or more people tried to take over and control the decision.
2. _____ Penetrating and challenging discussion; a very rewarding session to which we all were committed.
3. _____ Polite discussion, easygoing and pleasant, a very friendly session.
4. _____ The discussion was rather flat and lifeless; comments slid from point to point with little evidence of commitment.

Conflict

1. _____ There was considerable unnecessary and unprofitable disagreement; competitiveness resulted in win-lose conflict.
2. _____ Disagreements were explored to help the group produce the best possible decision; conflict was confronted and resolved.
3. _____ We were quite polite and pleasant; we took care to avoid conflict.
4. _____ There was very little open disagreement or conflict.

*This instrument was obtained by this author at the University of Massachusetts, School of Education, 1974. Author is unknown.

EXERCISE 9, WORKSHEET B (continued)

Communication

1. _____ Ideas and opinions were expressed to "win own point," there was little listening to conflicting points of view.
2. _____ Ideas and opinions were expressed openly and with candor; there was close attention paid to both majority and minority opinions so that we could fully understand all points of view.
3. _____ Ideas and opinions were expressed politely; we listened to all contributions attentively; no feelings were hurt.
4. _____ Ideas and opinions were expressed with little conviction and people listened with little evidence of concern.

Decision-Making

1. _____ To complete the task, decisions were "railroaded" by one or a few.
2. _____ After understanding all points of view, work group agreement resulted in a decision to which all were committed.
3. _____ Decisions were made in such a way to give maximum consideration to all people; we didn't want to "rock the boat."
4. _____ Compromise was the key to decision making; the traditional decision resulted from majority rule.

Commitment to Objectives

1. _____ We attempted to stay directly with the problem and we solved it as quickly and efficiently as possible.
2. _____ There was an attempt to look at the problem as broadly and deeply as possible. Involvement and creativity characterized the discussion.
3. _____ We often seemed to be more interested in harmony than in getting the job done.
4. _____ There was little consistent focus on the problem; we solved the problem as rapidly as possible based on past precedent.

EXERCISE 10
Self-Diagnoses of Behavior in a Small Group

PURPOSES
1. To raise one's consciousness of personal small group behavior.
2. To self-diagnose learning needs regarding small group functioning.

FACILITY
None; Homework Assignment.

MATERIALS
Worksheets A and B.

TIME REQUIRED
Fifteen to thirty minutes.

GROUP SIZE
Individual Homework Assignment.

DESIGN
1. Using Worksheet A, have class members respond to the items in terms of the categories represented.
2. Ask that they consider the following:
   A. Why do they take certain functions most often?
   B. Why are certain functions never or rarely carried out?
   C. How can they experience functions they would like to practice? What assistance, if any, is needed?

VARIATIONS
Self-diagnosis can be discussed within small groups; familiar members can offer feedback on their perceptions.

SELF-DIAGNOSIS OF SMALL GROUP BEHAVIOR

Listed below are functions which are performed by members of discussion groups. Considering each category, check the columns which apply to you.

Behavior	Behavior(s) I perceive myself to use most often	Behavior(s) I seldom use	Behavior(s) I never use	Behavior(s) I would like to practice
TASK FUNCTIONS 1. Initiator				
2. Information Seeker				
3. Evaluator				
4. Coordinator				
5. Recorder				
6. Procedural Technician				
GROUP MAINTENANCE FUNCTIONS 1. Harmonizer				
2. Encourager				
3. Gate Keeper				
4. Standard Setter				
5. Compromisor				
SELF-ORIENTED FUNCTIONS 1. Aggressor				
2. Blocker				
3. Recognition- Seeker				
4. Playboy				
5. Dominator				
6. Help-Seeker				

SELF-DIAGNOSIS OF SMALL GROUP BEHAVIOR

A. Why do I use certain functions most often?

B. Why are certain functions never or rarely carried out?

C. How can I experience functions that I would like to practice? What assistance, if any, is needed?

Bibliography

The following are suggested as sources of further humanistic exercises on topics from Part II.

Finch, F., Jones, H., and Litterer, J. Managing for organizational effectiveness: An experiential approach. New York: McGraw-Hill Books, Inc., 1976.

Gazda, G., Asbury, F., Balzer, F., Childers, W., and Walters, R. Human Relations development: A manual for educators. Boston: Allyn and Bacon, 1977.

Grove, T. Experiences in interpersonal communication. Englewood Cliffs, N.J.: Prentice-Hall, 1976.

Johnson, D. Reaching out: Interpersonal effectiveness and self-actualization. Englewood Cliffs, N.J.: Prentice-Hall, 1972.

Johnson, D., and Johnson, F. Joining together: Group theory and group skills. Englewood Cliffs, N.J.: Prentice-Hall, 1975.

Krupar, K. Communication games. New York: Free Press, 1973.

Maier, N., Solem, A., and Maier, A. The role-play technique: A handbook for management and leadership practice. La Jolla, Calif.: University Associates, Inc., 1975.

Napier, R., and Gershenfeld, M. Groups: Theory and experience. Boston: Houghton-Mifflin, 1973.

Pfeiffer, J., and Jones, J. Structured experiences for human relations training. Vols. I–VI. Iowa City, Iowa: University Associates Press, Press, 1973–1977.

Pfeiffer, J., and Jones, J. (eds.) The annual handbook for group facilitators. Iowa City, Iowa; University Associates Press, 1972–1978.

Vaughn, J., and Deep, S. Program of exercises for management and organizational behavior. Beverly Hills, Calif.: Glencoe Press, 1975.

PART III

QUALITY SYSTEMS IN NURSING PRACTICE

13

Problem Oriented Records

Thus far, the content of this book has been directed toward the individual nursing practitioner and those efforts which maintain quality within the caregiver's and care-receiver's systems. Building nursing actions around the needs of the client, the nurse, and the specific environment were stressed.

Part III expands this book's focus to capture the larger system of nursing practice by discussing procedural trends which can affect the quality of care. Problem oriented records, the nursing audit, and patient rights are discussed in this Part as valuable aspects of quality care delivery.

This chapter is devoted to the definition and description of problem oriented records. The steps of the problem oriented record system are parallel to the steps of the nursing process and scientific method, underscoring the importance of this system in insuring quality health care for the consumer. In using the problem oriented record, the methods discussed in Part I of this book are essential. Data collection, data processing, nursing diagnoses, and nursing orders all become elements of the problem oriented record. The nurse takes these methods, combines them with skills and competencies, and follows a specific format to yield a problem oriented record designed to enhance individualized quality client care. In this chapter, the protocol for the problem oriented system is elaborated, followed by the advantages and disadvantages of its usage. The problem oriented record method presented in this chapter is used in many health facilities. Even if this specific method is not used in your facility, it is a valuable device to be acquainted with.

PROBLEM ORIENTED RECORDS DEFINED

There can be some debate as to whether the problem oriented approach is simply a procedure for record keeping or whether it is a scientific and philosophic approach in health care. The term "problem oriented records" seems to connote the former—a procedure for record keeping—but a careful study of the concept behind the system connotes the latter—a scientific and philosophic approach. In actuality, the problem oriented record system constitutes a combination of both schools of thought. Lawrence Weed (1970) developed a method of using the problem oriented record (POR) which aptly captures the combination of record keeping and philosophy. Weed began with the scientific method, applied it to medical/health care, and delineated a standard, written format for communicating with colleagues. The POR is new neither in nursing nor any other science. What is new, however, is the standardized procedure for communicating in writing and the instant association of POR as a formalized procedure. Anyone who is familiar with and committed to using Weed's method follows a specific protocol using proper language; it is designed for universal understanding. Perhaps this can be considered a milestone in health care record keeping, and specifically nursing record keeping.

Problem oriented records involve both an application of the scientific method in health care as well as a logical, succinct system of record keeping. The POR incorporates a philosophic base mandating that clients be helped systematically and holistically. It defies fragmentation of care or the studying of patient problems as mutually exclusive. Built into the record keeper system, moreover, it is the means by which different professionals can concern themselves with select problems; the interaction of the many facets of client care is portrayed directly and clearly in the charting procedure.

In addition to being a landmark in coordinating care for patients, POR is also revolutionizing the education of health practitioners and the evaluation of health services (Schell and Campbell, 1972). Properly used, the POR method permits a learner to visualize the inductive and deductive reasoning that leads a health practitioner to particular conclusions; to conceptualize the rationale for all actions; and to study a whole person. Evaluation of care can be based on complete retrospective data as well as the alleviation of client problems through specific actions.

Even though the term "problem oriented records" is a descriptive phrase coined by Lawrence Weed for the medical profession, the procedural system has been applied to include all health care-givers. The specific POR system developed by Weed has been adapted for use on nursing records in hospitals and other community agencies (Bloom, Dressler, Kenny, Molbo, and Pardee, 1971; Bonkowsky, 1972), and is used in private and group professional offices and outpatient clinics with all professionals writing on one record.

Parallels between the nursing process, the scientific method, and the POR can be drawn as shown in Table 13-1.

All these methods are dynamic, and the evaluative facets of each create new data that begin the process again.

TABLE 13-1

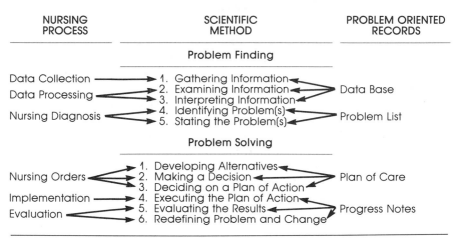

NURSING PROCESS	SCIENTIFIC METHOD	PROBLEM ORIENTED RECORDS
Problem Finding		
Data Collection	1. Gathering Information	
Data Processing	2. Examining Information	Data Base
	3. Interpreting Information	
Nursing Diagnosis	4. Identifying Problem(s)	
	5. Stating the Problem(s)	Problem List
Problem Solving		
	1. Developing Alternatives	
Nursing Orders	2. Making a Decision	Plan of Care
	3. Deciding on a Plan of Action	
Implementation	4. Executing the Plan of Action	
	5. Evaluating the Results	Progress Notes
Evaluation	6. Redefining Problem and Change	

PROTOCOL OF PROBLEM ORIENTED RECORDS

The procedure used in POR and developed by Weed (1970) has four essential parts: data base, problem list, initial plans, and progress notes. These four dimensions form the client's whole chart.

Data Base   The data base parallels the assessment phase of the nursing process. According to Weed (1970), the data base section includes the client's profile, history, physical, and laboratory reports. Usually, these four aspects are standardized. They are predefined as essential and it is guaranteed that these data will be obtained for every client.

The nature of the nurse's input on this record varies, depending on the structure of the organization. If a nurse is a practitioner in a group practice, the nurse may have the responsibility for obtaining all aspects of data on the client's initial visit to the facility. Should POR be used in nursing units only by nurses, then the record is adapted only to address areas of nursing responsibility. The responsibilities of the professional nurse, therefore, reflect the purpose for which the POR is used plus the structure of the group using it.

Problem List   The problem list corresponds to the nursing diagnoses, the first part of the planning phase in the nursing process. The problem list is a numbered and titled list on which is included every problem the client has or ever has had. Weed (1970) defines the problem list as anything that requires management or diagnostic work-up, including social and psychologic problems. It is a dynamic list with problems being resolved, added, or clarified.

This part of the chart provides a quick reference to the client's overall health state. As can be seen, Weed's definition is interpreted to include nursing problems or diagnoses. Recalling the definition of nursing diagnoses—that with which the client needs assistance—one can see a close parallel to the problem list.

Depending again on the purposes for which the POR is used, nursing and medical diagnoses should be included in the problem list unless the record is only for nursing use. Then only nursing diagnoses are charted.

Initial Plans   The initial plans of the POR parallel the planning phase of the nursing process. The plans contain items corresponding in identifying number with the problems listed on the POR; plans include diagnostic, therapeutic (drugs and procedures), and educational aspects of care, relative to each problem. The plans are, in essence, the orders—medical and nursing.

When medicine and nursing professionals are using the same chart, orders relative to each problem are listed together. This provides an easy guide to integrated care, assuring that comprehensiveness is maintained and relevant expertise is unified. All health workers' input follows this pattern.

Progress Notes   The progress notes of the POR parallel the implementation and evaluation phases of the nursing process. These notes, as are the others, are written by everyone involved in the client's care and are identified by a number which corresponds to the problem and plan in focus. A specific format is followed with the writer stating the date, time, problem name, and number. Each problem is communicated on, as seen in Table 13-2, based on the client from Part I.

The progress notes have thus been "SOAPed." Emphasis is placed on unresolved problems with those resolved being evaluated briefly (Weed, 1970). Progress notes provide the base for adding, altering, or deleting items from the problem list and orders (plan). Flow sheets and discharge notes relative to each problem are contained in this section.

Advantages of POR

The attributes of the POR system and method are many. Weed (1970) focuses benefits primarily on medical dimensions; this author adapts them to nursing:

1. Schools of learning are integrated with the outcomes of health care, focusing on the entire client and system.
2. The POR parallels a dictionary with all individuals involved in the care having quick access to all aspects of the plan.
3. Nurses, allied health workers, and physicians can see what they have done and learn from what others have done and observed—education is underscored.

TABLE 13-2

PROBLEM: BALANCED DIET, RESPECTIVE OF DIABETIC CONDITION

STEP	EXAMPLES OF EACH STEP
S Subjective Information Description of symptoms by client Feelings of client Concerns of client	Client does not like the food sent by kitchen; he refuses to eat meals since they are not in line with his usual eating patterns. Client seems anxious.
O Objective Information Observations of nurse, physician, others What was done for client Results of tests and objective parameters	Client has a daily caloric deficit. Insulin administration is not regulated; urine sugar and acetone levels fluctuate considerably.
A Assessment Record of judgment, thinking, and opinion on the problem by the professional	Client is not eating a balanced diet; given diabetic condition; unregulated insulin administration program.
P Projected course that should be followed Determination of whether consultation is necessary	1. Request that his meals be sent up or kept warm until client wants to eat—9-2-7; make special arrangements with the department head in food services. 2. Explain diabetes and the importance of eating well-balanced meals. 3. Tell client that you will help in any way you can so that he receives foods that are in accordance with his likes. 4. Obtain food exchange lists from dietician and plan meals with client. 5. Be aware if plan is not working and change accordingly. 6. Test urine for S/A, AC and HS. Give insulin as indicated. 7. Record I&O.

4. Clinical research is facilitated by the completeness of the records.

5. Quality of care is easily audited with deficiencies, if any, surfacing clearly.

6. All aspects of the client and system are respected and receive attention.

7. Satisfaction regarding outcomes is increased due to the visibility of progress.

8. Health team members are able truly to work as a team—collaboratively.

9. Client data are shared by all involved health workers.

Disadvantages of POR

Though the disadvantages are few in comparison with the advantages, they are worthy of mention:

1. Education of all involved health care workers regarding the procedures of POR can be lengthy.
2. The record system may expose practitioners to criticism from colleagues (Schnell and Campbell, 1972). Even though auditing is educative, it can also be threatening.
3. The system is only as good as the practitioners; if the client is viewed as a "problem" or "disease," the POR systm will do nothing to change this fragmentation of a person.

Careful use of the POR as well as careful respect and attention paid to all involved persons can minimize or eliminate these disadvantages, however.

SUMMARY

Chapter 13 looked at the problem oriented record, both as a scientific method of health care and as a standard procedure for record keeping. The protocol of the POR was delineated, followed by discussion of the advantages and disadvantages of the system.

REFERENCES

Bloom, J., Dressler, J., Kenny, M., Malbo, D., and Pardee, G. Problem oriented charting. *American Journal of Nursing* 71: 2144–2148, 1971.

Bonkowsky, M. Adapting the POMR to community child health care. *Nursing Outlook* 20: 515–518, 1972.

Schell, P., and Campbell, A. POMR—Not just another way to chart. *Nursing Outlook* 8: 510–514, 1972.

Weed, L. *Medical records, medical education, and patient care.* Cleveland: Press of Case Western Reserve University, 1970.

14

Nursing Audit

The purpose of Chapter 14 is to discuss the nursing audit, a program having the primary goal of assuring quality of nursing practice. In this chapter, the historical development of the audit is briefly traced followed by a definition of the audit. Characteristics of an effective audit (quality assurance) system are discussed. The chapter closes with methods for executing an audit, followed by a discussion of the benefits for the consumer and nurse.

HISTORICAL DEVELOPMENT

Pioneering work in medical assessment dates back to 1918 (Deeken, 1960) when the American College of Surgeons concluded that reliable and valid methods of evaluation did not exist. Prior to this time, however, the audit concept had been introduced by managers of industrial corporations who felt objective criticism of their fiscal status was important (McGuire, 1968).

With health care audit seeds primarily beginning in medicine, application to the field of nursing was first addressed in the middle fifties (Blanche, 1955; Deeken, 1960). This occurred in nursing despite Finer's (1952) earlier caution. Finer devoted an entire book to this caution and rather convincingly portrayed nursing care as quality that could not be quantified. Nevertheless, writings on the nursing quality assurance program flourished (Lesnik and Anderson, 1955; McGuire, 1968; Phaneuf, 1964, 1966, 1968, 1972; Rubin, Rinaldi, and Dietz, 1972). Multidisciplinary audit is now a requirement mandated by the Joint Commission on Accreditation and Hospitals and nurses have been highly creative in applying the concept of quality assurance to specific settings and groups in which nurses function.

322

NURSING AUDIT DEFINED

The term "audit" usually connotes an objective check on the balancing of accounts as well as a check on financial appropriations and expenditures. Nursing audit is similarly objective, yet differs because of the non-financial operations to which it is applied.

The nursing audit is a program used to assist nurses and nursing in assessing the quality of services provided. It is designed relative to the functions of nursing as well as established standards that define quality care. By definition, the term "audit" means a formal, methodical examination of a record by objective, outside observers. This is followed by a written report of the findings. In nursing audit, the procedure takes many forms (discussed in the methods portion of this chapter) and parallels the care given to clients with nursing standards. It is done by an objective observer. Its purposes are simple (Tinubu, 1976):

1. To constitute a tool for evaluating, verifying, and improving the quality of nursing practice;
2. To provide a basis for client and staff educational programs;
3. To provide a self-evaluative means for developing and improving nursing records;
4. To reveal specific areas of strengths and weaknesses in nursing care, measured against standards;
5. To reduce the incidence of medical/nursing/legal complications arising from inaccurate or incomplete records and practices.

NURSING AUDIT IN OPERATION

Characteristics of an Effective Evaluation System

The Joint Commission on Accreditation of Hospitals (JCAH) (1964) explicates the following as the essential requirements for an acceptable client care evaluation. These are:

1. *Objectivity.* In measuring whether care-givers are functioning at an appropriate level, standards and criteria must be established prior to the evaluation.
2. *Clinically sound.* Given the expertise and resources available, the standards and criteria must reflect optimum care for the client, achievable by the system of care-givers.
3. *Efficient.* Professional nursing time must be used when necessary; non-professional time should be allocated to those parts of a program which require no professional judgment.

4. *Flexible.* In the evaluation, variations from standards and criteria are permitted, with reported, good cause.
5. *Documented.* All decisions and evaluations must be written, signed, and reported to the responsible person(s) of quality care.
6. *Action-oriented.* Confirmed deficiencies which may result from an audit must be analyzed and appropriate corrective interventions built.

The JCAH further delineates seven components or steps of a quality assurance program; the author adds an eighth (step 2—Standards), based on the eloquent words of Hagen (1975):*

1. *Criteria*—The kind of variables which are to be appraised (Hagen, 1975).
2. *Standards*—Established expected performance levels of nursing care (Hagen, 1975).
3. *Measurement*—The retrieval of and methods for collecting patient and nursing data to show conformance with the preestablished criteria and standards.
4. *Evaluation*—The analysis of variations between collected data and standards; deduction of deficiencies and probable rationale for same.
5. *Action*—Specified corrective measures or programs to eradicate deficiencies.
6. *Follow-up*—Evaluation of the effectiveness of actions (step 5).
7. *Report*—Written, signed rendition of the entire audit, sent to appropriate, responsible, accountable leaders of the client care system.
8. *Repeat of the process*

It is obvious to denote the progressive quality of the nursing audit, the interaction of all steps, and the scientific, methodical approach to the problem of securing quality in care.

General Criteria for the Nursing Audit

The nursing audit must reflect the goals of the organization and the expertise within the organization relevant to care rendered. In other words, the audit must be personalized by the system in which it is to be used. For the purpose of learning, however, general variables which are common subjects of the audit can be delineated. Phaneuf (1966) specifies seven functions with 50 descriptive statements as a basis for an audit. Her list is not meant to be inclusive of every system, but provides a foundation upon which agencies can elaborate. Tucker, Breeding, Canobbio, Jacquet, Paquette, Wells, and

---

*Dr. Elizabeth Hagen's complete presentation on evaluation can be found in the selected reading portion of Chapter 6.

Willman (1975) provide a complete itemization of variables that may be used when developing audit criteria. Phaneuf's (1966) audit criteria follow:*

1. Application and execution of physician's legal orders
   a. Medical diagnosis complete
   b. Orders complete
   c. Orders current
   d. Orders promptly executed
   e. Evidence that nurse understood cause and effect
   f. Evidence that nurse took medical history into account
2. Observations of symptoms and reactions
   a. Related to course of above disease(s) in general
   b. Related to the course of above disease(s) in this patient
   c. Related complications due to therapy (each medication and treatment)
   d. Vital signs
   e. Patient to his condition (attitude)
   f. Patient to his course of disease(s)
3. Supervision of the patient
   a. Evidence that initial nursing diagnosis was made
   b. Safety of patient
   c. Security of patient
   d. Adaptation (support of patient in reactions to condition and care)
   e. Continuing assessment of patient's condition and capacity
   f. Nursing plans changed in accordance with assessment
   g. Interaction with family and with others considered
4. Supervision of those participating in care (except the physician)
   a. Care taught to patient, family, or other nursing personnel
   b. Physical, emotional, mental capacity to learn considered
   c. Continuity of supervision to those taught
   d. Support of those giving care
5. Reporting and recording
   a. Facts on which further care depended were recorded
   b. Essential facts reported to physician
   c. Reporting of facts included evaluation thereof
   d. Patient or family alerted as to what to report to physician
   e. Record permitted continuity of intramural and extramural care
6. Application and execution of nursing procedures and techniques
   a. Administration and/or supervision of medications
   b. Personal care (bathing, oral hygiene, skin, nail care, shampoo)
   c. Nutrition (including special diets)

*Reprinted with permission from *Nursing Outlook*. Copyright 1966 by American Journal of Nursing Company.

d. Fluid balance
e. Elimination
f. Rest or sleep
g. Physical activity
h. Irrigations (including enemas)
i. Dressings and bandages
j. Formal exercise program
k. Rehabilitation (other than formal exercises)
l. Prevention of complications and infections
m. Recreation, diversion
n. Clinical procedure—urinalysis, B/P
o. Special treatments (such as care of tracheostomy, use of oxygen, colostomy or catheter care, etc.)
7. Promotion of physical and emotional health by direction and teaching
a. Plans for medical emergency evident
b. Emotional support to patient
c. Emotional support to family
d. Teaching preventive health care
e. Evaluation of need for additional resources (such as, spiritual, social service, homemaker service, physical or occupational therapy)
f. Action taken in regard to needs identified.

It is noted that all of Phaneuf's components relate to the areas of responsibility of nurses discussed in Part I of this book. *Nurses are accountable for each and every one.*

JCAH (1964), in association with the Associated Hospital Service of New York (Blue Cross), specifies three recommended parts of the nursing audit report and inclusive items of each:

Part 1: Patient identification data and key administrative policy questions intended to safeguard the rights of patients and institutions; this part can be completed by a trained clerk.

Part 2: Judgment entry made by the nursing audit committee member who reviewed the chart.

Part 3: Specific comments on the functions of professional nurses, according to criteria and standards, in the care of patient(s) in focus.

Nursing Audit Methods

The most widely used method of collecting data for a nursing audit is the retrospective method. In this, the charts of clients are studied and measured against established criteria and standards. Client care outcome is the primary focus even though specific processes such as catheterization may be pointedly studied.

A variety of methods may be used in the audit, however, and it is important to be aware of them in each specific organization. Even though the term audit connotes retrospective study, reality says that neither is this always the case, nor is it indicated. Methods chosen for evaluation must reflect the purpose for which used, the time given for the project, and the availability of data. Given all three, the best method for achieving goals should be chosen. For more information on methods, the reader is referred to Thorndike and Hagen (1977) for a complete discussion of testing methods and evaluation procedures.

Benefits of a Nursing Quality Assurance Program

Aside from the fact that a multidisciplinary quality assurance program is required by JCAH, it must be recognized as valuable for nurses and clients.

With public officials' and consumer demands for health care quality reaching an all time high, standards and criteria must be shared and accepted by all. A quality assurance program in nursing suggests clarity and agreement between all parties on nursing care. It determines the extent to which standards are met and points out needed improvements. Elimination of poor practices is also facilitated through the documentation which occurs during the audit.

Toward the goal of quality in nursing practices, the audit lends reliability and validity to the changes in procedures, policies, educational priorities, staffing needs, and other aspects which may result as suggestions or needs from the auditing process. In other words, documentation through the nursing audit using a sound research method, is a firm basis for pointing out needed changes in the system.

SUMMARY

Chapter 14 discussed the nursing audit as the quality assurance program in professional nursing practice. The protocol for an effective evaluation system was delineated followed by explicit criteria applicable in nursing. The usual method for executing the audit was described and a discussion of the benefits of the program concluded the chapter.

REFERENCES

Blanche, Sr. A nursing audit. *Hospital Progress* 37: 67–68, 1955.

Deeken, Sr. M. *Guide for nursing service audit.* St. Louis, Mo.: Catholic Hospital Association of the United States and Canada, 1960.

Finer, H. *Administration and the nursing services.* New York: Macmillan Co., 1952.

Hagen, E. Conceptual issues in the appraisal of the quality of care. In *Assessment of Nursing Services.* Bethesda, Md. U.S.D.H.E.W., Publication No. (HRA) 75-40, May, 1975.

Joint Commission on Accreditation of Hospitals. *Five basic publications.* Chicago, Ill.: The Commission, 1964.

Lesnik, M. and Anderson, E. *Nursing practice and the law.* Philadelphia: J. B. Lippincott, 1955.

McGuire, R. Bedside nursing audit. *American Journal of Nursing* 68: 2146-2148, 1968.

Phaneuf, M. A nursing audit method. *Nursing Outlook* 12: 42-45, 1964.

Phaneuf, M. The nursing audit for evaluation of patient care. *Nursing Outlook* 14: 51-54, 1966.

Phaneuf, M. Analysis of a nursing audit. *Nursing Outlook* 16: 57-60, 1968.

Phaneuf, M. *The nursing audit: Profile for excellence.* New York: Appleton-Century-Crofts, 1972.

Rubin, C., Rinaldi, L., and Dietz, R. Nursing audit—nurses evaluating nursing. *American Journal of Nursing* 72: 916-921, 1972.

Thorndike, R., and Hagen, E. *Measurement and evaluation in psychology and education.* New York: John Wiley and Sons, 1977.

Tinubu, A. Nursing audit. Unpublished paper. Teachers College, Columbia University, New York, 1976.

Tucker, S., Breeding, M., Canobbio, M., Jacquet, G., Paquette, E., Wells, M., and Willman, M. *Patient care standards.* St. Louis: C. V. Mosby, 1975.

15

Patient Rights

The decade between the years 1965 and 1975 involved increasing attention to the rights of health care consumers. This trend was amplified as public awareness grew regarding health care activities and the health care-giver's response in desiring more effective, humanistic, care with greater client satisfaction. Besides client benefits, all members of the health system also reaped benefits: physician, client, nurse, allied health workers, and organizations which provide services.

The most important work accomplished in securing patients' rights was delivered by the American Hospital Association's Board of Trustees' Committee on Health Care for the Disadvantaged. This group has long been recognized as an advocate on behalf of the health care consumer population. On February 6, 1973, the AHA House of Delegates approved the original Patient's Bill of Rights, a revised statement of which is presented in this chapter (American Hospital Association, 1975). In addition, Chapter 15 discusses the advocacy role of the nurse in putting this document into operation in all health care settings. Both concepts—patient rights and advocacy—point out the amplified goal of increased humanism in health practices.

DEFINITION OF ADVOCACY

Advocacy is defined by Webster as an active act of pleading for, supporting, or recommending. The advocate is the person who fills this role. The advocate is one who pleads for or in behalf of another—an intercessor.

It should be obvious that the pure concept of advocacy does not merely imply a hierarchical structure such as a mother defending her child or nurse interceding for a client in a hospital system. Peers can be advocates of one another and children can be advocates for parents. Advocacy includes any necessary direction between involved people in any area of life.

A PATIENT'S BILL OF RIGHTS

The American Hospital Association Board of Trustees' Committee on Health Care for the Disadvantaged, which has been a consistent advocate on behalf of consumers of health care services, developed the Statement on a Patient's Bill of Rights, *which was approved by the AHA House of Delegates February 6, 1973. The statement was published in several forms, one of which was the S74 leaflet in the Association's S series. The S74 leaflet is now superseded by this reprinting of the statement.*

The American Hospital Association presents a Patient's Bill of Rights with the expectation that observance of these rights will contribute to more effective patient care and greater satisfaction for the patient, his physician, and the hospital organization. Further, the Association presents these rights in the expectation that they will be supported by the hospital on behalf of its patients, as an integral part of the healing process. It is recognized that a personal relationship between the physician and the patient is essential for the provision of proper medical care. The traditional physician-patient relationship takes on a new dimension when care is rendered within an organizational structure. Legal precedent has established that the institution itself also has a responsibility to the patient. It is in recognition of these factors that these rights are affirmed.

1. The patient has the right to considerate and respectful care.
2. The patient has the right to obtain from his physician complete current information concerning his diagnosis, treatment, and prognosis in terms the patient can be reasonably expected to understand. When it is not medically advisable to give such information to the patient, the information should be made available to an appropriate person in his behalf. He has the right to know, by name, the physician responsible for coordinating his care.
3. The patient has the right to receive from his physician information necessary to give informed consent prior to the start of any procedure and/or treatment. Except in emergencies, such information for informed consent should include but not necessarily be limited to the specific procedure and/or treatment, the medically significant risks involved, and the probable duration of incapacitation. Where medically significant alternatives for care or treatment exist, or when the patient requests information concerning medical alternatives, the patient has the right to such information. The patient also has the right to know the name of the person responsible for the procedures and/or treatment.
4. The patient has the right to refuse treatment to the extent permitted by law and to be informed of the medical consequences of his action.

5. The patient has the right to every consideration of his privacy concerning his own medical care program. Case discussion, consultation, examination, and treatment are confidential and should be conducted discreetly. Those not directly involved in his care must have the permission of the patient to be present.
6. The patient has the right to expect that all communications and records pertaining to his care should be treated as confidential.
7. The patient has the right to expect that within its capacity a hospital must make reasonable response to the request of a patient for services. The hospital must provide evaluation, service, and/or referral as indicated by the urgency of the case. When medically permissible, a patient may be transferred to another facility only after he has received complete information and explanation concerning the needs for and alternatives to such a transfer. The institution to which the patient is to be transferred must first have accepted the patient for transfer.
8. The patient has the right to obtain information as to any relationship of his hospital to other health care and educational institutions insofar as his care is concerned. The patient has the right to obtain information as to the existence of any professional relationships among individuals, by name, who are treating him.
9. The patient has the right to be advised if the hospital proposes to engage in or perform human experimentation affecting his care or treatment. The patient has the right to refuse to participate in such research projects.
10. The patient has the right to expect reasonable continuity of care. He has the right to know in advance what appointment times and physicians are available and where. The patient has the right to expect that the hospital will provide a mechanism whereby he is informed by his physician or a delegate of the physician of the patient's continuing health care requirements following discharge.
11. The patient has the right to examine and receive an explanation of his bill regardless of source of payment.
12. The patient has the right to know what hospital rules and regulations apply to his conduct as a patient.

No catalog of rights can guarantee for the patient the kind of treatment he has a right to expect. A hospital has many functions to perform, including the prevention and treatment of disease, the education of both health professionals and patients, and the conduct of clinical research. All these activities must be conducted with an overriding concern for the patient, and, above all, the recognition of his dignity as a human being. Success in achieving this recognition assures success in the defense of the rights of the patient.

SOURCE: Reprinted with permission from "A Patient's Bill of Rights," published by the American Hospital Association.

ROLE OF THE NURSE AS A PATIENT ADVOCATE

On pages 330–331 is the text of the Patient's Bill of Rights. Since the American Hospital Association passed the Patient's Bill of Rights, hospitals and other community agencies have paid closer attention to this matter. Many hand out brief versions of the rights of clients in pamphlet form upon admission; others post the rights in frequented client areas of the facility. The intent is to make the public aware and to elaborate on the client's control of care by enabling the client to perceive rights and then have avenues through which to insure them.

Large hospitals are beginning to employ someone in the position of "Patient Advocate" or "Ombudsman." The latter term is often more familiar in academic settings; the philosophic framework of both, however, is congruent. This person is employed primarily for the consumer and acts as liaison between consumer problems and organizational structure, clarifying and, it is hoped, satisfying all involved people regarding their rights.

Even with someone specifically designated as the advocate, a responsibility of advocacy always rests with nursing personnel because they are most closely in contact with clients. This contact and relationship can be the source of frequent questions, expression of fears, and teaching activity with the client. It is, therefore, necessary for the nurse to assume the coordinator role in carrying out the advocacy function in response to a system. If a designated Patient Advocate is available, questions of clients may be referred. Should diagnostic medical information be requested, the physician should be notified and a written notation made by the nurse. In any area that a professional nurse feels comfortable with knowledge and experience in answering questions and informing the clients—within the confines of the nurse's legal responsibility—the nurse should and must do so. Informed consent and the protection of human subjects are an *ethical* right of all consumers.

Since the Patient's Bill of Rights very often involves interpretation in application to the unique consumer, any questions which the professional nurse has must be answered. Peer teaching and discussion is often necessary and advice from colleagues with more experience and knowledge should be sought whenever a question exists in interpretation of application. Ethical standards of the nursing profession must *always* be followed.

Annas (1975) has elaborated on the Patient's Bill of Rights in his recent publication entitled *The Rights of Hospitalized Patients*. He specifies that in addition to the AHA items, clients should:

1. Have round-the-clock telephone access to an advocate who can answer their questions;
2. Participate in all decisions regarding their health care program;
3. Be knowledgeable of research and experimental protocols involved in their care;

4. Have access to an interpreter if they do not speak English;
5. Consult a specialist at their request and expense;
6. Have legal rights to refuse treatments performed on them with primary emphasis on educational purposes rather than direct personal benefits; and
7. Have a right to access of visitors and a telephone—parents and family of terminally ill clients should be able to come and go totally at their will.

Annas (1975) does not deviate from the AHA (1975) statements but does become more specific.

SUMMARY

Client rights have been discussed with emphasis on the role of the professional nurse in carrying out the statements on rights passed by the American Hospital Association in 1975. The responsibility of the nurse varies within the institution in which the nurse is employed and depends on the complement of personnel attending to this function. Coordination of all aspects of this facet of client care, however, rests with the nurse—the nurse must ensure that all client needs in this area are met.

REFERENCES

American Hospital Association. A patient's bill of rights. Chicago: American Hospital Association, 1975.

Annas, G. *The rights of hospital patients.* New York: Avon Books, 1975.

HUMANISTIC EXERCISES

PART III
QUALITY SYSTEMS IN NURSING PRACTICE

EXERCISE 1
Problem Oriented Nursing Records

EXERCISE 2
Evaluation of the Course

EXERCISE 3
Self-Evaluation and Diagnosis

EXERCISE 4
The Advocacy Role of the Nurse

EXERCISE 1
Problem Oriented Nursing Records

PURPOSE   To gain experience in using the problem oriented system
                    of charting.

FACILITY   Access to traditionally-charted client records.

MATERIALS   Worksheets A, B, C, D.

TIME REQUIRED   Two hours.

GROUP SIZE   This is a homework assignment.

DESIGN   1. Students should choose a client in a health care
                       setting where problem oriented nursing records are
                       not routinely used.
                    2. Using Worksheets A, B, C, and D, the regular chart
                       should be adapted to the problem oriented system.
                       Nursing care should be the focus.

VARIATIONS   1. The instructor can prepare a case data base and
                       groups of four to six students can adapt the case to
                       the problem oriented method in class. In a large
                       (total class) group, each smaller group can then
                       report to each other. Differences should be
                       discussed.
                    2. This exercise can be a class report assignment for
                       several students. The teaching experience will be also
                       then an objective.
                    3. The worksheets can be used as a basis for the
                       structure of POR and nursing care planning on a
                       continual basis.
                    4. The records can be used to include total health care
                       planning (physician's diagnoses and orders, etc.).

DATA BASE

Family Name

Family Roster

Family/Household Member	Sex	Birth Date	Comments: Relationship, Occupation, etc.
1.			
2.			
3.			
4.			
5.			

History (Sign and date entries): physical, functional, nutritional, etc.

*Guidelines for Worksheets A, B, C, and D have been adapted from those published by the National League for Nursing, New York, 1974.

EXERCISE 1, WORKSHEET A (continued)

Environment: housing, sanitation, transportation, safety, etc.

Adjustments: social, emotional, cultural, vocational, religious, etc.

EXERCISE 1
WORKSHEET B

PATIENT/FAMILY PROBLEM INDEX

Date	Problem No.	Problems Current–Potential	Date of Onset	Date Resolved	Past Problems Inactive

PATIENT CARE PLAN—FLOW SHEET

Date	Problem Number	Plan; Actions to Be Taken	Flow Sheet Date				

PROGRESS NOTES

Date	Problem Number	Progress Notes Subjective(S) Objective(O) Assessment(A) Plans(P)

EXERCISE 2
Evaluation of the Course

PURPOSE   To provide feedback to the course planner/instructor.

FACILITY   Regular classroom setting.

MATERIALS   Evaluations A, B, and/or C.

TIME REQUIRED   Approximately 10 minutes.

GROUP SIZE   Unlimited.

DESIGN   The course evaluations may be used when the instructor desires feedback from the learners. Each can be administered in class or taken home for completion.

EVALUATION A
Usable at any point during the semester in which the class is given. It provides a means for evaluating the needs of students midway through the semester in order for adjustments to be made as indicated by the responses.

Instructors must list in the left hand column the broad content areas covered to date of the evaluation.

EVALUATION B
This is a short, end-of-course evaluation.

EVALUATION C
Evaluation C provides a more descriptive end-of-course report.

All evaluations can be either anonymous or identifiable with the students and/or openly discussed or not with relevant participants or the entire group.

EXERCISE 2
EVALUATION A

COURSE CONTENT EVALUATION

Please circle the appropriate number that best describes each
content area.

COURSE CONTENT AREAS	Too Little	Just Right	Too Much
	1	2	3
	1	2	3
	1	2	3
	1	2	3
	1	2	3
	1	2	3
	1	2	3
	1	2	3
	1	2	3
	1	2	3
	1	2	3
	1	2	3
	1	2	3
	1	2	3
	1	2	3
	1	2	3
	1	2	3
	1	2	3
	1	2	3
	1	2	3
	1	2	3
	1	2	3
	1	2	3
	1	2	3
	1	2	3
	1	2	3
	1	2	3
	1	2	3
	1	2	3
	1	2	3
	1	2	3
	1	2	3
	1	2	3

EXERCISE 2
EVALUATION B

END-OF-COURSE EVALUATION

Mark an "X" on the line that best describes your evaluation of each item:

		Poor 1 2 3	Average 4 5 6 7	Excellent 8 9 10
I.	Subject Content			
	A. Interesting in terms of new knowledge	__ __ __	__ __ __ __	__ __ __
	B. Valuable in practice	__ __ __	__ __ __ __	__ __ __
	C. Applications in nursing practice were alive	__ __ __	__ __ __ __	__ __ __
II.	Instructor			
	A. Organization	__ __ __	__ __ __ __	__ __ __
	B. Ability to communicate	__ __ __	__ __ __ __	__ __ __
	C. Coverage of topic	__ __ __	__ __ __ __	__ __ __
	D. Effectiveness of teaching strategies	__ __ __	__ __ __ __	__ __ __
	E. Overall evaluation	__ __ __	__ __ __ __	__ __ __
III.	General			
	A. Overall evaluation of course	__ __ __	__ __ __ __	__ __ __

B. What was of most value to you in this course? _____

_____

_____

C. What was of least value? _____

_____

_____

D. How would you improve this course? _____

_____

_____

EXERCISE 2, EVALUATION B (continued)

E. Reflecting on the best instructor you have had, how did
your present instructor compare? _____

_____

_____

Why? _____

_____

_____

EXERCISE 2
EVALUATION C*

END-OF-COURSE EVALUATION

Course Number & Title:

Professor:

Date:

Using the scale provided, rate each item on the overall idea which runs through the item rather than the specific parts.

	Strongly disagree	Moderately disagree	Slightly disagree	Slightly agree	Moderately agree	Strongly agree
CONTENT						
1. Objectives are appropriate for course content	1	2	3	4	5	6
2. Objectives were met through class seminars, clinical practicum, and course design.	1	2	3	4	5	6
3. The course has provided me with extensive knowledge in the content area, and is applicable in my professional practice.	1	2	3	4	5	6
4. Course requirements cover essential aspects of the course and were of learning value.	1	2	3	4	5	6
5. This course has increased my learning, given me new viewpoints and appreciation, and increased my capacity to think and formulate questions.	1	2	3	4	5	6
6. Contrasting viewpoints, current developments and related theory were integrated into class topics.	1	2	3	4	5	6

*Adapted from a Faculty Evaluation Form used at the University of Massachusetts, 1975.

	Strongly disagree	Moderately disagree	Slightly disagree	Slightly agree	Moderately agree	Strongly agree

PROCESS

1. The instructor is clear, states objectives, summarizes major points, presents material in an organized manner and has extensive knowledge of subject. 1 2 3 4 5 6

2. The instructor is sensitive to the response of the class, encourages student participation and facilitates questions and discussion. 1 2 3 4 5 6

3. The instructor is available to students, conveys a genuine interest in students, and recognizes their individuality in learning. 1 2 3 4 5 6

4. The instructor enjoys teaching, is enthusiastic and makes the course content stimulating and alive. 1 2 3 4 5 6

5. The instructor has provided a class environment which increases my motivation to do my best, and acquired knowledge independently. 1 2 3 4 5 6

6. This course, as taught by this instructor, is one that I would recommend. On the whole, the course was excellent. 1 2 3 4 5 6

What was of most value in the course?

What was of least value in the course?

Other suggestions/comments.

EXERCISE 3
Self-Evaluation and Diagnosis

PURPOSES
: 1. To diagnose one's own areas of strength relevant to nursing practice.
  2. To diagnose one's own learning needs relevant to nursing practice.

FACILITY
: None.

MATERIALS
: Self-Evaluation and Diagnosis Form.

TIME REQUIRED
: One and one-half hours.

GROUP SIZE
: Homework Assignment.

DESIGN
: 1. Request that learners respond to the instrument out of class.
  2. Set up individual appointments with instructor and learner to discuss the responses.

VARIATIONS
: Both the teacher and learner can respond to the instrument. The teacher will be evaluating the learner and offering suggestions on ways to meet the indicated learning needs which he or she perceives. Differences in perceptions by self and others could form a basis for discussion.

EXERCISE 3
WORKSHEET A

SELF-EVALUATION AND DIAGNOSIS FORM*

Part I:

Directions: Select the **three** areas in which you feel you perform the best. Then select the **three** areas in which you comparatively perform the poorest. This is an evaluation of **your** comparative strengths and weaknesses, **not** one comparing you with others. Indicate in the column on your right your comments regarding your choices. (You may comment on as many other areas as are important to you.)

Area of Competency	Best	Poorest	Comment
A. Nursing Process			
1. Data collection			
a. Nursing histories			
b. Interviewing			
c. Interpretation of clinical data			
d. Consultation with other professionals			
e. Talking with families			
f. Physical assessment			
2. Processing data			
3. Nursing diagnosis			
a. Determining diagnosis			
b. Setting priorities			
4. Writing nursing orders			
5. Evaluating outcomes			

*This form is a modification of the original used by Professor Virginia Earles at the University of Massachusetts, Division of Nursing, 1975.

EXERCISE 3, WORKSHEET A (continued)

Area of Competency	Best	Poorest	Comment
B. Providing Care			
1. Direct physical care			
2. Effective use of inter-personal processes			
3. Technical skills			
4. Teaching			
5. Being an advocate of the client/family			
6. Making referrals			
7. Coordinating care			
8. Supervising nursing personnel			

Part II:
Discuss ways in which your thinking has developed about the nursing process and its role in nursing practice this semester.

EXERCISE 3, WORKSHEET A (continued)

Part III:
What do you plan to do about poorest areas?

Part IV:
What are you planning to do about further development of your strengths?

EXERCISE 3, WORKSHEET A (continued)

Part V:

List your personal course objectives and how you originally intended on meeting them. Describe how you actually met them with an evaluation of same.

Objectives	How you intend-ed to meet them	How you met them	Evaluation

EXERCISE 4
The Advocacy Role of the Nurse

PURPOSES
1. To raise consciousness on the various implications for nurses regarding patients' rights.
2. To become aware of various perceptions of the said role.
2. To identify major nursing implications of the Patients' Bill of Rights.
4. To identify and discuss problem areas relative to the topic.

FACILITY
Classroom to accommodate groups of ten.

MATERIALS
Patients' Bill of Rights (Chapter 15).
Paper and pencils.
Worksheets A and B.

TIME REQUIRED
Two hours.

GROUP SIZE
Unlimited groups of ten.

DESIGN
1. Ask group members to individually read the Patients' Bill of Rights and write down five areas or instances in which there are direct implications in nursing practice.
2. Have individuals then write down three problems relative to being a patients' advocate.
   Steps 1 and 2 can use Worksheet A (allow 20 minutes).
3. In the group of ten, have members share their individual implications and problem areas (20 minutes).
4. Then request that the group compile a list of ten major implications and five most significant problem areas from individual presentations (Worksheet B). Discussion should focus on possible solutions to the problem areas; that is, what would alleviate the problem; is the problem relative to my personality/position or can it be generalized and what do I/we need to do; etc. (45 minutes).
5. The balance of time can be used by having each group share with the total class their major impli-

cations, problems, and solutions. Someone could
write responses on the blackboard.
6. Discuss findings.

VARIATIONS   Each group could write their major implications,
problems, and solutions on large newsprint paper with
magic markers. These could be displayed during
Step 4.

INDIVIDUAL DIAGNOSIS

Implications in Nursing Practice

1.

2.

3.

4.

5.

Problem Areas

1.

2.

3.

EXERCISE 4
WORKSHEET B

GROUP DIAGNOSIS

Major Implications in Nursing Practice
  1.

  2.

  3.

  4.

  5.

  6.

  7.

  8.

  9.

10.

Problem Areas | Solutions

  1.

  2.

  3.

  4.

  5.

  6.

PART IV

THEORY AND STRATEGIES FOR FACILITATING PRACTICE IN THE CLINICAL ENVIRONMENT

16

Leadership in Nursing

Part IV is devoted to a discussion of leadership theory and its application in nursing environments. Models of nursing care delivery systems are described; this aspect involves the organizational structure in which nurses operate in delivering their services. The importance of leadership throughout nursing practice is described:

> Recognition that nurses need to become effective managers, supervisors, and administrators has pervaded the writings of nursing theorists over the years. The methods for providing nursing care have moved from case to functional, followed by establishment of the team concept, and then primary nursing. Styles of leadership have varied in each: autocratic, democratic, or *laissez-faire* behavior of the leader in any given situation.
> The variety of environments in nursing practice have expanded concurrently with the various preparations provided by educational institutions for prospective nurses. It has become increasingly apparent that nurse leaders must broaden their views, their knowledge, and their experience of leader behavior to accommodate the added responsibility placed on them by their organizational administration, by the specific goals of the faculty, and by the individual experiences, backgrounds, and needs of their nurses. (Hersey, Blanchard, and La Monica, 1976a, p. 17)

PURPOSE

The purpose of this chapter is to provide the prospective nurse leader with a brief study of one leadership theory*; this is intended to be of assistance in

*It must be noted that a complete study of leadership and management in nursing would fill several volumes. Situational leadership theory is only presented because of its pertinence in the span of theory and because it has previously been addressed in other portions of this book.

determining situational demands. It follows the same model of theory presented in Chapter 5 with the focus on implementing nursing care. In Chapter 5, the nurse was defined as the leader of nursing care. This chapter takes a broader view of the nurse manager as one who also leads other nurses and health care personnel as they deliver direct care to clients. The theory is designed to provide a conceptual framework enabling nurse leaders to maximize their effectiveness in working with individuals and environments within the health care system. The systems approach is again underscored with leadership style depending on the nurse leader, followers, superiors, and the environment.

The balance of this chapter is presented in the form of an article written by Paul Hersey, Kenneth Blanchard, and the author of this book; it was previously published in *Supervisor Nurse* (Hersey, Blanchard, and La Monica, 1976a). The journal ran a sequel to the above article (Hersey, Blanchard, and La Monica, 1976b) in which readers were given the opportunity to diagnose their own leadership style based on the theory presented in the first article.

REFERENCES

Hersey, P., Blanchard, K., and La Monica, E. A situational approach to supervision: Leadership theory and the supervising nurse. *Supervisor Nurse* 7:17–22, 1976a.

Hersey, P., Blanchard, K., and La Monica, E. A look at your supervisory style: Rationale and analyses. *Supervisor Nurse* 7:27–40, 1976b.

A Situational Approach to Supervision: Leadership Theory and the Supervising Nurse

Paul Hersey
Kenneth Blanchard
Elaine La Monica

A "BEST" STYLE OF LEADERSHIP?

The quest for an ideal type of leadership has appeared in management literature ever since the apparent conflict between the Scientific Management and the Human Relations schools of thought. The scientific management school emphasized a concern for task (production), while the human relations movement stressed concern for relationships (people).

The recognition of task and relationship as two different styles of leader behavior has pervaded the works of management theorists[2] over the past several decades. These styles have been defined as:

Task Behavior *The extent to which a leader organizes and defines the roles of individuals and members of her group by explaining what activities each is to do as well as when, where and how tasks are to be accomplished. It is further characterized by the extent to which a leader defines patterns of organization, formalizes channels of communication, and specifies ways of getting jobs accomplished.*

Relationship Behavior *The extent to which a leader engages in personal relationships with individuals or members of her group; the amount of socioemotional support and psychological strokes provided by the leader as well as the extent to which the leader engages in interpersonal communications and facilitating behaviors.[3]*

These two styles have been variously labeled, including such popular terminology as *autocratic vs democratic, employee-oriented or production-oriented, and goal achievement or group maintenance.*

For some time, it was believed that task and relationship were *either/or* styles of leader behavior and, therefore, could be depicted on a single dimension, a continuum, moving from very authoritarian (Task) leader behavior at one end to very democratic (Relationship) leader behavior at the other.[4]

Reprinted with permission from *Supervisor Nurse*, Vol. 7 (1976).

In more recent years, the feeling that task and relationship were *either/or* leadership styles has been dispelled. In particular, the leadership studies initiated in 1945 by the Bureau of Business Research at Ohio State University questioned this assumption.[5]

Observing the actual behavior of leaders in a wide variety of situations, the Ohio State staff found that leadership styles tended to vary considerably from leader to leader. The behavior of some was characterized mainly by structuring activities of followers in terms of task accomplishments, while others concentrated on providing socio-emotional support in terms of personal relationships among themselves and their followers. Other leaders had styles characterized by both task and relationship behavior. There were even some individuals in leadership positions whose behavior tended to provide little structure or consideration.

No dominant style appeared. Instead, various combinations were evident. Thus, it was determined that task and relationship are not *either/or* leadership styles as an authoritarian-democratic continuum suggests. Instead, these patterns of leader behavior can be plotted on two separate axes as shown in Figure 1.

Tri-Dimensional Model   After identifying task and relationship as the two central aspects of leader behavior, numerous practitioners and writers tried to determine which of the four basic styles depicted was the "best" style of leadership, that is, the one which would be successful in most situations. At one point, high task/high relationship (quadrant 2) was considered the "best" style while low task/low relationship (quadrant 4) was considered the "worst" style.[6]

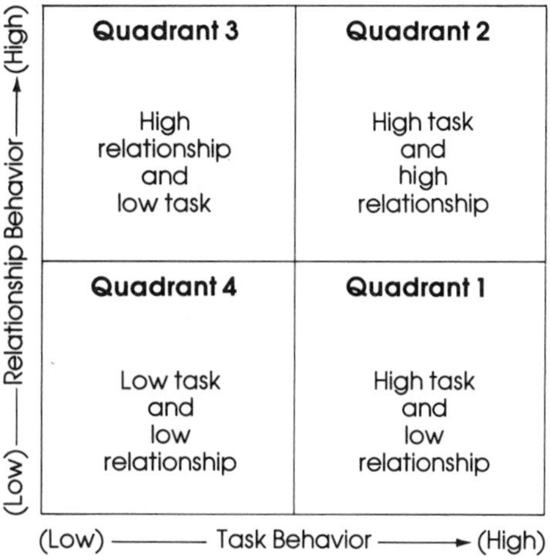

FIGURE 1
THE BASIC LEADER BEHAVIOR STYLES

Yet, evidence from research in the last decade clearly indicates that there is no single all-purpose leadership style.[7] Successful leaders are those who can adapt their behavior to meet the demands of their own unique environment.

If the effectiveness of a leader behavior style depends on the situation in which it is used, it follows that any of the four basic styles in Figure 1 may be effective or ineffective depending on the situation. *The difference between the effective and the ineffective styles is often not the actual behavior of the leader but the appropriateness of this behavior to the situation in which it is used.* In an attempt to illustrate this concept and build on previous work in leadership, an effectiveness dimension was added to the task and relationship dimensions of earlier leadership models to create the Tri-Dimensional Leader Effectiveness Model[8] presented in Figure 2.

The middle quadrants represent the four basic leader behavior styles; the left quadrants illustrate the four basic styles when they are ineffective (used in an inappropriate situation); and the right quadrants illustrate the four basic styles when they are effective (used in an appropriate situation).

The Tri-Dimensional Leader Effectiveness Model is distinctive because it does not depict a single ideal leader behavior style which is suggested to be appropriate in all situations. In essence, an effective leader must be able to *diagnose* the demands of the environment, and then *adapt* her leader style to fit these demands, or develop the means to change some of the other variables or all of them.

SITUATIONAL LEADERSHIP THEORY

Even nursing supervisors who realize that they must adapt their style of leadership to meet the demands of their environment are frustrated by the conclusion that the type of leader behavior needed "depends on the situation." They find little practical value in theory unless they can begin to see HOW leadership depends on the situation and, therefore, WHAT style tends to be effective with particular individuals and groups in changing environments. Yet, few theoretical frameworks have been developed to help supervisors diagnose the demands of their situation. This scarcity of practical situational leadership theories was one of the forces which motivated Hersey and Blanchard to develop *Life Cycle Theory of Leadership.*[9] This situational theory is based on a relationship among (1) the amount of direction (Task Behavior) a leader gives; (2) the amount of socio-emotional support (Relationship Behavior) a leader provides; and (3) the "maturity" of her followers or group. Followers in any situation are vital, not only because individually they accept or reject the leader, but also because as a group they actually determine whatever personal power she may have. Maturity is defined in Life Cycle Theory as the capacity to set high but attainable goals (achievement-motivation),[10] willingness and ability to take responsibility, and the education and the experience of an individual or a group. These variables of maturity should be considered in relation to a specific task to be performed. That is to say, an individual or a group is not mature or immature in any global sense,

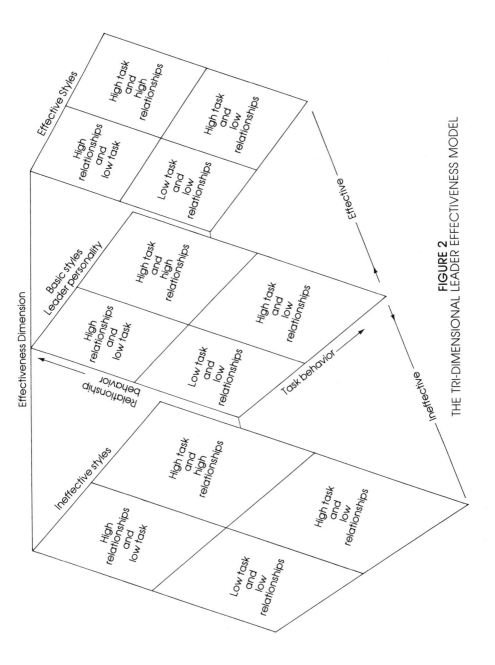

FIGURE 2
THE TRI-DIMENSIONAL LEADER EFFECTIVENESS MODEL

but is mature or immature only in terms of a specific task. Thus a new graduate may be very responsible in providing care for three or four individual patients, but not experienced in leading a team who care for sixteen patients.

According to Life Cycle Theory, as the level of maturity of one's followers continues to increase in terms of accomplishing a specific task, leaders should begin to *reduce* their task behavior and *increase* relationship behavior until the individual or group is sufficiently mature for the leaders to decrease their relationship styles according to the level of maturity of the followers. This cycle can be illustrated by the bell-shaped curve going through the four leadership quadrants as shown in Figure 3.

As can be seen in Figure 3, the curvilinear function of the cycle would be portrayed on the effective side of the Tri-Dimensional Leader Effectiveness Model. To determine what style is appropriate with what individual or group, some benchmarks of maturity have been provided for determining appropriate leadership style by dividing the maturity continuum into three categories— low, moderate, and high.

This theory of leadership states that when working with people who are low in maturity in terms of accomplishing a specific task, a high task style (quadrant 1) has the highest probability of success; whereas in dealing with people who are of average maturity on a task, moderate structure and moderate-to-high socio-emotional style (quadrants 2 and 3) appear to be most appropriate and a low task and low relationship style (quadrant 4) has the highest probability of success working with people of high task maturity.

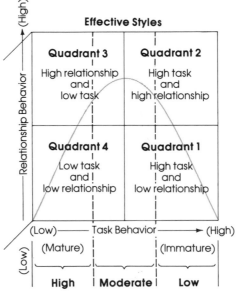

FIGURE 3
LIFE CYCLE THEORY OF LEADERSHIP

Modifying Levels of Maturity   In attempting to help a staff nurse or a group to mature, *i.e.*, to get them to take more and more responsibility for performing a specific task, a nursing leader must be careful not to delegate responsibility or to increase socio-emotional support too rapidly. If the leader does this, the individual nurse or group may take advantage and view the leader as a "soft-touch." Thus the leader must develop the maturity of followers slowly on each task that they must perform, using less task behavior and more relationship behavior as they mature and become more willing and able to take responsibility. When a staff nurse's performance is low on a specific task, one cannot expect drastic changes overnight. For a desirable behavior to be obtained, a supervisor must reward as soon as possible the slightest behavior exhibited by the nurse in the desired direction and continue this process as the individual's behavior comes closer and closer to the nursing leader's expectations of good performance. This is a behavior modification concept called *positively reinforcing successive approximations*[11] *of a desired behavior.* For example, a head nurse might want to move a new graduate through the cycle so that she would assume significantly more responsibility as a team member. If the new graduate is normally dependent on her head nurse for clarification and direction regarding the care of her four assigned patients, the head nurse can reduce the close supervision by asking the new graduate what she thinks needs to be done and adding to this only when quality care will not be provided for the patient. This will allow the staff nurse to begin to trust her own experience and knowledge. If this responsibility is well-handled, the head nurse should reinforce this behavior with increases in socio-emotional support or relationship behavior. This is a two-step process: first, a reduction in structure, and second, if adequate performance follows, an increase in socio-emotional support as reinforcement. This process should continue until the new graduate is carrying out all phases of patient care as a mature individual. This does not mean that the nurse's work will have less structure, but rather that the structure now will be internally provided by the individual instead of being externally imposed by the head nurse. When this happens, the cycle as depicted by Life Cycle Theory of leadership in Figure 3 begins to become a backward bending curve and to move toward Quadrant 4 (low task behavior and low relationship behavior). The staff nurses are able not only to structure many of the activities in which they engage while working on a specific task, but also are able to provide their own satisfaction for interpersonal and emotional needs. At this stage of maturity staff nurses are positively reinforced for their accomplishments by the supervisor not looking over their shoulders on a specific task and by the supervisor leaving them more and more on their own. It is not that there is less mutual trust and friendship but rather that less overt behavior is needed to prove it.

Although this theory suggests a basic style for different levels of task maturity, it is not a one-way street. When people begin to behave less maturely for whatever reason, *i.e.*, crisis at home, change in unit assignment, etc., it becomes appropriate for the supervisor to adjust behavior backward through the curve to meet the present maturity level of her group. For example, take the staff nurse who is presently working well on her own. Suppose, suddenly, the nurse faces a family crisis which begins to affect her performance on the job. In this situation, it may be appropriate for the supervisor moderately to increase structure and socio-emotional support until the individual regains his or her composure.

In summary, it is important for nursing supervisors to be aware of any progress of their subordinates so that they are in a position appropriately to reinforce improved performance. It must be remembered that change through the cycle from Quadrant 1 to Quadrant 2, 3, and 4 must be gradual. This process by its very nature cannot be revolutionary but must be evolutionary— it requires gradual developmental changes, a result of planned growth and the creation of mutual trust and respect.

REFERENCES

1. As examples see the following: L. Douglass. *Review of Team Nursing.* St. Louis: C. V. Mosby Co., 1973; L. Douglass and E. Bevis. *Team Leadership in Action: Principles and Application to Staff Nursing Situations.* St. Louis: C. V. Mosby C., 1970; Grace Eckelberry. *Administration of Comprehensive Nursing Care.* New York: Appleton-Century-Crofts, 1971; T. Kron. *The Management of Patient Care.* Phila.: W. B. Saunders Co., 1971.

2. As examples see the following: Robert F. Bales, "Task Roles and Social Roles in Problem-Solving Groups," in *Readings in Social Psychology,* E. E. Maccoby, T. M. Newcomb and E. L. Hartley (eds.). New York: Holt, Rinehart and Winston, 1958; Chester I. Bernard. *The Functions of the Executive.* Cambridge, Massachusetts: Harvard University Press. 1938; Dorwin Cartwright and Alvin Zander (eds.). *Group Dynamics: Research and Theory,* second edition. Evanston, Illinois: Row, Peterson and Company, 1960; D. Katz, N. Maccoby, and Nancy C. Morse. *Productivity, Supervision, and Morale in an Office Situation.* Detroit, Michigan: The Darel Press, Inc., 1950; Talcott Parsons. *The Social System.* Glencoe, Illinois: The Free Press, 1951.

3. These definitions have been adapted from The Ohio State definitions of "Initiating Structure" and "Consideration," Andrew W. Halpin, *The Leadership Behavior of School Superintendents.* Chicago: Midwest Administration Center, The University of Chicago, 1959, p. 4; and Roger M. Stogdill and Alvin E. Coons (ed.), *Leader Behavior: Its Description and Measurement,* Research Monograph No. 88. Columbus, Ohio: Bureau of Business Research, The Ohio State University, 1957.

4. Robert Tannenbaum and Warren H. Schmidt, "How to Choose a Leadership Pattern," *Harvard Business Review,* March-April, 1957, pp. 95–101.

5. Stogdill and Coons, *Op. cit.,* note 3.

6. See Andrew W. Halpin, *op. cit.,* note 3. Robert R. Blake and Jane S. Mouton. *The Managerial Grid.* Houston, Texas: Gulf Publishing, 1964; and Rensis Likert. *New Patterns of Management.* New York: McGraw-Hill Book Company, 1961.

7. As examples see A. K. Korman, " 'Consideration,' 'Initiating Structure,' and Organization Criteria—A Review," *Personnel Psychology: A Journal of Applied Research,* XIX, No. 4, Winter 1966, pp. 349–361; and Fred E. Fiedler. *A Theory of Leadership Effectiveness,* New York: McGraw-Hill Book Company, 1967.

8. Paul Hersey and Kenneth Blanchard. *Management of Organizational Behavior: Utilizing Human Resources.* Englewood Cliffs, New Jersey: Prentice Hall, Inc., pp. 81–87. For a discussion of an early attempt to add an effectiveness dimension to the task and relationships dimensions see William J. Reddin, "The 3-D Management Style Theory," *Training and Development Journal,* April 1967, pp. 8–17; see also Reddin, *Management Effectiveness.* New York: McGraw-Hill Book Company, 1970.

9. This theory was first published in Paul Hersey and Kenneth H. Blanchard, "Life Cycle Theory of Leadership," *Training and Development Journal,* May, 1969, and was further refined in Hersey and Blanchard, *Management of Organizational Behavior, op. cit.,* note 8.

10. David C. McClelland, J. W. Atkinson, R. A. Clark, and E. L. Lowell. *The Achievement Motive.* New York: Appleton-Century-Crofts, Inc., 1953, and *The Achieving Society.* Princeton, New Jersey: D. Van Nostrand Co., 1961.

11. The most classic discussions of behavior modification, or operant conditioning, have been done by B. F. Skinner. See Skinner. *Science and Human Behavior.* New York: The Macmillan Company, 1953.

17

Models of Nursing Care Delivery

There are five basic models for delivering nursing care in any health care setting. These involve the organizational structure of a unit and how a group of nurses and other health workers coordinate their expertise and efforts in taking care of a group of clients.

The focus of Chapter 17 is to discuss each model in terms of its definition, values, and disadvantages. The reader should be aware that nursing systems may apply the pure model to their setting or adapt one or more models as their individual systems warrant. The purpose of this discussion is to provide a basic framework by which the nurse can understand the model for delivering nursing care in any setting and/or design one that meets the particular needs of a group of health care-givers and clients. The individual delivery model, of course, should be built on theory and understanding.

The five models to be presented are: (1) case method, (2) functional method, (3) team nursing, (4) progressive client care, and (5) primary nursing.

All models have the possibility of resulting in quality, individualized care; the nurse implementors set the stage. The reader should note, however, that certain models lend more ease to accomplishment of nursing's ultimate goal, respective of the reality of our present health care system. These models are: team nursing and primary nursing.

Definition The case method is probably the oldest method of nursing care delivery. It involves the assignment of one or more clients to a nurse for a specific period of time, such as a shift (Douglass and Bevis, 1974). Complete care, including treatments, medication administration, and nursing care planning, is the assigned nurse's responsibility.

Even though the case method is one of the earliest developed and communicated through written sources, its usage remains in contemporary practice. Students most frequently learn within this model, private duty nurses practice with this design, and specialty units, such as intensive and coronary care areas, most often use this framework.

Values The values of the case method are:

1. The nurse can better see and attend to the total needs of clients due to the time and proximity of interactors. Coordination of all aspects of care is the responsibility of the nurse: physical, emotional, medical regimen, teaching, and all other aspects.
2. Continuity of care can be facilitated with ease.
3. Client/nurse interaction/rapport can be developed due to the intensity of time and proximity of those involved.
4. Client may feel more secure knowing that one person is thoroughly familiar with the needs and the course of treatment.
5. Educational needs of clients can be closely monitored.
6. Family and friends may become better known by nurse and more involved in the care of the client.
7. Workload for the unit can be equally divided among available staff.
8. Nurses' accountability for their functions is built-in.

Disadvantages The disadvantages of the case method are:

1. Many clients do not require the intensity of care inherent in this type of service.
2. The method must be modified if non-professional health workers are to be used effectively.
3. There are not enough nurses to fill the demand of this model; cost-effectiveness must be considered.
4. It is difficult for nurses using this model to become involved in long-term planning and evaluation of care.

FUNCTIONAL METHOD

Definition The functional method is a technical approach to nursing care that emphasizes the dependent functions of nursing practice (Kron, 1976). The available staff on a unit, for a particular period of time, are assigned to selected functions such as vital signs, treatments, medications. These functions are carried out for the entire group of clents on a unit. All the responsibilities of the unit are assigned to selected people in accordance with their expertise. The only person who has complete responsibility of the client is the head nurse or nurse acting in that role.

Values The values of the functional method are:

1. One person can become particularly skilled in performing assigned tasks; it can be efficient and economical.

2. The best utilization may be made of a person's aptitudes, experience, and desires.
3. Less equipment is needed and what is available is usually better cared for when used only by a few personnel.
4. This method saves time because it lends itself to strict organizational protocol.
5. The potential for development of technical skills is amplified.
6. There is a sense of productivity for the task-oriented nurse.
7. It is easy to organize the work of the unit and staff.

Disadvantages The disadvantages of the functional method are:

1. Client care may become impersonal, compartmentalized, and fragmented.
2. There is a tremendous risk for diminishing continuity of care.
3. Staff may become bored and have little motivation to develop self and others. Work may become monotonous.
4. The staff members are accountable for the task; only the nurse in charge of the unit has accountability for the individual, whole client.
5. There is little avenue for staff development, except as it relates to tasks.
6. Clients may tend to feel insecure, not knowing who is their own nurse.
7. Only parts of the nursing care plan are known to personnel.
8. It is difficult to establish client priorities and operationalize the care plan reflecting same.
9. It is only safe when the head nurse can coordinate the activities of all members of the staff and make certain that nothing essential in client care is overlooked or forgotten. This is a tremendous responsibility for one person who probably has to think of approximately thirty or more clients, plus the staff.

TEAM NURSING

Definition Team nursing was developed under a grant from the W. K. Kellogg Foundation in the early 1950s, directed by Eleanor Lambertsen at Teachers College, Columbia University, in New York City. It was designed to accommodate several categories of personnel in meeting the comprehensive nursing needs of a group of clients (Donovan, 1975).

Team nursing is based on a philosophy (Kron, 1976) in which a *group* of professional and non-professional personnel *work together* to identify, plan, implement, and evaluate comprehensive client-centered care. The key concept is a *group that works together* toward a common goal—providing quality, comprehensive nursing care.

Team nursing involves decentralization of a nursing unit and head nurse's authority. For example, instead of a Head Nurse directing three registered nurses, four licensed practical nurses and five nurse's aides in caring for 60 clients, the unit is divided into three teams. Each team is composed of the following:

- •Team Leader (RN)
- •Team Members (RN, LPN, aide)
- •Patients

Staff and clients are usually divided evenly, often within unit proximity such as a wing of a floor.

Comprehensive nursing care for the clients is the responsibility of the entire team, but is led by the team leader who should be a registered nurse, experienced in providing nursing care and in leadership (Kron, 1976). Team members comprise everyone else on the team; that is, graduate nurses, auxiliary personnel, LPNs, orderlies, and others. Assignments are made according to the capabilities of the members and respond to the needs of the group of clients.

There is no protocol for how a team leader assigns the members to care for the clients. Total care is the responsibility of the *team*, not any particular person; the team leader is the head. What follows in assignments reflects the expertise of team members as well as the needs of the clients. All of the work that needs to be done is accomplished by the *team*, in the best way and maintaining quality care. This method heavily relies on the use of the nursing care plan and the team conference in discussing and evaluating the care plans as well as the needs of the team (Kron, 1961; Lambertsen, 1953; Newcomb, 1953).

Values   The values of team nursing are:

1. It includes all health care personnel in the group's functioning and goals.
2. Feelings of participation and belonging are facilitated with team members.
3. Workload can be balanced and shared.
4. Division of labor allows members the opportunity to develop leadership skills.
5. Every team member has the opportunity to learn from and teach colleagues.
6. There is a variety in the daily assignments.
7. Interest in clients' well-being and care is shared by several people; reliability of decisions is increased.
8. Nursing care hours are usually cost-effective.
9. The client is able to identify personnel who are responsible for his care.
10. All care is directed by a registered nurse.
11. Continuity of care is facilitated, especially if teams are constant.
12. Barriers between professional and non-professional workers can be minimized; the group effort prevails.
13. Everyone has the opportunity to contribute to the care plan.

Disadvantages   The disadvantages of team nursing are:

1. Establishing the team concept takes time, effort, and constancy of personnel. Merely assigning people to a group does not make them a "group" or "team."
2. Unstable staffing patterns make team nursing difficult.
3. All personnel must be client-centered.
4. The team leader must have complex skills and knowledge: communication, leadership, organization, nursing care, motivation, and other skills.
5. There is less individual responsibility and independence regarding nursing functions.

PROGRESSIVE CLIENT CARE

Definition   Progressive client care is a method in which client-care areas or units provide various levels of care. Examples include: (1) intensive care unit for the critically ill, (2) post-intensive care unit, (3) regular care unit, (4) convalescent unit, (5) self-care unit. Clients are evaluated with respect to the level (intensity) of care needed. As they "progress" towards increased self-care (as they become less critically ill or in need of intensive care or monitoring) they are moved to units staffed to best provide the type of care needed.

Values   Values of progressive care are:

1. Efficient use is made of personnel and equipment.
2. Clients are in the best place to receive the care they require.
3. Use of nursing skills and expertise are maximized due to different staffing patterns in each unit.
4. Clients are moved toward self-care; independence is fostered when indicated.
5. Efficient use and placement of equipment is possible.
6. Personnel have greater probability to function toward their fullest capacity.

Disadvantages   Disadvantages of progressive care are:

1. There may be discomfort to clients who are moved often.
2. Continuity of care is difficult, even though possible.
3. Long-term nurse/client relationships are difficult to arrange.
4. Heavy emphasis is placed on comprehensive, written care plans.
5. There is oftentimes difficulty in meeting administrative need of the organization: staffing, evaluation, accreditation.

PRIMARY NURSING

Definition   Primary nursing involves total nursing care, directed by a nurse on a 24-hour basis as long as the client is under care. One specific nurse is the client's nurse, at all times, directing, planning, evaluating, and teaching. The primary nurse is essentially on call all the time and arranges coverage when away. Even though the primary nurse is the director of care for clients, segments of care are often delegated.

This method is the latest in development, receiving increasing attention within the past decade (Manthey, 1973; Manthey and Kramer, 1970; Marram, et al., 1976). It is often confused with the case method, which was discussed earlier. The difference exists in the fact that the case method involves a specified segment of time (such as a shift). Primary nursing is 24-hour responsibility for as long as care is needed by the client.

Values   Values of primary nursing are:

1. There is opportunity for the nurse to see the client and family as one system.
2. Nursing accountability, responsibility, and independence are increased.
3. The nurse is able to use a wide range of skills, knowledge, and expertise.
4. The method potentiates creativity by the nurse; work satisfaction may increase significantly.
5. The scene is set for increased trust and satisfaction by the client and nurse.

Disadvantages   Disadvantages of primary nursing are:

1. The nurse may be isolated from colleagues.
2. There is little avenue for group planning of client care.
3. Nurses must be mature and independently competent.
4. It may be cost-ineffective even though recent articles indicate otherwise.
5. Staffing patterns may necessitate a heavy client load.

SUMMARY

Chapter 17 discussed five models for nursing care delivery. Each was addressed in terms of its definition, values, and disadvantages. Even though any model can be as effective as the implementation of the model, primary nursing and team nursing emerge as the most facilitative models for individualized care. Each group of health care personnel, however, must respond to its own needs, the environmental demands, and clientele. All should be directed toward quality, individualized care.

REFERENCES

Donovan, H. *Nursing service administration.* St. Louis: C. V. Mosby, 1975.

Douglass, L., and Bevis, E. *Nursing leadership in action.* St. Louis: C. V. Mosby, 1974.

Kron, J. *Nursing team leadership.* Philadelphia: W. B. Saunders, 1961.

Kron, J. *The management of patient care.* Philadelphia: W. B. Saunders, 1976.

Lambertson, E. *Nursing team—organization and functioning.* New York: Columbia University Press, 1953.

Manthey, M. Primary nursing is alive and well in the hospital. *American Journal of Nursing* 73:83–87, 1973.

Manthey, M., and Kramer, M. A dialogue on primary nursing. *Nursing Forum* 9:356–379, 1970.

Marram, G., Schlegel, M., and Bevis, E. *Primary nursing.* St. Louis: C. V. Mosby, 1974.

Newcomb, D. *The team plan.* New York: G. P. Putnam's Sons, 1953.

HUMANISTIC EXERCISES

PART IV
THEORY AND STRATEGIES FOR FACILITATING PRACTICE IN THE CLINICAL ENVIRONMENT

EXERCISE 1
Self-Diagnosis of Leadership Style and Effectiveness

PURPOSES

1. To diagnose one's personal leadership style and the effectiveness of the style in a given situation.
2. To understand the implications of one's leadership style.

FACILITY

Classroom.

MATERIALS

Worksheet A: Leader Behavior (Self) Questionnaire
Worksheet B: Scoring Key for "Initiating Structure"
Worksheet C: Scoring Key for "Consideration"
Worksheet D: Ideal Leader Behavior Questionnaire (What You Expect of a Leader)
Worksheet E: Locating Scores on the Ohio State Leadership Studies Model
Pencil

TIME REQUIRED

Forty-five minutes.

GROUP SIZE

Unlimited.

DESIGN

1. Instruct members to individually respond to the items in Worksheet A. Follow directions on the instrument.
2. After completing step 1, go to Worksheets B and C and follow the directions for scoring.
3. Repeat steps 1 and 2 for items in Worksheet D (What You Expect of a Leader).
4. Go to Worksheet E and interpret scores on model.
5. Discuss findings. Compare self with expectations.

VARIATIONS

Worksheet A can be given to an associate, a superior, and a follower. Their task is to rate you on how they feel you behave. Instruments can then be scored and compared with perceptions of self. Since behavior is as perceived by others, ratings scales filled out on your behavior lend reliability to your perceptions of self. A discussion of differences in perceptions among raters can be an excellent consciousness-raising activity.

EXERCISE 1
WORKSHEET A

LEADER BEHAVIOR (SELF) QUESTIONNAIRE

This questionnaire is determine your leadership style. Following is a list of items that may be used to describe your behavior as you think you act. This is not a test of ability. It simply asks you to describe how you believe you act as a leader of a group.

Directions
a. READ each item carefully.
b. THINK about how frequently you engage in the behavior described by the item.
c. DECIDE whether you **always, often, occasionally, seldom,** or **never** act as described by the item.
d. DRAW A CIRCLE around one of the five letters following the item to show the answer you have selected: A=always, B=often, C=occasionally, D=seldom, E=never.

When acting as a leader, I:

1.	Do personal favors for group members.	A	B	C	D	E
2.	Make my attitudes clear to the group.	A	B	C	D	E
3.	Do little things to make it pleasant to be a member of the group.	A	B	C	D	E
4.	Try out my new ideas with the group.	A	B	C	D	E
5.	Act as the real leader of the group.	A	B	C	D	E
6.	Be easy to understand.	A	B	C	D	E
7.	Rule with an iron hand.	A	B	C	D	E
8.	Find time to listen to group members.	A	B	C	D	E
9.	Criticize poor work.	A	B	C	D	E
10.	Give advance notice of changes.	A	B	C	D	E
11.	Speak in a manner not to be questioned.	A	B	C	D	E
12.	Keep to myself.	A	B	C	D	E
13.	Look out for the personal welfare of individual group members.	A	B	C	D	E
14.	Assign group members to particular tasks.	A	B	C	D	E
15.	Be the spokesman of the group.	A	B	C	D	E
16.	Schedule the work to be done.	A	B	C	D	E

SOURCE: Copyright Ohio State University. Developed by staff members of the Ohio State Leadership Studies, Center for Business and Economic Research, Division of Research, College of Administrative Science, Ohio State University, Columbus, Ohio. Reproduced by permission.

17. Maintain definite standards of performance. A B C D E
18. Refuse to explain my actions. A B C D E
19. Keep the group informed. A B C D E
20. Act without consulting the group. A B C D E
21. Back up the members in their actions. A B C D E
22. Emphasize the meeting of deadlines. A B C D E
23. Treat all group members as my equals. A B C D E
24. Encourage the use of uniform procedures. A B C D E
25. Get what I ask for from my superiors. A B C D E
26. Be willing to make changes. A B C D E
27. Make sure that my part in the organization is understood by group members. A B C D E
28. Be friendly and approachable. A B C D E
29. Ask that group members follow standard rules and regulations. A B C D E
30. Fail to take necessary action. A B C D E
31. Make group members feel at ease when talking with them. A B C D E
32. Let group members know what is expected of them. A B C D E
33. Speak as the representative of the group. A B C D E
34. Put suggestions made by the group into operation. A B C D E
35. See to it that group members are working up to capacity. A B C D E
36. Let other people take away my leadership in the group. A B C D E
37. Get my superiors to act for the welfare of the group members. A B C D E
38. Get group approval in important matters before going ahead. A B C D E
39. See to it that the work of group members is coordinated. A B C D E
40. Keep the group working together as a team. A B C D E

SCORING KEY FOR "INITIATING STRUCTURE"

Scoring Instructions

On the LEADER BEHAVIOR (Self) questionnaire draw a circle (2) around the questionnaire item numbers noted below (2, 4, 7, 9, etc.) Beside each such item write the score you get for each item. The appropriate score is determined by noting, as indicated below, the points for the response you made on the questionnaire. For example, if your response to question 2 was "seldom" you would put a "1" by question number 2 on your questionnaire. Do this for each of the 15 questions below. Add these 15 scores together. The total is your score for **Initiating Structure.** Transcribe this score in the space provided on Worksheet E.

Item No.	Always	Often	Occasion-ally	Seldom	Never
2	4	3	2	1	0
4	4	3	2	1	0
7	4	3	2	1	0
9	4	3	2	1	0
11	4	3	2	1	0
14	4	3	2	1	0
16	4	3	2	1	0
17	4	3	2	1	0
22	4	3	2	1	0
24	4	3	2	1	0
27	4	3	2	1	0
29	4	3	2	1	0
32	4	3	2	1	0
35	4	3	2	1	0
39	4	3	2	1	0

SCORING KEY FOR "CONSIDERATION"

Scoring Instructions

On the LEADER BEHAVIOR (Self) questionnaire circle the question-naire item numbers noted below (1, 3, 5, 8, etc.). On the left side of the questionnaire, beside each circled item, write the score you get for each item. The appropriate score is determined by noting, as indicated below, the points for the response you made on the questionnaire. For example, if your response to question 1 was "often" you would put a "3" by question number 1 on your questionnaire. Do this for each of the 15 questions below. Add the 15 scores. The total is your score for **Consideration.** (Note that there are 10 questions "left over" which are not scored. These are in the questionnaire in order to maintain conditions comparable to when the questionnaire was standardized.) Transcribe this score in the space provided on Worksheet E.

Item No.	Always	Often	Occasion-ally	Seldom	Never
1	4	3	2	1	0
3	4	3	2	1	0
6	4	3	2	1	0
8	4	3	2	1	0
12	0	1	2	3	4
13	4	3	2	1	0
18	0	1	2	3	4
20	0	1	2	3	4
21	4	3	2	1	0
23	4	3	2	1	0
26	4	3	2	1	0
28	4	3	2	1	0
31	4	3	2	1	0
34	4	3	2	1	0
38	4	3	2	1	0

EXERCISE 1
WORKSHEET D

IDEAL LEADER BEHAVIOR QUESTIONNAIRE (WHAT YOU EXPECT OF A LEADER)

Following is a list of items that may be used to describe the behavior of a supervisor, as you think he or she **should** act. This is not a test of ability. It simply asks you to describe what an ideal leader **ought to do** in supervising a group.

Directions
a. READ each item carefully.
b. THINK about how frequently the leader SHOULD engage in the behavior described by the item.
c. DECIDE whether he SHOULD **always, often, occasionally, seldom,** or **never** act as described by the item.
d. DRAW A CIRCLE around one of the five letters following the item to show the answer you have selected: A = always, B = often, C = occasionally, D = seldom, E = never.

What the IDEAL leader SHOULD do:

1. Do personal favors for group members. A B C D E
2. Make his attitudes clear to the group. A B C D E
3. Do little things to make it pleasant to be a member of the group. A B C D E
4. Try out his new ideas with the group. A B C D E
5. Act as the real leader of the group. A B C D E
6. Be easy to understand. A B C D E
7. Rule with an iron hand. A B C D E
8. Find time to listen to group members. A B C D E
9. Criticize poor work. A B C D E
10. Give advance notice of changes. A B C D E
11. Speak in a manner not to be questioned. A B C D E
12. Keep to himself. A B C D E
13. Look out for the personal welfare of individual group members. A B C D E
14. Assign group members to particular tasks. A B C D E
15. Be the spokesman of the group. A B C D E
16. Schedule the work to be done. A B C D E

SOURCE: Copyright Ohio State University. Developed by staff members of the Ohio State Leadership Studies, Center for Business and Economic Research, Division of Research, College of Administrative Science, Ohio State University, Columbus, Ohio. Reproduced by permission.

EXERCISE I, WORKSHEET D (continued)

17. Maintain definite standards of performance.   A   B   C   D   E
18. Refuse to explain his actions.   A   B   C   D   E
19. Keep the group informed.   A   B   C   D   E
20. Act without consulting the group.   A   B   C   D   E
21. Back up the members in their actions.   A   B   C   D   E
22. Emphasize the meeting of deadlines.   A   B   C   D   E
23. Treat all group members as his equals.   A   B   C   D   E
24. Encourage the use of uniform procedures.   A   B   C   D   E
25. Get what he asks for from his superiors.   A   B   C   D   E
26. Be willing to make changes.   A   B   C   D   E
27. Make sure that his part in the organization is understood by group members.   A   B   C   D   E
28. Be friendly and approachable.   A   B   C   D   E
29. Ask that group members follow standard rules and regulations.   A   B   C   D   E
30. Fail to take necessary action.   A   B   C   D   E
31. Make group members know what is expected of them.   A   B   C   D   E
32. Let group members know what is expected of them.   A   B   C   D   E
33. Speak as the representative of the group.   A   B   C   D   E
34. Put suggestions made by the group into operation.   A   B   C   D   E
35. See to it that group members are working up to capacity.   A   B   C   D   E
36. Let other people take away his leadership in the group.   A   B   C   D   E
37. Get his superiors to act for the welfare of the group members.   A   B   C   D   E
38. Get group approval on important matters before going ahead.   A   B   C   D   E
39. See to it that the work of group members is coordinated.   A   B   C   D   E
40. Keep the group working together as a team.   A   B   C   D   E

SCORING: Use same scoring method and keys as you did for the Leader Behavior (Self) questionnaire. Place your scores in the spaces provided on Worksheet E.

EXERCISE 1
WORKSHEET E

LOCATING SCORES ON THE OHIO STATE
LEADERSHIP STUDIES MODEL

	Self	Ideal Leader
Initiating Structure Score	————	————
Consideration Score	————	————

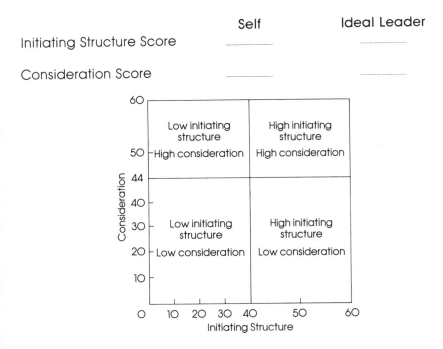

Directions:

In scoring both instruments, Worksheets A and D, indicate where your initiating structure score places on that continuum, followed by your consideration score. Draw the horizontal and vertical line from each axis until both meet. The box in which lines meet indicates your leadership style and what you expect from others as leaders with regard to leader behavior. Scores above 40 on the initiating structure dimension indicate you are above the mean. If you scored above 44 on the consideration dimension, you would also be above the mean.

SOURCE: Copyright Ohio State University. Developed by staff members of the Ohio State Leadership Studies, Center for Business and Economic Research, Division of Research, College of Administrative Science, Ohio State University, Columbus, Ohio. Reproduced by permission.

EXERCISE I, WORKSHEET E (continued)

The purpose for using this instrument is to begin the process of studying the congruence or differences between your leader behavior and your expectations of leader behavior. The Leader Behavior (Self) questionnaire is a rough indicator. If your scores conform to your experience in dealing with others and their perception of you, then the instrument provides an excellent basis for further self-study. Discrepancies between your perceptions of self and expectations of others should also provide questions for further exploration.

EXERCISE 2
Leadership: Diagnosing a Situation

PURPOSE
To gain experience in diagnosing the leadership styles and effectiveness of members within a situation.

FACILITY
Large room to accommodate learners working in groups of eight.

MATERIALS
Case from Urban City Hospital.
Diagnostic Skills Worksheet.

TIME REQUIRED
One and one-half hours.

GROUP SIZE
Unlimited groups of eight.

DESIGN
1. Each individual working alone is to assess the actions of the assigned leaders (George Jones and May Conte) as to their Task Behavior and Relationship Behavior, identify their dominant styles, and their effectiveness. In assigning these styles and determining effectiveness, develop reasons for your determinations. These reasons will serve as the basis for discussion in reaching work group consensus (step 3).
2. Record individual determinations on the Diagnostic Skills Worksheet (steps 1 and 2—20 minutes).
3. Each work group of eight should then reach consensus as to the basic leader behavior styles of the characters and their effectiveness. A group recorder must be chosen to record the group decisions (45 minutes).
4. Reform into a total group and have each recorder share their group's decisions and rationale. Record decisions on the blackboard. The following format for this step is suggested:

	Leadership Style		Effectiveness	
	Jones	Conte	Jones	Conte
Group 1				
Group 2				
Group 3				

5. Refer to the discussion section and share the experts'*
   interpretations.
6. Discuss the experience.

URBAN CITY HOSPITAL†

Janis Monroe, Executive Director of Urban City Hospital, was concerned by reports of absenteeism among some of the staff at the hospital. From reliable sources she had learned that some of the staff were punching the timecards of fellow workers who were arriving late or leaving early. Monroe had only recently been appointed to head Urban City Hospital. She judged from conversations with the previous Director and other administrators that people were, in general, pleased with the overall performance of the hospital.

Urban City Hospital has a reputation for quality medical care with a particularly good reputation in the areas of coronary unit, special care, and emergency room. Located in the center of Urban City, the hospital draws many of its patients from lower socio-economic families but does service extensively patients from the suburban areas. The staff with various educational backgrounds and training was generally from the small state in which Urban City is located. In fact, a number of nurses are graduates of the hospital's nursing program.

It is thought that patients usually enter Urban Hospital for one of the following reasons:

- high quality of care
- somewhat lower costs than other nearby facilities
- variety of medical care available.

George Jones, a long-time employee in the hospital, was administrator of Urban City Hospital. He generally left the staff alone, spending most of his time with personnel scheduling, procuring funds and supplies, overseeing budget matters, and related issues. Jones had an assistant, Rudy Lucas. When he needed to communicate with people in a particular area, George would just call them together or talk to an individual in the area and ask him to "pass the word." The latter was his usual approach.

*The experts are P. Hersey and K. Blanchard. Oral presentation, University of Massachusetts, School of Education, 1974.

† The author of this case is unknown; it was received by the author at the University of Massachusetts, School of Education, 1974.

Work situations at the hospital were quite varied. Some laboratories were cramped and less than adequate by some standards for the job required, whereas others more than met minimum criteria. Work efficiency did not seem to be related to these circumstances.

It should be noted that as far as hospitals are concerned, Urban City Hospital was one of the finest in the area. Patients generally liked their care and spoke highly of the facility.

The pay scale for the staff was low compared to other similar facilities. The average starting salary for a nurse was about $130 per week and the age of the building made working conditions generally more difficult than might be desirable.

Judy Mulry, a first year administrative assistant to the Director, provided the data for this case. After she had been working at the hospital for a month or so, Mulry noted that certain members of the staff tended to seek each other out during free time and after hours. She then observed that these informal associations were enduring, built upon common activities and shared ideas about what was and what was not legitimate behavior in the hospital. Her estimate of these associations is diagrammed in Exhibit 1. The hospital responsibility for each person is given.

The Conte group, so named because May Conte was its most respected member and the one who seemed to take responsibility for maintaining good relations within the group, was the largest. The group invariably tried to eat lunch together and operated as a team, regardless of the differences in individual assignments. Off the job, Conte group members often joined parties or got together for weekend trips. Conte's summer camp was a frequent rendezvous.

Conte's group was also the most cohesive one in the hospital in terms of its organized punch-in punch-out systems. The time clock system for the staff had been started three years before by the Board of Trustees which had been taken over by a conservative element. There might be times, however, when an individual staff member would have completed any specific responsibilities from one-half to three-quarters of an hour prior to the scheduled time to leave. If there were errands or other things to do that extra free time would help, another member of the group would punch out for the one who left early. The "right" to leave early was informally balanced among the members of the group. In addition, the group members would punch a staff member "in" if he/she were unavoidably late.

Conte explained the logic behind the system to Mulry.

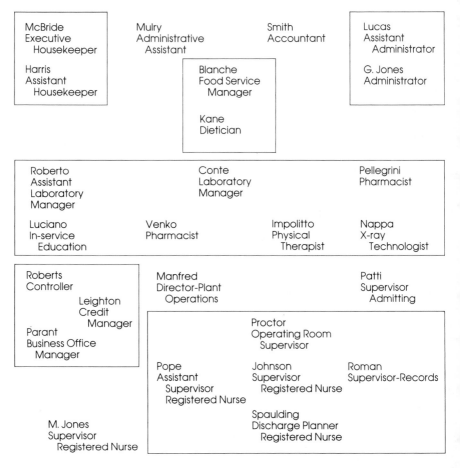

| McBride
Executive
Housekeeper | Mulry
Administrative
Assistant | Smith
Accountant | Lucas
Assistant
Administrator |
| Harris
Assistant
Housekeeper | Blanche
Food Service
Manager | | G. Jones
Administrator |

Kane
Dietician

Roberto
Assistant
Laboratory
Manager

Conte
Laboratory
Manager

Pellegrini
Pharmacist

Luciano
In-service
Education

Venko
Pharmacist

Impolitto
Physical
Therapist

Nappa
X-ray
Technologist

Roberts
Controller

Leighton
Credit
Manager

Parant
Business Office
Manager

Manfred
Director-Plant
Operations

Patti
Supervisor
Admitting

Proctor
Operating Room
Supervisor

Pope
Assistant
Supervisor
Registered Nurse

Johnson
Supervisor
Registered Nurse

Roman
Supervisor-Records

M. Jones
Supervisor
Registered Nurse

Spaulding
Discharge Planner
Registered Nurse

EXHIBIT 1
URBAN CITY HOSPITAL STAFF, INFORMAL GROUPINGS

"You know we don't get paid as well here as in other hospitals," she said. "What makes this the best hospital to work in is that we are not continually bothered by administrators. When things are under control, as they are now, and the patients are satisfied, the top brass seems to be happy. It seems silly to have to stay to punch out on those few occasions when a little extra free time would be of help to you. Of course, some people abuse this sort of thing. . . like Marsha. . . but the members of our group get the job done and it all averages out.

"When there is extra work, naturally I stay as late as necessary. So do a lot of others. I believe that if I stay until the work is done and everything is in order, that's all the administration expects of us. They leave us alone and expect the job to get done . . . and we do."

When Mulry asked Conte if she would not rather work at a newer hospital at a higher salary, she just laughed and said: "Never."

The members of Conte's group were explicit about what constituted a good job. Customarily, they cited Marsha Jones, who happened to be the administrator's sister, as a woman who continually let others down. Mulry received an informal orientation from Marsha during her first few days at the hospital. As Marsha put it: "I've worked at his hospital for years, and I expect to stay here a good many more. You're just starting out and you don't know the 'lay of the land' yet. Working in a hospital is tough enough without breaking your neck. You can wear yourself out fast if you're not smart. Look at Manfred, the Director of Plant Operations. There's a guy who's just going to burn himself out and for what? He makes it tough on everybody and on himself, too."

Mulry reported further on her observations of the group activities:

> May and her group couldn't understand Marsha. While Marsha arrived late a good deal of the time, May was usually early. If a series of emergency situations had created a backlog of work, almost everyone but Marsha would spend extra time to help catch up. May and members of her group would always stay later. While most of the staff seemed to find a rather full life in their work, Marsha never got really involved. No wonder they couldn't understand each other.
>
> There was quite a different feeling about Bob Manfred, the Director of Plant Operations. Not only did he work his full shift, but he often scheduled meetings with maintenance and other plant personnel on other shifts to consider better ways of getting their jobs done. He is also taking courses in the evening to complete the requirements for a degree. He often worked many Saturdays and Sundays . . . and all for "peanuts." He hardly got paid a cent extra. Because of the tremendous variance in responsibilities, it was hard to make comparisons, but I'm sure I wouldn't be far wrong in saying that Bob worked twice as hard as Marsha and 50 percent more than almost anyone else in the hospital. No one but Marsha and a few old-timers criticized him for his efforts. May and her group seemed to feel a distant affection for Bob, but the only contact they or anyone else had with him consisted of brief greetings.

To the members of May's group, the most severe penalty that could be inflicted was exclusion. This they did to both Manfred and Marsha. Manfred, however, was tolerated; Marsha was not. Evidently, Marsha felt her exclusion keenly, though she answered it with derision and aggression. Marsha kept up a steady stream of stories concerning her attempt to gain acceptance outside working hours. She wrote popular music which was always rejected by publishers. She attempted to join several social and literary clubs, mostly without success. Her favorite pastime was attending concerts. She told me that "music lovers" were friendly, and she enjoyed meeting new people whenever she went to a concert. But she was particularly quick to explain that she preferred to keep her distance from the other people on the staff at the hospital.

May's group emphasized more than just effort in judging a person's work. Among them had grown a confidence that they could develop and improve on the efficiency of any responsibility. May herself symbolized this. Before her, May's father had been an effective laboratory manager and helped May a great deal. When problems arose, the Director and other staff would frequently consult with May and she would give counsel willingly. She had a special feeling for her job. For example, when a young lab technician couldn't seem to get off the ground, May was the only one who successfully stepped in and probably saved a promising young technician. To a lesser degree, the other members of the group were also imaginative about solving problems which arose in their own areas.

Marsha, for her part, talked incessantly about her accomplishments. As far as I could tell during the year I worked in the hospital, there was little evidence to support these stories. In fact, many of the other staff members laughed at her. What's more, I never saw anyone seek Marsha's help.

Willingness to be of help was a trait the staff associated with Conte and was prized. The most valued help of all was a personal kind, though the jobs were also important.

The members of Conte's group were constantly lending and borrowing money, cars, and equipment among themselves and, less frequently, with other members of the hospital staff.

On the other hand, Marsha refused to help others in any way. She never tried to aid those around her who were in the midst of a rush of work, though this was customary throughout most of the hospital. I can distinctly recall the picture of the 7–3 Supervisor trying to handle an emergency situation at about 3 p.m. one day while Marsha continued a casual telephone conversation. She acted as if she didn't even notice the supervisor. She, of course, expected me to act this same way, and it was this attitude in her I found virtually intolerable.

More than this, Marsha took little responsibility for breaking in new nurses, leaving this entirely to the Assistant Supervisor. There had been four new nurses on her shift in the space of a year. Each had asked for a transfer to another shift, publicly citing personal reasons associated with the 7-3 shift but privately blaming Marsha. May was the one who taught me the ropes when I first joined the staff.

The staff who congregated around Pat Johnson were primarily nursing supervisors, but as a group tended to behave similar to the Conte group, though they did not quite approach the creativity or the amount of helping activities that May's group did. They were, however, all considered "good" in their jobs. Sometimes the Johnson group sought outside social contact with the Conte group. Even though they worked in different areas, both groups seemed to respect each other; and several times a year, the two groups went out "on the town" together.

The remainder of the people in the hospital stayed pretty much to themselves or associated in pairs or triplets. None of these people were as inventive, as helpful, or as productive as Conte's or Johnson's groups, but most of them gave verbal support to the same values as those groups held.

The distinction between the two organized groups and the rest of the hospital was clearest in the punching-out routine. McBride and Harris, Blanche and Kane, and Roberts, Parant, and Leighton arranged within their small groups for any early punch-outs. George Jones was frequently out of the building during any punch-outs and he didn't seem to pay attention to such things like the time clock anyway. His assistant Lucas, although always in the hospital, wasn't seen by many people. He seemed to "hide" in his office. Marsha Jones and Patti had no early punch-out organization to rely upon. Marsha was reported to have established an arrangement with Patti whereby the latter would punch Marsha out for a fee. Such a practice was unthinkable from the point of view of Conte's group. Marsha constantly complained about the dishonesty of other members of the staff in the hospital.

Just before I left Urban City to take another position, I casually met Ms. Monroe on the street. She asked me how I had enjoyed my experience at Urban City Hospital. During the conversation I learned that she knew of the punch-out system. What's more, she told me she was wondering if she ought to "blow the lid off the whole mess."

EXERCISE 2

DIAGNOSTIC SKILLS WORKSHEET

LEADER BEHAVIOR STYLE—Indicate dominant style with a checkmark for each character.

LEADERSHIP STYLE	INDIVIDUAL DIAGNOSIS		GROUP DIAGNOSIS	
	George Jones	May Conte	George Jones	May Conte
High Task & Low Relationship				
High Task & High Relationship				
High Relationship & Low Task				
Low Task & Low Relationship				

EFFECTIVENESS DIMENSION—Indicate by a checkmark your determination of the degree of effectiveness or ineffectiveness for each character in the case.

	+4	+3	+2	+1	−1	−2	−3	−4
Individual Diagnosis: George Jones								
May Conte								
Group Diagnosis: George Jones								
May Conte								

DISCUSSION

LEADERSHIP STYLES

George Jones
May Conte

EFFECTIVENESS

George Jones
May Conte

EXPERTS' DIAGNOSIS

(Remember that this is as perceived by others)

Low Task & Low Relationship
High Task & High Relationship, or High Relationship & Low Task

(Remember that for everything that occurs in the environment, the good reflects his or her effective leadership as well as the bad.)

+2 and going up
+2 and going up

EXERCISE 2 WORKSHEET (continued)

Leader Effectiveness should be evaluated on the following four variables (Hersey and Blanchard, 1977, pp. 117–119):

1. **Casual variables:** those things which have influence on the development, results and accomplishments of an organization, that is, strategies, policies, procedures, etc.
2. **Intervening variables:** these are the conditions, morale, motivational-levels of the human resources in an organization.
3. **Output variables:** reflect the achievements of the organization, such as the quality of care and reactions or feelings about the health environment.
4. **Long-term goals versus short-term goals:** this aspect involves long-term versus short-term planning. One example is whether workers can function effectively without their leader. Since the effective leader helps people mature, Low-Task, Low-Relationship behavior is a goal.

It is easy to create a halo effect and judge a leader's effectiveness on one trait; the leader then will be either good (+4) or bad (−4). This must be avoided and can be done by looking at all four evaluative dimensions.

EXERCISE 3
Models in Nursing Care Delivery

PURPOSES

1. To study the advantages of the five models of nursing care delivery.
2. To experience group processes when external motivations are in force.

FACILITY

Large classroom to accommodate learners working in five groups.
Bargaining table in the front of the room.

MATERIALS

Basket or cup.

TIME REQUIRED

One hour.

GROUP SIZE

The entire class divided into five equal groups. Groups under 10 in number are ideal.

DESIGN

1. Explain the experience. The task is for each group to compete against one another for a prize. The focus of competition is to sell to a Director of Nursing their method of nursing care delivery, which is considered to be the best. The entire group will prime and meet with their self-selected bargainer. Following this period, the bargainer will convene at the bargaining table with the competitors and the Director. Group members can no longer talk but are solely represented by their bargainer.

The situation is:
I am a new Nursing Director charged with setting up a new acute-care, 50-bed hospital. Our focus is on major surgical problems involving everything except open-heart surgery. Our estimated average hospital stay is seven days. I would like to hear from the experts on what model of nursing care delivery I should employ. Then I will make a decision and reward those representative experts.
Each bargainer will have five minutes to sell the Director on the model selected. Order will be randomly chosen.
After all representatives have talked once, each will be given another two minutes for final words.
The Director will then choose. The group of winners

will be given the cup of money (10¢ from each participant) to do with as they please.
2. Ask for an unbiased, volunteer Director. This person will not participate in the groups.
3. Divide into equal groups.
4. List the five models and five numbers on ten separate pieces of paper. Put the models in one cup and the numbers in another. Have one member of each group choose one slip of paper from each cup. Numbers indicate order of selling the Director.

Five Models: Case
                     Functional
                     Team
                     Primary
                     Progressive

5. Collect 10¢ each (or whatever the group uniformly desires) from everyone in the groups.
6. The groups should convene for 20 minutes to prime their bargainer. First, they must choose this person. Groups must keep in mind that this person represents them and the prestige of winning rests on him or her.
7. Groups should then engage in what they desire to have said or offered to the Director. Creativity in offerings is encouraged but groups should not promise more than can be delivered.
8. Following the allotted time, bargainers and the Director convene. The bargaining starts; each representative has five minutes followed by a two-minute closing statement.
9. The Director chooses a model and rewards the group.
10. Groups should re-form and discuss the experience.
11. In a total group, the instructor can discuss the experience in light of the following suggested areas:
   a. How did the leaders feel? Was it difficult being responsible for your groups?
   b. Did the external motivation have any effects on your functioning? If so, what effects?
   c. What were the reactions of the losing groups? To themselves? To their leaders?
   d. Would you have done things differently? If so, what?
   e. Were rebuttals needed? Why?
   f. Is there a best model of nursing care delivery? If yes, why? If no, why?

PART V

NURSING:
A HELPING PROFESSION

18

Helping

As we have seen in this book, the nursing process is the scientific foundation upon which all nursing practice is built. It is applicable to any client population in any setting and provides the framework in which the art and science of nursing can be carried out so as to assure individualized, quality, nursing care. To facilitate fuller understanding of what the nursing process means today, Part V views the present and future development of nursing, as well as the theoretical concepts which provide the foundation for humanistic nursing.

PROFESSIONS

This past decade has brought continuous and seemingly unending conflict over who or what a "profession" is. Since everyone from pest controllers to building contractors currently advertise services as "professional," it is not surprising that nurses, as well as other dedicated humanists, are in the process of defining their services explicitly in an attempt to discern the meaning of this commonly used term. Nursing literature abounds with authors who have defined professionalism in nursing, and one has only to look in the nursing indices to discover an array of existing beliefs, all similar, yet different. The strongest common bond is the conclusion that being a professional means different things to different people. This is based on the individual backgrounds, experiences, expectations, and practices of varied nurses. Yet in respect to scholarship, it becomes necessary to be able to state beliefs in concrete terms usable by growing professionals as each builds his or her own theory of nursing.

General review of writings on professions portray three essential components:

Area of responsibility   +   Authority   +   Autonomy

The content of the area of responsibility depends solely upon the profession; the area of responsibility carries with it the legal authority to set standards and administer services. All professions are based on an extensive body of knowledge, both pure and applied. Perhaps the key difference between the nursing profession and the rest of the "professional" world is that nursing is based on directly assisting and supporting the total individual.

According to Flexner (1975) there are six distinct attributes which qualify an occupation as a profession:

1. Possession of a body of knowledge relevant to problems in its area;
2. Conjoining knowledge and skills in an intellectual enterprise;
3. Applying knowledge in response to an area of human need;
4. Striving to acquire and improve the knowledge bank through research efforts;
5. Acquiring knowledge and experience developed primarily through formal university educational systems culminating with an earned academic degree; and
6. Formulating a code of ethics and character of the profession.

Other theorists would argue that a full commitment of time and energy is essential (Moore, 1975), as well as a licensing mechanism and independent practice design (Wilson, 1975).

Items one through five of Flexner's (1975) criteria feature knowledge, which can be derived in three ways: (1) applied theory from other disciplines; (2) pure theory from research discoveries in the specific area; and (3) experimental knowledge developed through individual practice. Adding to Flexner's fifth attribute, a mode for knowledge acquisition implies a definitive, transferable method that can be taught and learned. The nursing process provides such a method.

A profession becomes an integral part of one's existence. The personality of the profession is reflected in the personality of the professional. This person is a scholar who is seen as continuously learning. Mandated by the profession, nursing must be based on all the scientific and human knowledge available. Because knowledge is the necessary base, the roots of the profession are in formalized educational systems.

In viewing the nursing profession today, it remains implicit that the study and elaboration of nursing attributes and components must continue. Three essential learning and practice dimensions become evident: cognitive, psychomotor, and affective. Cognitive learning involves the theory and knowledge base; psychomotor learning involves the skills; and affective learning involves the process and feelings associated with each of the first two. The humanistic approach in learning encompasses all three dimensions and will be addressed more fully in a subsequent chapter. It becomes necessary, however, to study the theory of helping in order to understand fully the concepts of a *helping profession.*

Helping Models

A generally accepted viewpoint is that most of human behavior is learned; it evolves as a consequence of persons interacting with all facets of their environment. In essence, one learns to be the kind of being one is through past and present relationships. It is through furthering such relationships that one grows into tomorrow's self (Otto, 1970).

The conceptual model of helping upon which this book is based stems primarily from the writings of Carl Rogers. As will be noted, several authors have extended his original work and also conducted substantiating investigations. Foremost in this amplification are the studies by Robert Carkhuff.

Carkhuff (1973) uses the analogy of an infant and an aging person to emphasize that the way in which one's environment and one's relationships with important people evolve largely determines one's self-perception. An infant who is totally dependent would likely not live more than a few hours if left alone. An aging person seizes life's last opportunity to understand, be understood, and to develop meaning for self at that point in time. Each one then depends on self and others in the environment, together and at the same time. A crisis in one's life may lead to greater growth or greater deterioration, depending on what is done by the individuals involved and the skills available to them in helping one another. Weigand (1971, p. 247) wrote: "How we interact, relate and transact with others, and the reciprocal impact of this phenomenon, form the single most important aspect of our existence."

Carl Rogers (1961) developed a general hypothesis regarding the facilitation of personal growth based on what he had learned during his experiences and encounters in all human relationships. The essence of this hypothesis involved his ability as a helper to create a relationship characterized by genuineness, warmth, and sensitivity. With this environment, the other individual would then be able to grow effectively. Moreover, the degree toward which he could create relationships that facilitated the growth of others as individuals would be a measure of the growth he himself had achieved. This was based on his hypothesis that the optimal helping relationship is that created by a psychologically mature person.

Based on this general hypothesis, Rogers (1961, p. 41) further posed the questions: "What are the characteristics of those relationships which do help, which do facilitate growth?" and "Is it possible to discern those characteristics which make a relationship unhelpful, even though it was the sincere intent to promote growth and development?"* There was not a large amount of

---

*Reprinted with permission. Copyright 1961 by Houghton Mifflin Company.

empirical research that would give objective answers at the time Rogers asked these questions (1957–1958). Most of the following studies focused on the attitudes of the helper, which either promoted or inhibited growth.

Baldwin, Kalhorn, and Breese (1945) made a careful study of parent/child relationships. They concluded that of the various attitudes exhibited by parents toward children, the "acceptant-democratic" one seemed most growth-facilitating. These children showed accelerated intellectual development, more originality, and emotional security. In direct contrast to this, children whose parental attitudes were classified as "actively rejectant" showed opposite effects.*

Rogers (1961) suggested that these findings most likely apply in other relationships as well. Stated Rogers (1961, p. 42): "The counselor or physician or administrator who is warmly emotional and expressive, respectful of the individuality of himself and of the other, and who exhibits a nonpossessive caring, probably facilitates self-realization much as does a parent with these attitudes."† He drew the analogy from parental attitudes to helper attitudes and added that the helper must express "acceptant-democratic" attitudes in his behavior. He did not clearly distinguish attitudes from behavior. It is important to point out that Hersey and Blanchard (1977) addressed the attitudes or predispositions of the helper/manager as different from behavior, which tend to be actions perceived by others. Attitudes of empathy, respect, warmth, and concern can then be viable only if the behavior of the helper is perceived as such by the helpee.

Whitehorm and Betz (1954) investigated the degree of success physicians found while working with schizophrenic patients on a psychiatric ward. They found that helpful physicians primarily made use of active personal participation. They tended to see the schizophrenic client in terms of the personal meaning which various behaviors had to the client and worked towards goals rooted in the personality of the client. They developed a rapport in which the client felt trust and confidence in the physician. These approaches were in contrast to those of the physician who used procedures such a interpretation, instruction, advice, or emphasis on practical care.

Another study investigated the way in which a person being helped perceived the relationship. Heine (1950) studied the individuals who had undergone psychotherapeutic treatment. The clients reported similar changes in themselves regardless of the orientation of the therapist. The major elements they found helpful in their environment centered on the trust they had felt for the therapist, the feelings of being understood, and the independence they had in making decisions. The therapy procedure found to be most helpful was

---

*"Acceptance-democratic" and "actively rejectant" were phrases used by the authors to describe the dichotomy between open, loving parents who listened to the individual aspects of their children versus rigid, controlling parents who saw their children only as extensions of themselves.

†Reprinted with permission. Copyright 1961 by Houghton Mifflin Company.

clarification and the open stating of feelings that the client had approached hesitantly. The identified unhelpful elements included lack of interest, remoteness, superfluous sympathy, and emphasis on past history rather than on present problems.

Fiedler (1953) found that expert therapists, regardless of their orientation, formed similar elements that characterized their relationships. These included empathy, a sensitivity to the client's attitudes, and a warm interest minus emotional overinvolvement. Seeman (1954) noted that psychotherapeutic success is closely tied to a mutual liking and respectful interaction between the client and therapist. Rogers (1961, p. 44) discovered that "it is the attitudes and feelings of the therapist, rather than his theoretical orientation, which is important."* It is also "the way in which his attitudes and procedures are perceived which makes a difference (Rogers, 1961, p. 44)." Halkides (1958) also affirmed that a high degree of empathic understanding was significantly associated with successful therapy, as were a high degree of unconditional positive regard and the counselor's genuineness.

It was with this background that Carkhuff (1969) went on to state and empirically document the core conditions necessary to promote facilitative human relationships, namely: empathy, respect, warmth, genuineness, self-disclosure, concreteness, confrontation, and immediacy of relationship.

Carkhuff's (1969) work stemmed from the basic assumption that counseling and psychotherapy are aspects of interpersonal and relearning processes or, generally, human relations. From this assumption, research has documented that human encounters may have constructive or destructive effects and that all effective processes share a common bond of conditions that are conducive to facilitative human experiences (Berenson and Carkhuff, 1967; Berenson and Mitchell, 1968; Carkhuff and Berenson, 1967; Rogers, Gendlin, Kiesler and Truax, 1967).

Effective and Ineffective Cycles   This research led Carkhuff (1969) to a model for effective and ineffective functioning. At each point in one's life during which one has contact with another person, the encounter either enables one to grow further or to deteriorate; there is no neutrality. The severely deteriorated person who seems to be functioning ineffectively in all relationships can be viewed as a product of prolonged, non-helpful relationships that hinder growth. By comparison, the person who has experienced a series of facilitative relationships will function at high or effective levels in most areas of the person's existence. Those persons who are neither totally effective nor ineffective in coping with life's processes are those who have had a series of mixed rela-

*Reprinted with permission. Copyright 1961 by Houghton Mifflin Company.

tionships—some effective, some harmful. According to Carkhuff (1969, p. 22): "Each significant encounter, then, between more knowing and less knowing persons* may be considered a crisis in the lives of both groups. Whether an individual grows or deteriorates is dependent in large part upon the interaction of the activities of both the more knowing and the less knowing persons."† A person's basic direction—toward growth or toward deterioration—depends a great deal upon what happens at each critical stage in the person's development, even though different resources and predispositions of individuals are involved (Carkhuff, 1969). This can be equated to Hersey and Blanchard's (1977) effective and ineffective cycles.

The *effective cycle* in organizational theory is one of which high expectations by leaders produce high performance of followers. This process spirals upward and builds upon itself. The ineffective cycle is one during which low expectations imposed on followers produce low performance; it spirals downward (Hersey and Blanchard, 1977). Human relationships can be analyzed in the same way if one would add to the effective/ineffective cycles the variable of the leader's ability to communicate. Constructive and facilitative experiences with other persons during crisis points in one's life produce a spiral upward and provide a new level from which to continue growth. Ineffective or deteriorating experiences produce the opposite effects, spiraling downward, thus placing a person on a lower level of functioning from which the person must then regrow. It is possible to project then that a series of helpful relationships reinforces one at an elevated level, whereas a series of ineffective relationships can be extremely harmful.

Going back to Hersey and Blanchard's (1977) theory, it appears logical to conclude, therefore, that if a leader's high expectations of followers are coupled with facilitative communication skills, this may catalyze an effective cycle. Likewise, if one joined low expectations with poor communicative skills, a deleterious downward cycle might result. High expectations/ ineffective communications and low expectations/facilitative skills could act similar to an acid/base buffer system. They might neutralize each other, thereby retarding outcome. It follows that effective process must be synchronized with realistic goals. This same point also confirms Beck's (1963) existential view that the total human organism reacts to any situation. One cannot react either intellectually or emotionally to the exclusion of the other. Humans also behave in terms of their subjective view of reality, not according to some externally defined objective. Each person has heredity and experiences unique to that person. From these, it is to be expected that each will behave differently from others whose experiences are different.

---

*"More knowing and less knowing persons" refers to the relationship between a helper/ helpee, parent/child, teacher/student, etc.

†Reprinted with permission. Copyright 1969 by Holt, Rinehart and Winston, Inc.

Facets of the Helping Relationship

Carkhuff provides a description of facets in a helping relationship: helper, helpee, and environmental variables.

The Helper The helper's contribution can be divided broadly into two phases —understanding and action. Phase I, understanding, enables the helpee to probe inwardly by exploring and experiencing the core of his existence. The facilitative conditions of empathy, respect, warmth, and self-disclosure employed during this phase offer the helpee both stimulus and reinforcement. In turn, this serves to lower the helpee's defenses, thereby enabling the helper to elicit more meaningful material (Carkhuff, 1969). "High levels of facilitative conditions enable the helper to understand the helpee and the helpee to experience the feeling of being understood (Carkhuff, 1969, p. 42)."*

The second phase is correlated with the action oriented dimension. Carkhuff and Berenson (1967) call this the upward phase, or period of "emergent directionality." After having explored self, the distressed person experiences a need to act on the world in a more effective manner than in previous encounters. Since trust and understanding have previously been established in Phase I, the helper can now be a guide in this action oriented dimension (Carkhuff, 1969).

It is important to note that studies of helper trainee characteristics have suggested that traditional feminine response patterns have been demonstrated in helper trainees.† Farson (1954), McClain (1968), and Patterson (1967) have discovered that helpers tend to get high scores on social service interests and nurturant inclinations as well as on indexes of more traditionally feminine personality dispositions such as restraint, friendliness, deference, and affiliation. Low scores were observed on more aggressive, assertive, and achievement oriented traits. A comprehensive model for the helping process should be viewed as containing both types. Carkhuff (1969, p. 34) expressed this succinctly in his following statements: "The effective helper is both mother and father. The whole person has incorporated both the responsive and assertive components. He (or she) can understand his internal and external physical, emotional, and intellectual world with sensitivity and can act upon these worlds with responsibility."*

The two phases of helping have been shown to be essential components of a comprehensive helping model. They may not be sequential and distinctive but they must be self-contained. The helper must be functioning at a level in which the helper is established by the helpee as a model for effective living (Carkhuff, 1969).

*Reprinted with permission. Copyright 1969 by Holt, Rinehart and Winston, Inc.

†The use of a "feminine" description of any trait refers only to usage of the term by the authors cited.

The Helpee Since an interaction involves a minimum of two people, it becomes necessary to look at the *helpee*. According to Carkhuff (1969), contributions made by the helpee can be delineated as follows: (1) what the helpee brings to the experience; (2) how the helpee reacts within the process; and (3) what changes are elicited in the helpee as a result of the process.

The first set of factors—what a helpee brings to the situation—are divided into (1) the demographic characteristics of the helpee's system and (2) its level of functioning. There is little or no research relating helpee demographic characteristics to treatment outcome. Social class and racial variables have been studied, however. Banks, Berenson, and Carkhuff (1967) found that the counselors who either were similar or could generate perceived similarity were seen by black college students as more effective change agents. Anderson and Anderson (1963), Banks (1972), Carkhuff and Pierce (1967) and Correll (1955) found that racial similarity was a source of increased client self-exploration while social class had no statistical significance. Winder and Hersko (1955) and Hollingshead and Redlich (1958) reported that both counselors and psychologists, themselves middle class, facilitated self-exploration in clients of similar social status and discouraged it in clients of lower social status. Gardner (1972) investigated the variables of race, education, and experience as significant factors in the degree in which counselors are perceived as effective by black college students. He found all three to be significant sources of effect for student ratings. The implications of the research are that counselors with similar backgrounds to the client are most effective. However, the works of Rogers et al (1967) and Truax and Carkhuff (1967) gave evidence that helpees who were seen by motivated helpers, regardless of social class or demographic characteristics, had an opportunity for constructive change.

The helpee's level of functioning is the second division of what the helpee brings to the relationship. There is little evidence to indicate that assessments of levels of functioning are in any way correlated with differential treatment (Carkhuff, 1968; Carkhuff and Berenson, 1967, Pagell, Carkhuff, and Berenson, 1967; Spiegel and Spiegel, 1967; Thorne, 1967; Truax and Carkhuff, 1967). "Traditional diagnosis does not make a difference (Carkhuff, 1969, p. 50)."* In other words, the theoretic framework on which a helper bases practice and diagnosis is far less important to counseling outcome than is the helper's level of functioning in communication skills.

The second set of factors of the helpee's contribution to the counseling relationship is how the helpee reacts within the relationship. This includes the helpee's sets, expectancies, motivation, and process variables. These variables are internal in the helpee. What a helpee perceives (sets) plus the expectations of therapy produce motivation. The energy resulting from motivation affects the process of counseling itself. Carkhuff (1969, p. 52) stated that "basically

---

*Reprinted with permission. Copyright 1969 by Holt, Rinehart and Winston, Inc.

what the helpee expects and, indeed, needs are a high level of understanding in his life."* Helping process variables, which include helpee self-exploration, problem expression, and the immediacy of experiencing, are essential to constructive helpee change or gain (Carkhuff, 1969; Carkhuff and Berenson, 1967). States Carkhuff (1969, p. 54), "The degree to which the helpee can explore himself within the helping process is related to the degree to which he changes constructively."* Writings of Carkhuff and Berenson (1967) and Truax and Carkhuff (1967) confirm this point.

The last contribution of the helpee involves the changes the relationship elicited in the helpee. The outcome of the helping relationship is a reflection of the goals of counseling. The helpee must be autonomous (Carkhuff, 1969). Carkhuff states (1969, p. 62), "The helper's task is thus to serve as a guide on the helpee's journey toward finding himself and acting upon who he is. Through the helper's eyes and ears the helpee can come to see and hear the sights and sounds of life; with the helper's hands he can learn to touch and to act; through the helper's life he can come to find his own life."*

The Environment   The last set of variables that must be considered in the helping process includes environmental and contextual influences (Carkhuff, 1966; Carkhuff and Berenson, 1967). The helper and helpee do not interact in a vacuum. The setting in which helping takes place, as well as the environment and people to which the helpee must return, incorporate critical variables (Goffman, 1956, 1961; Jones, 1953; Rapaport, 1960; Scheff, 1966, 1967; Shibutani, 1961; Smelser and Smelser, 1963; Wesseu, 1964). Within the rationale for helping, Carkhuff (1969, p. 69) maintained, "what the helpee learns to do within the context of the helping relationship can be generalized to other significant areas of his life."*

Importance of Empathy

Writings of other authors have clarified the concept of empathy and its primary importance in a helping relationship. Combs, Avila, and Purkey (1971, p. 185) described empathy as "the capacity to place one's self in another's shoes, to perceive as he does." They further stated that helpers must be able to understand the private world of the helpee in terms of feelings, attitudes, wants, and goals. This requires reaching inside the skin of another person.

Blocher (1966) divided empathy into two components. The cognitive component involves psychologic understanding while the affective component is feeling *with* a person. Buchheimer (1963) addressed empathy within the context of several dimensions of the helping process:

*Reprinted with permission. Copyright 1969 by Holt, Rinehart and Winston, Inc.

1. The *tone* of the counseling relationship is an expressive and possibly non-verbal dimension based upon expressions of warmth and spontaneity.
2. The *pace* involves the appropriateness and the flow of the relationship.
3. The counselor's *perception* is related to the counselor's abilities to abstract the core of the client's concerns and respond to these in an accepable, constructive manner.
4. *Strategy* relates to the predictive or role-playing aspect of the relationship.
5. *Leading* involves the resourcefulness of the counselor in moving the relationship in the direction of the client's concerns.

Jourard (1971) correlated the helper's ability to effect constructive growth in helpees with what Foote and Cottrell (1955) called interpersonal competence. This is described as the ability of the helper to produce valued, desirable outcomes in transactions with people. Professionals who have achieved interpersonal competence are those who are able to achieve desirable outcomes in their encounters with their clients; outcomes are measured in terms of the signs exemplifying the quality of care given the helpees. Professionals must, therefore, possess and use empathy in the helping process as a vehicle to effect overt and measurable changes.

It has been shown that empathy involves more than a simple understanding and reflection of the client's verbalizations. Empathy operates throughout the helping process and signifies a central focus and feeling with and in the helpee's world.

The theory of two related, yet distinct, concepts have been portrayed: professions and helping models. Integration of these two areas forms the foundation for defining a helping profession. A helping profession, therefore, is one that has the following attributes:

1. A unique area of service that fills an area of human need
2. Data-based knowledge derived from research processes
3. Skills that build on knowledge
4. Formal educational avenues for acquisition of knowledge and experience
5. Authority to implement services according to standards set by the unique helping profession, and
6. Responsibility and accountability for all services provided by the profession.

NURSING AS A HELPING PROFESSION

In order to establish that nursing is a helping profession, it becomes necessary to define nursing. The literature is replete with descriptive and succinct nursing definitions: nursing concepts, roles, and actions. Among many other reasons, these definitions are necessary to set professional standards and also to provide a frame of reference for the learner as each begins the individual journey of practice. They are also helpful in increasing role awareness in the public sector.

For current purposes, it is necessary to look at established definitions and decide whether nursing qualifies as a helping profession. Perhaps the most widely used and current definition of nursing was written by Henderson (1966, p. 3),* who stated:

> The practice of professional nursing means the performance for compensation of any act in the observation, care, and counsel of the ill, injured, or infirm, or in the maintenance of health or prevention of illness of others, or in the supervision and teaching of other personnel, or the administration of medications and treatments as prescribed by a licensed physician or dentist; requiring substantial specialized judgment and skill and based on knowledge and application of the principles of biological, physical, and social science.

The simplest definition of a nurse as provided by Webster (1971), is that of a person educated to provide care and curative help or treatment to any in need. Florence Nightingale (1967) encompassed nursing as the care which put a patient in the best condition for nature to restore health, and the prevention and cure of injury or disease. Stressed throughout her definition was that nursing meant treating the *person*, not the disease.

Reiter (1966) focused professional nursing practice and clinical competence on three "Cs": care, cure, and coordination. These included promotion of health; counseling; responsibility for individuals, families and the community; supervision; teaching; directing care providers; collaborating and synchronizing health services. These require knowledge of high order and skill based on a broad framework of theory.

For the purposes of this book, the author defines a nurse as:

> A formally educated person who is a provider of knowledge, support, assistance, and/or care to any person who is in need, in any setting, on a twenty-four-hour basis, and in collaboration with other health professionals as appropriate and in conjunction with the current American Nurses' Association Standards of Practice.

It has been shown that nursing, by all of its own definitions, is indeed a helping profession. The attributes of a helping profession can be seen throughout nursing education and practice. Basically speaking, there are four parts of nursing education and practice:

1. **Knowledge.**   Our primary knowledge begins and ends with our client(s) and what is known about human behavior, health, sickness, and treatment. In formal and informal educational systems, applied theory from the pure

---

*Reprinted with permission. Copyright 1966 by Macmillan Publishing Company.

sciences, humanities, and behavioral sciences is integrated into client care. Nursing research, our pure segment, is studied and expanded throughout.
2. **Skills.** The skills and competencies necessary for the delivery of nursing care are basic in education and perpetual throughout practice. They include skills relative to nursing's responsibility including those reflective of helping processes. Service institutions are constantly providing programs for practitioners in which skills and concepts can be learned and/or updated.

   Skills and competencies are divided into two broad areas: attitudinal and behavioral learning. They include content and process and are discussed in Chapter 19.
3. **Code of Ethics.** The Code of Ethics in nursing practice is set by our professional organization, the American Nurses' Association (1976), and is followed by all nursing administrations and individual practitioners.
4. **Method.** The definitive transferable method in nursing is the nursing process. It is our own scientific method and forms the basis for all nursing care.

The helping model presents the helping concept as promoting growth and constructive change, whereas the nursing model features meeting the client's needs. It becomes crucial to visualize these two areas as harmoniously operating together and at the same time.

SUMMARY

This chapter has studied the attributes of a helping profession as well as the facets of the action of helping. Nursing is portrayed in terms of its components relative to the entire process. It becomes evident that the professional and helping aspects of practice are threads in the gestalt of nursing. The nursing process is the method that enables a practitioner to utilize a broad basework of knowledge and experience in the client/nurse interaction.

REFERENCES

American Nurses' Association. *Code for nurses.* New York: American Nurses Association, 1976.

Anderson, R., and Anderson, G. The development of an instrument for measuring rapport. *Personnel and Guidance Journal* 41: 18–24, 1963.

Baldwin, A., Kalhorn, J., and Breese, F. Patterns of parent behavior. *Psychological Monographs* 58: 1–75, 1945.

Banks, W. The differential effects of race and social class in helping. *Journal of Clinical Psychology* 28: 90–92, 1972.

Banks, G., Berenson, B., and Carkhuff, R. The effects of counselor race and training upon counseling process with negro clients in initial interviews. *Journal of Clinical Psychology* 23: 70–72, 1967.

Beck, C. *Philosophical foundations of guidance.* Englewood Cliffs, N. J.: Prentice-Hall, 1963.

Berenson, B., and Carkhuff, R. *Sources of gain in counseling and psychotherapy.* New York: Holt, Rinehart and Winston, 1967.

Berenson, B., and Mitchell, K. Confrontation in counseling and life. Mimeographed manuscript, American International College, Springfield, Massachusetts, 1968.

Blocher, D. *Developmental counseling.* New York: The Ronald Press, 1966.

Buchheimer, A. The development of ideas about empathy. *Journal of Counseling Psychology* 10: 61–71, 1963.

Carkhuff, R. Counseling research, theory and practice. *Journal of Counseling Psychology* 13: 467–480, 1966.

Carkhuff, R. The differential functioning of lay and professional helpers. *Journal of Counseling Psychology* 15: 117–126, 1968.

Carkhuff, R. *Helping and human relations: A primer for lay and professional helpers,* Vol. I. New York: Holt, Rinehart and Winston, 1969.

Carkhuff, R. *The art of helping.* Amherst, Massachusetts: Human Resource Development Press, 1973.

Carkhuff, R., and Berenson, B. *Beyond counseling and therapy.* New York: Holt, Rinehart and Winston, 1967.

Carkhuff, R., and Pierce, R. The differential effects of therapist race and social class upon patient depth of self-exploration in the initial clinical interview. *Journal of Consulting Psychology* 31:631–634, 1967.

Combs, A., Avila, D., and Purkey, W. *Helping relationships: Basic concepts for the helping professions.* Boston: Allyn and Bacon, 1971.

Correll, P. Factors influencing communication in counseling. Doctoral Dissertation, University of Missouri, 1955.

Farson, R. The counselor is a woman. *Journal of Counseling Psychology,* 1: 221–223, 1954.

Fiedler, F. Quantitative studies on the role of the therapists' feelings toward their patients. In O. H. Mowrer (ed.), *Psychotherapy: Theory and research.* New York: Ronald Press, 1953.

Flexner, A. Cited by: W. Metzer, What is a profession? *Seminar Reports.* New York: Columbia University, 1975.

Foote, N., and Cottrell, L. *Identity and interpersonal competence.* Chicago: University of Chicago Press, 1955.

Gardner, W. The differential effects of race, education, and experience in helping. *Journal of Clinical Psychology* 28: 87–89, 1972.

Goffman, E. *The presentation of self in everyday life.* Edinburgh: University of Edinburgh Social Sciences Research Centre, 1956.

Goffman, E. *Encounters: Two studies in the sociology of interaction.* New York: Bobbs-Merrill Company, 1961.

Halkides, G. An experimental study of four conditions necessary for therapeutic change. Unpublished doctoral dissertation, University of Chicago, 1958.

Heine, R. A comparison of patients' reports on psychotherapeutic experience with psychoanalytic, non-directive, and Adlerian therapists. Unpublished doctoral dissertation, University of Chicago, 1950.

Henderson, V. *The nature of nursing.* New York: The Macmillan Company, 1966.

Hersey, P., and Blanchard, K. *Management of organizational behavior: Utilizing human resources.* Englewood Cliffs, N. J.: Prentice-Hall, 1977.

Hollingshead, A., and Redlich, F. *Social class and mental illness.* New York: John Wiley and Sons, 1958.

Jones, M. *The therapeutic community.* New York: Basic Books, 1953.

Jourard, S. *The transparent self.* New York: Van Nostrand Reinhold Company, 1971.

McClain, E. Is the counselor a woman? *Personnel and Guidance Journal* 46: 444–448, 1968.

Moore, W. Cited by W. Metzger, What is a profession? *Seminar Reports.* New York: Columbia University, 1975.

Nightingale, F. *Notes on nursing: What it is and what it is not.* New York: Dover Publications, 1967.

Otto, H. *Group methods to actualize human potential: A handbook.* Beverly Hills, Calif.: Holistic Press, 1970.

Pagell, W., Carkhuff, R., and Berenson, B. The predicted differential effects of the level of counselor functioning upon the level of functioning of outpatients. *Journal of Clinical Psychology* 23: 510–512, 1967.

Patterson, C. The selection of counselors. Paper presented at the Conference on Research Problems in Counseling, Washington University, St. Louis, Missouri, 1967.

Rapaport, R. *The community as a doctor.* Chicago: Charles C. Thomas, 1960.

Reiter, F. The nurse-clinician. *American Journal of Nursing* 66: 274–280, 1966.

Rogers, C. *On becoming a person.* Boston: Houghton Mifflin Company, 1961.

Rogers, C., Gendlin, E., Kiesler, D., and Truax, C. (eds.). *The therapeutic relationship and its impact: A study of psychotherapy with schizophrenics.* Madison, Wisconsin: University of Wisconsin Press, 1967.

Scheff, T. *Being mentally ill: A sociological theory.* Chicago: Aldine Publishing Company, 1966.

Scheff, T. *Mental illness and social processes.* New York: Harper and Row, 1967.

Seeman, J. Counselor judgments of therapeutic processes and outcome. In C. Rogers and R. Dymond (eds.), *Psychotherapy and personality change.* Chicago: University of Chicago Press, 1954.

Shibutani, T. *Society and personality: An interactional approach to social psychology.* Englewood Cliffs, N. J.: Prentice-Hall, 1961.

Smelser, N., and Smelser, W. (eds.) *Personality and social systems.* New York: John Wiley and Sons, 1963.

Spiegel, P., and Spiegel, D. Perceived helpfulness of others as a function of compatible intelligence. *Journal of Counseling Psychology* 14: 61–62, 1967.

Thorne, K. The etiological equation. In R. Carkhuff and B. Benson, *Beyond counseling and therapy.* New York: Holt, Rinehart and Winston, 1967, Appendix A.

Truax, C., and Carkhuff, R. *Toward effective counseling and psychotherapy: Training and practice.* Chicago: Aldine Publishing Company, 1967.

Webster's Third International Dictionary. Springfield, Massachusetts: G. & C. Merriam Company, 1971.

Weigand, J. (ed.). *Developing teacher competencies.* Englewood Cliffs, N. J.: Prentice-Hall, 1971.

Wesseu, A. *The psychiatric hospital as a social system.* Chicago: Charles C. Thomas, 1964.

Whitehorn, J., and Betz, B. A study of psychotherapeutic relationships between physicians and schizophrenic patients. *American Journal of Psychiatry* 111: 321–331, 1954.

Wilson, L. Cited by W. Metzger, What is a profession? *Seminar Reports.* New York: Columbia University, 1975.

Winder, A., and Hersko, M. The effect of social class on the length and type of psychotherapy in a V.A. Mental Hygiene Clinic. *Journal of Clinical Psychology* 11: 77–79, 1955.

SELECTED READINGS

The selected readings for this chapter include a classic article by Carl Rogers (1958) on the characteristics of a helping profession. Writing as a psychologist, he amplifies and extends the theory and rationale for helping which has been presented in the chapter. Schlotfeldt (1974) is the author of the second reading and discusses nursing as a profession.

The Characteristics of a Helping Relationship

Carl R. Rogers

My interest in psychotherapy has brought about in me an interest in every kind of helping relationship. By this term I mean a relationship in which at least one of the parties has the intent of promoting the growth, development, maturity, improved functioning, improved coping with life of the other. The other, in this sense, may be one individual or a group. To put it in another way, a helping relationship might be defined as one in which one of the participants intends that there should come about, in one or both parties, more appreciation of, more expression of, more functional use of the latent inner resources of the individual.

Now it is obvious that such a definition covers a wide range of relationships which usually are intended to facilitate growth. It would certainly include the relationship between mother and child, father and child. It would include the relationship between the physician and his patient. The relationship between teacher and pupil would often come under this definition, though some teachers would not have the promotion of growth as their intent. It includes almost all counselor-client relationships, whether we are speaking of educational counseling, vocational counseling, or personal counseling. In this last-mentioned area it would include the wide range of relationships between the psychotherapist and the hospitalized psychotic, the therapist and the troubled or neurotic individual, and the relationship between the therapist and the increasing number of so-called "normal" individuals who enter therapy to improve their own functioning or accelerate their personal growth.

These are largely one-to-one relationships. But we should also think of the large number of individual-group interactions which are intended as helping relationships. Some administrators intend that their relationship to their staff groups shall be of the sort which promotes growth, though other administrators would not have this purpose. The interaction between the group therapy leader and his group belongs here. So does the relationship of the community consultant to a community group. Increasingly the interaction between the industrial consultant and a management group is intended as a helping relationship. Perhaps this listing will point up the fact that a great many of the relationships in which we and others are involved fall within this category of interactions in which there is the purpose of promoting development and more mature and adequate functioning.

Reprinted with permission from *Personnel and Guidance Journal*, Vol. 37. Copyright 1958 by American Personnel and Guidance Association. This article also appears in Dr. Roger's book *On Becoming a Person*, Boston: Houghton Mifflin Company, 1961, pp. 39–58.

THE QUESTION

But what are the characteristics of those relationships which *do* help, which do facilitate growth? And at the other end of the scale is it possible to discern those characteristics which make a relationship unhelpful, even though it was the sincere intent to promote growth and development? It is to these questions, particularly the first, that I would like to take you with me over some of the paths I have explored, and to tell you where I am, as of now, in my thinking on these issues.

THE ANSWERS GIVEN BY RESEARCH

It is natural to ask first of all whether there is any empirical research which would give us an objective answer to these questions. There has not been a large amount of research in this area as yet, but what there is is stimulating and suggestive. I cannot report all of it but I would like to make a somewhat extensive sampling of the studies which have been done and state very briefly some of the findings. In so doing, over-simplification is necessary, and I am quite aware that I am not doing full justice to the researches I am mentioning, but it may give you the feeling that factual advances are being made and pique your curiosity enough to examine the studies themselves, if you have not already done so.

Studies of Attitudes

Most of the studies throw light on the attitudes on the part of the helping person which make a relationship growth-promoting or growth-inhibiting. Let us look at some of these.

A careful study of parent-child relationships made some years ago by Baldwin and others (1) at the Fels Institute contains interesting evidence. Of the various clusters of parental attitudes toward children, the "acceptant-democratic" seemed most growth-facilitating. Children of these parents with their warm and equalitarian attitudes showed an accelerated intellectual development (an increasing IQ), more originality, more emotional security and control, less excitability than children from other types of homes. Though somewhat slow initially in social development, they were by the time they reached school age, popular, friendly, non-aggressive leaders.

Where parents' attitudes are classed as "actively rejectant" the children show a slightly decelerated intellectual development, relatively poor use of the abilities they do possess, and some lack of originality. They are emotionally unstable, rebellious, aggressive, and quarrelsome. The children of parents with other attitude syndromes tend in various respects to fall in between these extremes.

I am sure that these findings do not surprise us as related to child development. I would like to suggest that they probably apply to other relationships as well, and that the counselor or physician or administrator who is warmly emotional and expressive respectful of the individuality of himself and of the other, and who exhibits a non-possessive caring, probably facilitates self-realization much as does a parent with these attitudes.

Let me turn to another careful study in a very different area. Whitehorn and Betz (2, 18) investigated the degree of success achieved by young resident physicians in working with schizophrenic patients on a psychiatric ward. They chose for special study the seven who had been outstandingly helpful, and seven whose patients had shown the least degree of improvement. Each group had treated about 50 patients. The investigators examined all the available evidence to discover in what ways the A group (the successful group) differed from the B group. Several significant differences were found. The physicians in the A group tended to see the schizophrenic in terms of the personal meaning which various behaviors had to the patient, rather than seeing him as a case history or a descriptive diagnosis. They also tended to work toward goals which were oriented to the personality of the patient, rather than such goals as reducing the symptoms or curing the disease. It was found that the helpful physicians, in their day by day interaction, primarily made use of active personal participation—a person-to-person relationship. They made less use of procedures which could be classed as "passive permissive." They were even less likely to use such procedures as interpretation, instruction or advice, or emphasis upon the practical care of the patient. Finally, they were much more likely than the B group to develop a relationship in which the patient felt trust and confidence in the physician.

Although the authors cautiously emphasize that these findings relate only to the treatment of schizophrenics, I am inclined to disagree. I suspect that similar facts would be found in a research study of almost any class of helping relationship.

Another interesting study focuses upon the way in which the person being helped perceived the relationship. Heine (11) studied individuals who had gone for psychotherapeutic help to psychoanalytic, client-centered, and Adlerian therapists. Regardless of the type of therapy, these clients report similar changes in themselves. But it is their perception of the relationship which is of particular interest to us here. When asked what accounted for the changes which had occurred, they expressed some differing explanations, depending on the orientation of the therapist. But their agreement on the major elements they had found helpful was even more significant. They indicated that these attitudinal elements in the relationship accounted for the changes which had taken place in themselves: the trust they had felt in the therapist; being understood by the therapist; the feeling of independence they had had in making choices and decisions. The therapist procedure which they had found most helpful was that the therapist clarified and openly stated feelings which the client had been approaching hazily and hesitantly.

There was also a high degree of agreement among these clients, regardless of the orientation of their therapists, as to what elements had been unhelpful in the relationship. Such therapist attitudes as lack of interest, remoteness or distance, and an over-degree of sympathy, were perceived as unhelpful. As to procedures, they had found it unhelpful when therapists had given direct specific advice regarding decisions or had emphasized past history rather than present problems. Guiding suggestions mildly given were perceived in an intermediate range—neither clearly helpful nor unhelpful.

Fiedler, in a much quoted study (7), found that expert therapists of differing orientations formed similar relationships with their clients. Less well known are the elements which characterized these relationships, differentiating them from the relationships formed by less expert therapists. These elements are: an ability to understand the client's meanings and feelings; a sensitivity to the client's attitudes; a warm interest without any emotional over-involvement.

A study by Quinn (15) throws light on what is involved in understanding the client's meanings and feelings. His study is surprising in that it shows that "understanding" of the client's meanings is essentially an attitude of *desiring* to understand. Quinn presented his judges only with recorded therapist statements taken from interviews. The raters had no knowledge of what the therapist was responding to or how the client reacted to his response. Yet it was found that the degree of understanding could be judge about as well from this material as from listening to the response in context. This seems rather conclusive evidence that it is an attitude of wanting to understand which is communicated.

As to the emotional quality of the relationship, Seeman (16) found that success in psychotherapy is closely associated with a strong and growing mutual liking and respect between client and therapist.

An interesting study by Dittes (4) indicates how delicate this relationship is. Using a physiological measure, the psychogalvanic reflex, to measure the anxious or threatened or alerted reactions of the client, Dittes correlated the deviations on this measure with judge's ratings of the degree of warm acceptance and permissiveness on the part of the therapist. It was found that whenever the therapist's attitudes changed even slightly in the direction of a lesser degree of acceptance, the number of abrupt GSR deviations significantly increased. Evidently when the relationship is experienced as less acceptant the organism organizes against threat, even at the physiological level.

Without trying fully to integrate the findings from these various studies, it can at least be noted that a few things stand out. One is the fact that it is the attitudes and feelings of the therapist, rather than his theoretical orientation, which is important. His procedures and techniques are less important than his attitudes. It is also worth noting that it is the way in which his attitudes and procedures are *perceived* which makes a difference to the client, and that it is this perception which is crucial.

"Manufactured" Relationships

Let me turn to research of a very different sort, some of which you may find rather abhorrent, but which nevertheless has a bearing upon the nature of a facilitating relationship. These studies have to do with what we might think of as manufactured relationships.

Verplanck (17), Greenspoon (8) and others have shown that operant conditioning of verbal behavior is possible in a relationship. Very briefly, if the experimenter says "Mhm," or "Good," or nods his head after certain types of words or statements, those classes of words tend to increase because of being reinforced. It has been shown that using such procedures one can bring about increases in such diverse verbal categories as plural nouns, hostile words, statements of opinion. The person is completely unaware that he is being influenced in any way by these reinforcers. The implication is that by such selective reinforcement we could bring it about that the other person in the relationship would be using whatever kinds of words and making whatever kinds of statements we had decided to reinforce.

Following still further the principles of operant conditioning as developed by Skinner and his group, Lindsley (12) has shown that a chronic schizophrenic can be placed in a "helping relationship" with a machine. The machine, somewhat like a vending machine, can be set to reward a variety of types of behaviors. Initially it simply rewards—with candy, a cigarette, or the display of a picture—the lever-pressing behavior of the patient. But it is possible to set it so that many pulls on the lever may supply a hungry kitten—visible in a separate enclosure—with a drop of milk. In this case the satisfaction is an altruistic one. Plans are being developed to reward similar social or altruistic behavior directed toward another patient, placed in the next room. The only limit to the kinds of behavior which might be rewarded lies in the degree of mechanical ingenuity of the experimenter.

Lindsley reports that in some patients there has been marked clinical improvement. Personally I cannot help but be impressed by the description of one patient who had gone from a deteriorated chronic state to being given free ground privileges, this change being quite clearly associated with his interaction with the machine. Then the experimenter decided to study experimental extinction, which, put in more personal terms, means that no matter how many thousands of times the lever was pressed, no reward of any kind was forthcoming. The patient gradually regressed, grew untidy, uncommunicative, and his ground privileges had to be revoked. This (to me) pathetic incident would seem to indicate that even in a relationship to a machine, trustworthiness is important if the relationship is to be helpful.

Still another interesting study of a manufactured relationship is being carried on by Harlow and his associates (10), this time with monkeys. Infant monkeys, removed from their mothers almost immediately after birth, are, in one phase of the experiment, presented with two objects. One might be termed the "hard mother," a sloping cylinder of wire netting with a nipple from which the baby may feed. The other is a "soft mother," a similar cylinder made of foam rubber and terry cloth. Even when an infant gets all his food from the "hard mother" he clearly and increasingly prefers the "soft mother." Motion pictures show that he definitely "relates" to this object, playing with it, enjoying it, finding security in clinging to it for venturing into the frightening world. Of the many interesting and challenging implications of this study, one seems reasonably clear. It is that no amount of direct food reward can take the place of certain perceived qualities which the infant appears to need and desire.

Two Recent Studies

Let me close this wide-ranging—and perhaps perplexing—sampling of re-search studies with an account of two very recent investigations. The first is an experiment conducted by Ends and Page (5). Working with hardened chronic hospitalized alcoholics who had been committed to a state hospital for 60 days, they tried three different methods of group psychotherapy. The method which they believed would be more effective was therapy based on a two-factor theory of learning; a client-centered approach was expected to be se-cond; a psychoanalytically oriented approach was expected to be least effi-cient. Their results showed that the therapy based upon a learning theory ap-proach was not only not helpful, but was somewhat deleterious. The outcomes were worse than those in the control group which had no therapy. The analytically oriented therapy produced some positive gain, and the client-centered group therapy was associated with the greatest amount of positive change. Follow-up data, extending over one and one-half years, confirmed the in-hospital findings, with the lasting improvement being greatest in the client-centered approach, next in the analytic, next the control group, and least in those handled by a learning theory approach.

As I have puzzled over this study, unusual in that the approach to which the authors were committed proved *least* effective, I find a clue, I believe, in the description of the therapy based on learning theory (13). Essentially, it consisted (1) of pointing out and labeling the behaviors which had proved un-satisfying, (2) of exploring objectively with the client the reasons behind these behaviors, and (3) of establishing through re-education more effective problem-solving habits. But in all of this interaction the aim, as they for-mulated it, was to be impersonal. The therapist "permits as little of his own personality to intrude as is humanly possible." The "therapist stresses personal anonymity in his activities, i.e., he must studiously avoid impressing the pa-tient with his own (therapist's) individual personality characteristics." To me this seems the most likely clue to the failure of this approach, as I try to inter-pret the facts in the light of the other research studies. To withhold one's self as a person and to deal with the other person as an object does not have a high probability of being helpful.

The final study I wish to report is one just being completed by Halkides (9). She started from a theoretical formulation of mine regarding the necessary and sufficient conditions for therapeutic change (14). She hypothesized that there would be a significant relationship between the extent of constructive personality change in the client and four counselor variables: (1) the degree of empathic understanding of the client manifested by the counselor; (2) the degree of positive affective attitude (unconditional positive regard) manifested by the counselor toward the client; (3) the extent to which the counselor is gen-uine, his words matching his own internal feeling; and (4) the extent to which the counselor's response matches the client's expression in the intensity of af-fective expression.

To investigate these hypotheses she first selected, by multiple objective criteria, a group of 10 cases which could be classed as "most successful" and a group of 10 "least successful" cases. She then took an early and late recorded interview from each of these cases. On a random basis she picked nine client-counselor interaction units—a client statement and a counselor response—from each of these interviews. She thus had nine early interactions and nine late interactions from each case. This gave her several hundred units which were now placed in random order. The units from an early interview of an unsuccessful case might be followed by the units from a late interview of a successful case, etc.

Three judges, who did not know the cases or their degree of success, or the source of any given unit, now listened to this material four different times. They rated each unit on a seven point scale, first as to the degree of empathy, second as to the counselor's positive attitude toward the client, third as to the counselor's congruence or genuineness, and fourth as to the degree to which the counselor's response matched the emotional intensity of the client's expression.

I think all of us who knew of the study regarded it as a very bold venture. Could judges listening to single units of interaction possibly make any reliable rating of such subtle qualities as I have mentioned? And even if suitable reliability could be obtained, could 18 counselor-client interchanges from each case—a minute sampling of the hundreds or thousands of such interchanges which occurred in each case—possibly bear any relationship to the therapeutic outcome? The chance seemed slim.

The findings are surprising. It proved possible to achieve high reliability between the judges, most of the inter-judge correlations being in the 0.80's or 0.90's, except on the last variable. It was found that a high degree of empathic understanding was significantly associated, at a 0.001 level, with the more successful cases. A high degree of unconditional positive regard was likewise associated with genuineness or congruence—the extent to which his words matched his feelings—was associated with the successful outcome of the case, and again at the 0.001 level of significance. Only in the investigation of the matching intensity of affective expression were the results equivocal.

It is of interest too that high ratings of these variables were not associated more significantly with units from later interviews than with units from early interviews. This means that the counselor's attitudes were quite constant throughout the interviews. If he was highly empathic, he tended to be so from first to last. If he was lacking in genuineness, this tended to be true of both early and late interviews.

As with any study, this investigation has its limitations. It is concerned with a certain type of helping relationship, psychotherapy. It investigated only four variables thought to be significant. Perhaps there are many others. Nevertheless it represents a significant advance in the study of helping relationships. Let me try to state the findings in the simplest possible fashion. It seems to indicate that the quality of the counselor's interaction with a client can be satisfactorily judged on the basis of a very small sampling of his behavior. It also means that if the counselor is congruent or transparent, so that his words are in line with his feelings rather than the two being discrepant—if the counselor likes the client, unconditionally, and if the counselor understands the essential feelings of the client as they seem to the client—then there is a strong probability that this will be an effective helping relationship.

Some Comments

These then are some of the studies which throw at least a measure of light on the nature of the helping relationship. They have investigated different facets of the problem. They have approached it from very different theoretical contexts. They have used different methods. They are not directly comparable. Yet they seem to me to point to several statements which may be made with some assurance. It seems clear that relationships which are helpful have different characteristics from relationships which are unhelpful. These differential characteristics have to do primarily with the attitudes of the helping person on the one hand and with the perception of the relationship by the "helpee" on the other. It is equally clear that the studies thus far made do not give us any final answers as to what is a helping relationship, nor how it is to be formed.

HOW CAN I CREATE A HELPING RELATIONSHIP?

I believe each of us working in the field of human relationships has a similar problem in knowing how to use such research knowledge. We cannot slavishly follow such findings in a mechanical way or we destroy the personal qualities which these very studies show to be valuable. It seems to me that we have to use these studies, testing them against our own experience and forming new and further personal hypotheses to use and test in our own further personal relationships.

So rather than try to tell you how you should use the findings I have presented I should like to tell you the kind of questions which these studies and my own clinical experience raise for me, and some of the tentative and changing hypotheses which guide my behavior as I enter into what I hope may be helping relationships, whether with students, staff, family, or clients. Let me list a number of these questions and considerations.

1. Can I *be* in some way which will be perceived by the other person as trustworthy, as dependable or consistent in some deep sense? Both research and experience indicate that this is very important, and over the years I have found what I believe are deeper and better ways of answering this question. I used to feel that I fulfilled all the outer conditions of trustworthiness—keeping appointments, respecting the confidential nature of the interviews, etc.—and if I acted consistently the same during the interviews, then this condition would be fulfilled. But experience drove home the fact that to act consistently acceptant, for example, if in fact I was feeling annoyed or skeptical or some other non-acceptant feeling, was certain in the long run to be perceived as inconsistent or untrustworthy. I have come to recognize that being trustworthy does not demand that I be rigidly consistent but that I be dependably real. The term congruent is one I have used to describe the way I would like to be. By this I mean that whatever feeling or attitude I am experiencing would be matched by my awareness of that attitude. When this is true, then I am a unified or integrated person in that moment, and hence I can *be* whatever I deeply *am*. This is a reality which I find others experience as dependable.

2. A very closely related question is this: Can I be expressive enough as a person that what I am will be communicated unambiguously? I believe that most of my failures to achieve a helping relationship can be traced to unsatisfactory answers to these two questions. When I am experiencing an attitude of annoyance toward another person but am unaware of it, then my communication contains contradictory messages. My words are giving one message, but I am also in subtle ways communicating the annoyance I feel and this confuses the other person and makes him distrustful, though he too may be unaware of what is causing this difficulty. When as a parent or a therapist or a teacher or an administrator I fail to listen to what is going on in me, fail because of my own defensiveness to sense my own feelings, then this kind of failure seems to result. It has made it seem to me that the most basic learning for anyone who hopes to establish any kind of helping relationship is that it is safe to be transparently real. If in a given relationship I am reasonably congruent, if no feelings relevant to the relationship are hidden either to me or the other person, then I can be almost sure that the relationship will be a helpful one.

One way of putting this which may seem strange to you is that if I can form a helping relationship to myself—if I can be sensitively aware of and acceptant toward my own feelings—then the likelihood is great that I can form a helping relationship toward another.

Now, acceptantly to be what I am, in this sense, and to permit this to show through to the other person, is the most difficult task I know and one I never fully achieve. But to realize that this *is* my task has been most rewarding because it has helped me to find what has gone wrong with interpersonal relationships which have become snarled and to put them on a constructive track again. It has meant that if I am to facilitate the personal growth of others in relation to me, then I must grow, and while this is often painful it is also enriching.

3. A third question is: Can I let myself experience positive attitudes toward this other person—attitudes of warmth, caring, liking, interest, respect? It is not easy. I find in myself, and feel that I often see in others, a certain amount of fear of these feelings. We are afraid that if we let ourselves freely experience these positive feelings toward another we may be trapped by them. They may lead to demands of us or we may be disappointed in our trust, and these outcomes we fear. So as a reaction we tend to build up distance between ourselves and others—aloofness, a "professional" attitude, an impersonal relationship.

I feel quite strongly that one of the important reasons for the professionalization of every field is that it helps to keep this distance. In the clinical areas we develop elaborate diagnostic formulations, seeing the person as an object. In teaching and in administration we develop all kinds of evaluative procedures, so that again the person is perceived as an object. In these ways, i believe, we can keep ourselves from experiencing the caring which would exist if we recognized the relationship as one between two persons. It is a real achievement when we can learn, even in certain relationships or at certain times in those relationships, that it is safe to care, that it is safe to relate to the other as a person for whom we have positive feelings.

4. Another question the importance of which I have learned in my own experience is: Can I be strong enough as a person to be separate from the other? Can I be a sturdy respecter of my own feelings, my own needs, as well as his? Can I own and, if need be, express my own feelings as something belonging to me and separate from his feelings? Am I strong enough in my own separateness that I will not be downcast by his depression, frightened by his fear, nor engulfed by his dependency? Is my inner self hardy enough to realize that I am not destroyed by his anger, taken over by his need for dependence, nor enslaved by his love, but that I exist separate from him with feelings and rights of my own? When I can freely feel this strength of being a separate person, then I find that I can let myself go much more deeply in understanding and accepting him because I am not fearful of losing myself.

5. The next question is closely related. Am I secure enough within myself to permit him his separateness? Can I permit him to be what he is—honest or deceitful, infantile or adult, despairing or over-confident? Can I give him the freedom to be? Or do I feel that he should follow my advice, or remain somewhat dependent on me, or mold himself after me? In this connection I think of the interesting small study by Farson (6) which found that the less well adjusted and less competent counselor tends to induce conformity to himself, to have clients who model themselves after him. On the other hand, the better adjusted and more competent counselor can interact with a client through many interviews without interfering with the freedom of the client to develop a personality quite separate from that of his therapist. I should prefer to be in this latter class, whether as parent or supervisor or counselor.

6. Another question I ask myself is: Can I let myself enter fully into the world of his feelings and personal meanings and see these as he does? Can I step into his private world so completely that I lose all desire to evaluate or judge it? Can I enter it so sensitively that I can move about in it freely, without tramping on meanings which are precious to him? Can I sense it so accurately that I can catch not only the meanings of his experience which are obvious to him, but those meanings which are only implicit, which he sees only dimly or as confusion? Can I extend this understanding without limit? I think of the client who said, "Whenever I find someone who understands a *part* of me at the time, then it never fails that a point is reached where I know they're *not* understanding me again. . . .What I've looked for so hard is for someone to understand."

For myself I find it easier to feel this kind of understanding, and to communicate it, to individual clients than to students in a class or staff members in a group in which I am involved. There is a strong temptation to set students "straight," or to point out to a staff member the errors in his thinking. Yet when I can permit myself to understand in these situations, it is mutually rewarding. And with clients in therapy, I am often impressed with the fact that even a minimal amount of empathic understanding—a bumbling and faulty attempt to catch the confused complexity of the client's meaning—is helpful, though there is no doubt that it is most helpful when I can see and formulate clearly the meanings in his experiencing which for him have been unclear and tangled.

7. Still another issue is whether I can be acceptant of each facet of this other person which he presents to me. Can I receive him as he is? Can I communicate this attitude? Or can I only receive him conditionally, acceptant of some aspects of his feelings and silently or openly disapproving of other aspects? It has been my experience that when my attitude is conditional, then he cannot change or grow in those respects in which I cannot fully receive him. And when—afterward and sometimes too late—I try to discover why I have been unable to accept him in every respect, I usually discover that it is because I have been frightened or threatened in myself by some aspect of his feelings. If I am to be more helpful, then I must myself grow and accept myself in these respects.

8. A very practical issue is raised by the question: Can I act with sufficient sensitivity in the relationship that my behavior will not be perceived as a threat? The work we are beginning to do in studying the physiological concomitants of psychotherapy confirms the research by Dittes in indicating how easily individuals are threatened at a physiological level. The psychogalvanic reflex—the measure of skin conductance—takes a sharp dip when the therapist responds with some word which is just a little stronger than the client's feelings. And to a phrase such as "My, you *do* look upset," the needle swings almost off the paper. My desire to avoid even such minor threats is not due to a hypersensitivity about my client. It is simply due to the conviction based on experience that if I can free him as completely as possible from external threat, then he can begin to experience and to deal with the internal feelings and conflicts which he finds threatening within himself.

9. A specific aspect of the preceding question but an important one is: Can I free him from the threat of external evaluation? In almost every phase of our lives—at home, at school, at work—we find ourselves under the rewards of punishments of external judgments. "That's good"; "that's naughty." "That's worth an A"; "that's a failure." "That's good counseling"; "that's poor counseling." Such judgments are a part of our lives from infancy to old age. I believe they have a certain social usefulness to institutions and organizations such as schools and professions. Like everyone else I find myself all too often making such evaluations. But, in my experience, they do not make for personal growth and hence I do not believe that they are a part of a helping relationship. Curiously enough a positive evaluation is as threatening in the long run as a negative one, since to inform someone that he is good implies that you also have the right to tell him he is bad. So I have come to feel that the more I can keep a relationship free of judgment and evaluation, the more this will permit the other person to reach the point where he recognizes that the locus of evaluation, the center of responsibility lies within himself. The meaning and value of his experience is in the last analysis something which is up to him, and no amount of external judgment can alter this. So I should like to work toward a relationship in which I am not, even in my own feelings, evaluating him. This I believe can set him free to be a self-responsible person.

10. One last question: Can I meet this other individual as a person who is in process of *becoming,* or will I be bound by his past and by my past? If, in

my encounter with him, I am dealing with him as an immature child, an ignorant student, a neurotic personality, or a psychopath, each of these concepts of mine limits what he can be in the relationship. Martin Buber, the existentialist philosopher of the University of Jerusalem, has a phrase, "confirming the other," which has had meaning for me. He says "Confirming means...accepting the whole potentiality of the other... I can recognize in him, know in him, the person he has been...*created* to become... I confirm him in myself, and then in him, in relation to this potentiality that...can now be developed, can evolve" (3). If I accept the other person as something fixed, already diagnosed and classified, already shaped by his past, then I am doing my part to confirm this limited hypothesis. If I accept him as a process of becoming, then I am doing what I can to confirm or make real his potentialities.

It is at this point that I see Verplanck, Lindsley, and Skinner, working in operant conditioning, coming together with Buber, the philosopher of mystic. At least they come together in principle, in an odd way. If I see a relationship as only an opportunity to reinforce certain types of words or opinions in the other, then I tend to confirm him as an object—a basically mechanical manipulable object. And if I see this as his potentiality, he tends to act in ways which support this hypothesis. If, on the other hand, I see a relationship as an opportunity to "reinforce" *all* that he is, the person that he is with all his existent potentialities, then he tends to act in ways which support *this* hypothesis. I have then—to use Buber's term—confirmed him as a living person, capable of creative inner development. Personally I prefer this second type of hypothesis.

CONCLUSION

In the early portion of this paper I reviewed some of the contributions which research is making to our knowledge *about* relationships. Endeavoring to keep that knowledge in mind I then took up the kind of questions which arise from an inner and subjective point of view as I enter, as a person, into relationships. If I could, in myself, answer all the questions I have raised in the affirmative, then I believe that any relationships in which I was involved would be helping relationships, would involve growth. But I cannot give a positive answer to most of these questions. I can only work in the direction of a positive answer.

This has raised in my mind the strong suspicion that the optimal helping relationship is the kind of relationship created by a person who is psychologically mature. Or to put it in another way, the degree to which I can create relationships which facilitate the growth of others as separate persons is a measure of the growth I have achieved in myself. In some respects this is a disturbing thought, but it is also a promising or challenging one. It would indicate that if I am interested in creating helping relationships I have a fascinating lifetime job ahead of me, stretching and developing my potentialities in the direction of growth.

I am left with the uncomfortable thought that what I have been working out for myself in this paper may have little relationship to your interests and your work. If so, I regret it. But I am at least partially comforted by the fact that all of us who are working in the field of human relationships and trying to understand the basic orderliness of that field are engaged in the most crucial enterprise in today's world. If we are thoughtfully trying to understand our tasks as administrators, teachers, educational counselors, vocational counselors, therapists, then we are working on the problem which will determine the future of this planet. For it is not upon the physical sciences that the future will depend. It is upon us who are trying to understand and deal with the interactions between human beings—who are trying to create helping relationships. So I hope that the questions I ask of myself will be of some use to you in gaining understanding and perspective as you endeavor, in your way to facilitate growth in your relationships.

REFERENCES

1. Baldwin, A. L., Kalhorn, Jr., and Breese, F. H. Patterns of parent behavior. *Psychol. Monogr.*, 1945, *58*, No. 268, 1–75.

2. Betz, G. J., & Whitehorn, J. C. The relationship of the therapist to the outcome of therapy in schizophrenia. *Psychiat. Research Reports #5. Research techniques in schizophrenia.* Washington, D. C.: American Psychiatric Association, 1956, 89–117.

3. Buber, M., & Rogers, C. Transcription of dialogue held April 18, 1957, Ann Arbor, Mich. Unpublished manuscript.

4. Dittes, J. E. Galvanic skin response as a measure of patient's reaction to therapist's permissiveness. *J. abnorm. soc. Psychol.*, 1957, *55*, 295–303.

5. Ends, E. J. and Page, C. W. A study of three types of group psychotherapy with hospitalized male inebriates. *Quar. J. Stud. Alchol.* 1957, *18*, 263–277.

6. Farson, R. E. Introjection in the psychotherapeutic relationship. Unpublished doctoral dissertation, University of Chicago 1955.

7. Fiedler, F. E. Quantitative studies on the role of therapists' feelings toward their patients. In Mower, O. H. (ed.). *Psychotherapy: theory and research.* New York: Ronald Press, 1953, Chap. 12.

8. Greenspoon, J. The reinforcing effect of two spoken sounds on the frequency of two responses. *Amer. J. Psychol.*, 1955, *68*, 409–416.

9. Halkides, G. An experimental study of four conditions necessary for therapeutic change. Unpublished doctoral dissertation, University of Chicago, 1958.

10. Harlow, H., and associates. Experiment in progress, as reported by Robert Zimmerman.

11. Heine, R. W. A comparison of patients' reports on psychotherapeutic experience with psychoanalytic, nondirective, and Adlerian therapists. Unpublished doctoral dissertation, University of Chicago, 1950.

12. Lindsley, O. R. Operant conditioning methods applied to research in chronic schizophrenia. *Psychiat. Research Reports #5. Research techniques in schizophrenia.* Washington, D.C.: American Psychiatric Association, 1956, 118–153.

13. Page, C. W., and Ends, E. J. A review and synthesis of the literature suggesting a psychotherapeutic technique based on two-factor learning theory. Unpublished manuscript, loaned to the writer.

14. Rogers, C. R. The necessary and sufficient conditions of psychotherapeutic personality change. *J. consult. Psychol.*, 1957, *21*, 95–103.

15. Quinn, R. D. Psychotherapists' expressions as an index to the quality of early therapeutic relationships. Unpublished doctoral dissertation, University of Chicago, 1950.

16. Seeman, J. Counselor judgments of therapeutic process and outcome. In Rogers, C. R. and Dymond, R. F., (eds.), *Psychotherapy and personality change.* Chicago: University of Chicago Press, 1954, Chap. 7.

17. Verplanck, W. S. The control of the content of conversation: reinforcement of statements of opinion. *J. abnorm. soc. Psychol.*, 1955, *51*, 668–676.

18. Whitehorn, J. C., and Betz, G. J. A study of psychotherapeutic relationships between physicians and schizophrenic patients. *Amer. J. Psychiat.*, 1954, *111*, 321–331.

On the Professional Status of Nursing

Rozella M. Schlotfeldt

Being by nature an optimist, and having had that optimism consistently enhanced over a professional career sufficiently long to be able to savor contributions that well-educated nurses have made and continued to make to the advancement of knowledge and to the improvement of society, I have found it difficult to give much credence to the purveyors of gloom with regard to nursing's survival. It is necessary, however, periodically to examine the assumptions upon which one operates and to appraise as objectively as possible, within one's own biased frame of reference, circumstances that exist. Perhaps I have been wrong in steadfastly maintaining my optimism relative to the growth, development, and perceived increasing significance of the contributions made by professionals known as nurses.

In preparing for this presentation, I continued to read widely, to examine data, to review my perceptions of nursing and its several publics, and to ideate about perceptions communicated by other professionals. I am prepared to make some generalizations about nursing at the beginning of 1974. I am prepared also to set forth some recommendations that, if accepted and implemented, hold promise of enhancing the contributions that nursing, as an emerging, learned, profession and scholarly discipline, can, must, and certainly will make to the work of the world. Quite obviously, the position here taken is that nursing must not only survive; it must also thrive.

The optimism that underlies this presentation stems from the well-established fact that it is within the nature of man to seek to improve his individual and collective positions through his quest to make advancements in knowledge and through the creative use of that knowledge to foster the betterment of his lot, and that of his fellows. Nursing, representing a corporate group of individuals having a mission to serve others, is no exception.

The evolution of the nursing profession mirrors the evolution of all other professions whose members are dedicated to the use of knowledge in particular ways to improve the services they render. Whether it is clergymen, committed to helping man in his quest for goodness; lawyers, committed to promoting justice; physicians, committed to eradicating or alleviating the sequelae of pathological agents; social workers, committed to helping people become socialized human beings; teachers, committed to helping students dispel ignorance; artists, dedicated to enhancing man's enjoyment; or nurses, committed to sustaining and improving man's effectiveness in attaining his highest

Reprinted from *Nursing Forum*, Vol. 13, No. 1, with permission of the author and of Nursing Publications, Inc., 194-B Kinderkamack Road, Park Ridge, New Jersey.

possible level of health, all are engaged in fields of work that have, sooner or later, achieved the characteristics of professions. Members of those occupational groups, in varying degrees and in altered proportions at different time periods, exemplify practices that characterize professionals. Each of those professions has emerged from being, in succession, trial and error operations, vocations having meager scientific rationale for functions accomplished, technologies, whose guild members held command of relatively firm bases of verified knowledge, and finally, professions whose practitioners were called upon to exercise exquisite judgment in the selective and artistic use of extensive knowledge in the execution of responsibilities having profound consequences. The point being made is that commitment of practitioners to rendering a needed social service that is valued by their fellows guarantees the emergence of professions. If there is a question, therefore, concerning whether or not nursing is to survive, let alone continue its emergence into becoming a full-fledged and learned profession, the point at issue is whether or not the services rendered by practitioners known by the term "nurse" are, in fact, valued by society. A concomitant, and perhaps even more penetrating question, is whether or not nursing care rendered by nurses is considered by them to be of value and worthy of continuous development and refinement. The latter question prompted some observations and generalizations that may illuminate some impediments to nursing's emergence to full professional status, and to identify some problems that must be resolved.

With some concern for overstating the circumstances as they exist universally, it seems useful to present observations that contrast what seems generally to prevail with that which should prevail, if nursing is to fulfill its mission to society. Although certainly not exhaustive, four generalizations will be presented, along with observations that seem to support them. They relate to nursing practice, nursing education, and nursing research. Either implicitly or explicitly, the observations to be made point up problems that need resolution. Some general directions for the future will be cited; hopefully, they will provoke discussion.

The first generalization is that nursing, as a corporate entity, represents personnel who manifest great concern with means and inadequate concern with ends. The unevenness of nursing's development to professional status by geographic region and even within geographic regions, makes it imperative to state the caveat that observations supporting this generalization may pertain all of the time in some regions, some of the time in all regions, and with varying degrees of certainty in all regions at any time.

A field of human endeavor concerned primarily with ends, rather than with means, implies certainty on the part of its practitioners with regard to the mission they are expected to accomplish. Its practitioners are generally unified in their belief that they have consequential contributions to make to the well-being of those they serve. They grasp the significance of their corporate mission and the enduring responsibility it entails; and they are willing to be held accountable for fulfilling their obligations to society. In short, practitioners' concern with ends, in contrast to overconcern with means, represents emergence of a field of work into full-fledged, professional status. It characterizes a profession whose mission is valued by society and one whose practitioners are held in high regard because they have command of particular knowledge, demonstrate unique competencies, and promote and uphold exemplary practices and ethical standards. What are the circumstances regarding nursing practice?

The uncertainties that prevail with regard to nursing's mission and nurses' role, responsibilities, and scope of practice are well known to those both within and outside the occupation. They were pointed up to me recently by a former colleague who, after stating disdain for the lack of good nursing care exemplified in the place of her current practice, poignantly questioned the meaning of the term, the "expanded nurse role," when no basic nursing role was identifiable.

Although some nurses may be reasonably clear about their role, nursing's literature is replete with evidence that nurses are not generally united with regard to their mission and the focus and scope of their responsibilities. The current debate concerning whether or not the nurse role is expanded, extended, or shrinking, and whether or not nurses must be transformed into "nurse practitioners" in order to be recognized as practicing nurses points up nursing's concern with means, rather than ends. Further evidence is supplied by policies and procedures within practice settings. They set forth in detail how rituals are to be performed in accomplishing the gamut of nursing tasks. Rarely do policies extant communicate confidence that each nurse professional understands her mission and has sufficient knowledge and skills to demonstrate the nurse role fully. The extent to which other health professionals and clients conceive nurses as doing things, rather than accomplishing worthwhile outcomes through their employment of a variety of means, each with individual style, lends further credence to this observation.

Nurse educators quite often exemplify their concern with means at the expense of their understanding the ends to be attained. Traditionally, nurse-teachers have been greatly concerned with teaching strategies, with curriculum structure and organization of learning opportunities, with observational guides to be used by students and by themselves, and with approaches to be used in arriving at decisions concerning whether or not students should be passed, and with the grades they should be awarded. They have been, in general, less concerned with delineation of the competencies graduates should uniformly possess, at least at the minimal level of acceptable performance, and certainly less concerned with the advancement of nursing's science. Certainly nurse educators' relatively high concern with means has delayed there being concensus concerning the knowledge practitioners about to enter general and specialty practice must master and be able to employ creatively in their work. One should be able to expect educators to lead the field with regard to delineating the nature and scope of nursing practice inasmuch as one must conceptualize the competencies graduates must possess before designing their learning opportunities. Only rare educators have given such definitive leadership.

Nursing, like other emerging professions, has placed considerable emphasis on teaching neophyte investigators the rules of the research game and on introducing them to research methodologies. These are worthy and needed endeavors. In contrast, however, relatively more mature professions and disciplines lead their neophyte investigators to focus intently on study of phenomena about which knowledge is inadequate, and to focus less intently on precise strategies through which to obtain that knowledge. This observation is made, not to denigrate emphasis on teaching students about research strategies, but rather to point up that nursing still focuses heavily on students' learning techniques and research strategies, often borrowed from other disciplines, in preference to their being motivated to seek answers to significant questions about the health-seeking behaviors of man, through whatever means are available, or can be developed.

The second generalization that seems warranted is that nursing is overconcerned with quantity and underconcerned with quality. Considerable evidence exists that in many nurse practice settings, concern is primarily with numbers of persons employed to carry out nursing tasks, rather than with the quality of services rendered. The widespread practice of substituting nursing technicians for nurse professionals and failure to require designated personnel to be competent in giving leadership with regard to nursing care supports this generalization. Inasmuch as most of those services are still led by nurses, the conclusion seems warranted that those nurses who support and even promote undesirable practices must condone emphasis on quantity, rather than quality. The paucity of peer review and quality assessment of nursing practices in hospitals and in other health care agencies lends further support to this generalization.

Nurse educators have characteristically acted to recruit and to produce increasing numbers of personnel, without thoughtful establishment of policy guides concerning the numbers of nurse professionals, nursing technicians, and nursing assistants actually needed. The recently established statewide planning agencies, whose efficacy is still to be assessed, may offer some needed change. The nursing profession urgently needs to address the question of how numbers of nursing personnel can and should be controlled through regulating inputs at the point of admissions into all types of nursing education programs. The well-recognized over-production of assisting and technical personnel and the relative paucity of professionals support this recommendation. Further, nursing has yet to delineate minimal standards that must be uniformly exemplified before nursing schools can be opened, and to have those standards prevail. The result is that there are large numbers of nursing schools, some of quite poor quality.

In spite of remarkable progress made in some settings, nurse educators still lament about the poor quality of practice exemplified in clinical learning environments, while they continue to grind out large numbers of students who learn poor practices from the models they emulate in those learning laboratories. Rarely does educators' concern for quality lead them to act to imrpove those practice settings; rarely does it lead them to restrict student admissions when inadequate numbers of qualified faculty are available to teach them. Are nurse educators sufficiently concerned with quality—or are they committed to continued, unrestrained production of large numbers of nursing personnel?

The relative scarcity of nursing research makes it impossible to make valid observations about the validity of the quantity versus quality generalization, as it relates to scientific inquiry. It does seem appropriate to observe, however, that the recent, immediate reaction of many administrators to cutbacks in federal funds supporting graduate training and research was to act as if neither has legitimate claim to support from tuition and endowment income and from general university funds and unrestricted gifts and grants that support undergraduate education. In the face of abundant data that demonstrate nursing's great need for research and for leadership personnel, such priority setting would seem to lend credence to the observation that the highest quality training and research are being short changed in the interest of continued production of large and increasing numbers of personnel trained at lower levels of sophistication. The extent to which university nursing school faculty members are supported to engage in inquiry, scholarly practice, contemplation, and publication, in contrast to teaching relatively large numbers of students also points up the quality-quantity dichotomy in nursing.

A third generalization about nursing that seems valid early in 1974, is that nursing is still over-committed to doing and under-committed to knowing. That observation reflects the fact that the balance is just beginning to tip toward an occupational orientation reflecting professionalism in contrast to technology. It is important to point out that technology is an important aspect of all professional practice and that professional practitioners are expected to be highly competent, technically. They are also expected, however, to be highly knowledgeable, to be able to use knowledge creatively, to exercise exquisite judgment, and to be visionary with regard to practice and research.

In settings where practitioners are responsible for execution of practice responsibilities, focus naturally is on doing. However, recognition must be given to the speed with which knowledge becomes obsolete and the extent to which practice settings must provide opportunities for practitioners' continuous learning. In institutions that provide learning laboratories for health profession students, opportunities for continuous learning should be relatively easy to provide. Regrettably, however, there is insufficient evidence in most practice settings that nurses are expected to engage in inquiry and in continuous learning. Indeed, enforcement of outdated institutional policies and denial of research evidence that should mandate change is, at times, antithetical to promoting the ethic of science and of continuous learning.

Some few practice settings now have a growing group of nurse specialists who practice, teach, and engage in inquiry. Even in those settings, the ethic of science has yet to be fully developed. I covet the day when each professional will routinely record her observations with a view toward systematically asking questions of that rich, clinical data. I covet the day when practitioners will routinely theorize as they make and record their observations. When that day comes nursing will be as committed to knowing as to doing; and the profession will have arrived.

Although the trend is certainly developing, nurse educators as yet do not uniformly reflect commitment to scholarship and to continuous learning. The ethic of commitment to science, to research, to publication, to contemplation, and to scholarly practice has yet to be uniformly exemplified in nursing schools. In most nursing schools, commitment to doing is reflected in faculty activities, some of which are quite ritualistic. When each university nursing faculty consistently provides for students, models of scientists engaged in inquiry relative to nursing practice, nursing education, and nursing administration, and models of theorists concerned with testing promising hypotheses concerning man's health-seeking behavior, it can be said with confidence that nursing is truly concerned with knowing as well as with doing. That day has not yet arrived.

There are some circumstances that militate against nursing's developing a commitment to science. The field has insufficient numbers of well-prepared leaders to fulfill all the demands placed upon them. Nurses who are best prepared are expected to do research, to theorize, to give leadership in nursing schools, to improve practice settings, to be spokesmen for nursing in civic and governmental arenas, to publish, to give leadership in professional societies, to serve on editorial boards, to give speeches, to write textbooks, to be administrators, and to serve as good models for the next generation of professionals. The point is made, I believe, that nursing is, indeed, committed to doing; but the truly remarkable thing is that nursing is also developing a growing commitment to knowing—when there is so much to be done, and all at once!

The fourth generalization that seems warranted is that individual and corporate self-consciousness seems to take precedence over individual and corporate self-confidence in the occupational field of nursing. Undoubtedly, nurses exemplify the self-consciousness characteristic of all women who have, throughout their lives, been duped into believing that they exist at and for the pleasure of others, rather than because of their inherent worth and the value of the contributions they have to make. The time is long overdue for nurses to assert their professional prerogatives, and with confidence, communicate and demonstrate the nature and value of their contributions. Nurses' own characteristics, self-effacing denial of their contributions to the health-care system and denial by other health professionals and by health-care planners of nurses' collaborative role in designing the system of health and sickness care are well known. An embarrassing plethora of putdowns could be cited by every nurse.

Perhaps the most vivid, recent example of nurses' self-consciousness is their acceding to the notion that it is only with the sanction of physicians that they have the right to assess the health status and potential of those they serve, in preparation for planning and effecting programs of nursing care. With sanction of some nurse leaders, nurses have self-consciously sought from physicians permission to make observations and to gather data essential to planning nursing regimens. The right to use a stethoscope or other instruments to sharpen the acuity of their observations has, in many circumstances, been self-consciously justified by nurses who see themselves as mere second-rate extenders of physicians' services. Some actually believe that they have no role to play as nurses, and that their reason for being exists only because of the created shortage and maldistribution of physicians.

Properly, nurses are concerned with their own inadequacies; and properly they act to correct them. Improperly, however, nurses allow their own responsibilities and contributions to go unnoticed by other professionals with whom they work and by those they serve. The time is long overdue for nurses, without embarrassment, to declare the scope of their responsibilities, demonstrate their competencies, and expect appropriate rewards—not only those that are intrinsic to their work, but also those that include recognition and compensation commensurate with their contributions to the health-care system.

The conspicuous absence of nurses among those planning for new, federal government and community sponsored systems of health care, and organized nursing's belated and self-conscious responses to being so ignored lends support to this generalization. The time is long overdue for nurses to seek and to gain the recognition they deserve for collaborative planning and effecting accessible, high quality, efficacious, cost-effective programs of health care. Without embarrassment, nurses should brag a little! They have made tremendous contributions in the face of almost unsurmountable odds. It is possible that when nurses gain in self-confidence, they will less frequently self-consciously engage in discussion with one another about the frustrations they experience from being routinely ignored.

Although nurse educators talk a great deal about professional colleague-ship relative to planning and effecting programs of education for future health professionals, meager accomplishments indicate that few nurses have exerted effective leadership in that regard. Rare is the circumstance in which nurse faculty confidently interact with faculty of the other health professions to demonstrate to future practitioners the collaborative roles they all must play, if society is to be served with a comprehensive system of care. It is possible that when nurse faculties gain more self-confidence in practice, they will be less self-conscious about their abilities to give leadership to colleagues in the other health professions. It is possible, also, that nurse educators will soon self-confidently give leadership in effecting changes in the perceptions of nursing held by citizens, most of whom still believe that nurses are self-effacing practitioners, whose every act is accomplished only upon order.

Until nurse investigators came to recognize that the prime focus of their research is the health-seeking behavior of man, they, too, exemplified self-consciousness in justifying their research endeavors. Thanks to the excellent example and leadership of a few nurse investigators, the focus of nursing research is now turning away from problems tangential to nursing's central reason for being; and increasingly, nurses are, with confidence, seeking to find answers to valid nursing questions and seeking to advance knowledge that, when applied in nursing practice, will improve those practices. No longer do nurse investigators and theorists self-consciously speak of their commitment to science; they now, with self-confidence and pride, proclaim their obligation to advance, verify, and continuously restructure the expanding body of knowledge known as nursing science. As their contributions are increasingly recognized and respected by investigators in nursing and in other fields, members of the nursing profession will grow in self-confidence and hopefully soon demonstrate that this generalization is totally invalid.

In order to make changes that hold promise of producing improved circumstances, deterrents to progress must be identified. Implicit or explicit in this discussion, I have suggested that nursing must enhance nurses' commitment to their mission goals and be accountable for their practices. They must delineate the scope of the profession's responsibility, and intensify endeavors to assure quality performance on the part of all practitioners. Educators must realistically balance concern for quantity with concern for quality. Nurses must place high priority on knowing, and on the advancement of knowledge through scholarly endeavors. They must effectively shed the mantle of self-consciousness and, instead, project justifiable self-confidence and pride in the accomplishments of nurses and in the contributions nursing has made and will continue to make to the society it serves.

Quite obviously, my confidence is placed in learning, scholarship, and the power of the disciplined mind in bringing about needed change. I believe that the nursing profession must make itself more visible through effective public relations and through colleagueship with people they serve. I believe that nurses must become politically astute and economically secure. I believe that nurses need to be cooperative and supportive of the work of their own colleagues. I believe that nurses should be encouraged to seek positions providing opportunities for professional and political influence. Quite obviously, I believe in nurses and in nursing.

There is no doubt in my mind that nursing will survive, and thrive. There is no doubt in my mind that society will support nursing. The need, as I see it, is for enlightened, visionary, courageous leadership that will be effective in releasing the tremendous potential possessed by nurses for improving the lot of their fellow man.

19

The Nursing Process

Throughout this book we have been working toward a complete understanding of the nursing process. Beginning in early chapters with basic parts, we have been moving—step by step—to a whole, progressing from basic component to integrated process. At the same time, we have been progressing toward understanding.

Part I presented the phases of the nursing process: assessment, planning, implementation, and evaluation. In addition, Part I discussed in detail each method involved in each phase of the nursing process: from data collection to nursing orders. The objective of the nursing process throughout each step has been to provide quality, individualized care—to assist the client to fullest health potential.

But methods do not stand alone, and methods do not create a process nor understanding of the process. In Parts II, III, and IV, other variables affecting the nursing process—skills, quality systems, and theories and strategies of health care delivery—were added to the foundation established in Part I. Thus, the seeds of the nursing process sown in earlier chapters have been cultivated, step by step and part by part, to yield a whole workable process.

Now, in Chapter 19, we arrive at a more complete picture. At this time, our discussion turns to the conceptual framework which holds all the parts of the nursing process together. This chapter presents the concepts guiding the nursing process, as well as a definition and statement of purpose. In the final chapter of this book, one final element—humanism—will be added to the nursing process to color it in the human tones of the future.

THE CONCEPTUAL FRAMEWORK

The conceptual framework upon which the nursing process is based employs general system theory. System theory was first presented in the

Introduction of this book, and parts of it have been discussed as it related to a particular method or phase. In the next section, however, we will combine the pieces already presented into a whole, workable theory which relates to nursing, health care, and all human life.

General System Theory

The general system theory framework provides a construct for studying people within an environment—and, indeed, as builders of their environment. General system theory mandates analysis of all the parts of a system, the relationship between these parts, and the purposes, reasons, or tasks of the system. Simply stated, this theory includes purpose, content, and process (Yura and Walsh, 1973).

General system theory is a model developed by von Bertalanffy (1968) that can be used to study designated phenomena, regardless of the properties contained within the event. Von Bertalanffy identifies assumptions of the general system theory:

1. *A system is more than a sum of its parts.* More explicitly, the system develops a character of its own, subsumed by collective goals of the parts.
2. It is *ever-changing,* since one change in any part affects the whole.
3. Boundaries are implicit in each system and are defined by its purpose. Closed systems end when a quantity needed for fulfillment is obtained. This phenomenon is not pertinent in human systems, as they are considered *open* and *dynamic.*
4. All systems must be *goal-directed,* otherwise they fall apart. Goals of the individual parts of the system may not be directly in line with the group goal; however, they should not be in conflict. Even though the goal is often most difficult to specify, it provides the core of a system's functioning.

The universe is perhaps our absolute outer system; all that goes on within the world falls into subsystems. However, it becomes necessary to realize that one system is always related to or a part of a larger whole. Logical, systematic pursuits of a problem require that boundaries be designated. Figure 19–1 provides one example of the nursing profession's boundaries and how the profession can be portrayed as a hierarchical subsystem.

The most direct way to identify a system is to state its purpose (Banathy, 1968). This becomes paramount when studying a problem systematically. The boundaries of any system must be circumscribed by the relevant parts of the environment as they pertain to the purpose. This answers the question: "What is the goal of a system and what are the important components for this purpose within the relevant environment?" The purpose and goal of health care systems, of course, is client care. It follows that each system is unique, developed from specified segments in a time and place. Therefore, what may

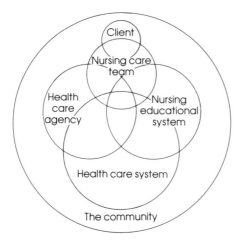

FIGURE 19-1
THE SYSTEM OF NURSING VIEWED FROM AN
OVERALL HEALTH CARE PERSPECTIVE

be important in the care of one client in a certain place will not be totally appropriate for another. The systems framework facilitates delivery of individualized nursing care, since only those areas and people relevant in a client's care are included in the system, with purposes broadly *and* specifically stated. This is general system theory, with importance being placed on diagnosing the environment (Hersey and Blanchard, 1977).

Using general system theory, the client becomes the focus of purpose— care—but all of the facets of the system, in essence, receive care. A hypothetical example can be observed in Figure 19-2.

As can be seen in the figure, the client is, of course, the major segment of the system. Since the client is seen as being largely influenced by many other people and environmental factors, all relevant aspects then become part of the system. Each person or aspect is felt to have a relationship with and in the client's care; each must be assessed and included in the care plan development, implementation, and evaluation. The size of the piece of the pie allotted to each facet of the system reflects the relative importance of the factor in the client's world. Nursing theorists have extensively applied general system theory in their study of nursing practice. This application is helpful in stressing the concept of individualized care in the nursing profession.

Rogers' Theoretical Basis of Nursing   Rogers (1970, p. 3) discussed the concern of nursing as being "man in his entirety, his wholeness. Nursing's body of scientific knowledge seeks to describe, explain, and predict about human beings."

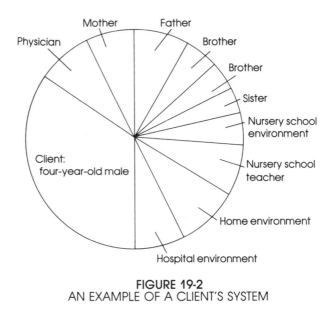

FIGURE 19-2
AN EXAMPLE OF A CLIENT'S SYSTEM

The theoretical model developed by Rogers (1970) rests on the following assumptions. These assumptions relate directly to that described in general system theory by von Bertalanffy (1968).

1. Each person is a unique, unified whole being whose characteristics are different from or greater than the sum of his or her parts (Rogers, 1970; Roy, 1974a).
2. Matter and energy constantly exchange in persons and their environment(s). The system of a person's being is, therefore, dynamic (Rogers, 1970; Roy, 1974a).
3. The process of life is developmental within the space-time continuum. It is irreversible and linear in direction (Rogers, 1970; Roy, 1974a).
4. There is pattern and organization reflected in the whole entity of each person (Rogers, 1970; Roy, 1974a). It is primarily through this assumption that study of human behavior is possible.
5. Each person's uniqueness is characterized by abstraction and behaviors that use language, emotion, feelings, and fantasy (Rogers, 1970; Roy, 1974a).

Rogers's (1970) belief about nursing implies a deep respect for the individuality of each person. This reflects study of the relationship between persons and their environment, with the goal of facilitating effective nursing care outcomes. Disease is low-keyed, with the unified person and human functioning taking priority. The well-being of society, as the suprasystem of persons, must also be a focal point.

Roy's Adaptation Model   Developed subsequently to Rogers's model, Roy's model (1974b) primarily uses the systems approach in patient care. Similarities between both theories become obvious as one looks at the assumptions presented by Roy (1974b, p. 136):

1. "Man is a bio-psycho-social being." Study of a human being must reflect all of these facets.
2. "Man is in constant interaction with a changing environment." The dynamic aspect of being is, therefore, portrayed.
3. Biologic, psychologic and sociologic facets are used by persons in coping with their ever-changing world.
4. The life experience of persons involves health and illness. Moreover, illness is not idiosyncratic in living.
5. Adaptation to the environment is requisite in living.
6. Guiding the process of adaptation for an individual are the stimuli available in the particular environment.
7. Positive adaptive responses result from stimuli that are within the individual's repertoire of response patterns.
8. The four basic adaptive modes of human beings are: physiologic needs, self-concept, role function, and interdependent relations.

These adaptive modes guide the nursing process. The ultimate concern of nursing is the total person, supporting and promoting adaptation of the individual within the context of the person's own health-illness pattern, environmental process, and stimuli available for use (Roy, 1974b).

Other Nursing Models Employing Systems Theory   Hall's (1964) philosophy of nursing thoroughly supports general system theory and the technical/professional position of the American Nurses' Association (1965). She describes nursing practice as moving from simple to complex such as that pictured in Figure 19-3.

The simple/complex dichotomy is illustrated in the following example: A client in an ambulatory care situation having a foot injury may state that she is cold. A blanket may be offered by the nurse. This simple function of nursing is different from caring for a post-operative client who is in a recovery room following abdominal surgery. Should the client express chill, many complex factors must be considered. These include low blood pressure, internal bleeding, reactions to transfusions, and so forth. It is the professional nurse's responsibility to do much more than simply offer the client a blanket.

The simple functions of nursing practice require few factors for consideration prior to a discrimination or nursing judgment; as one moves outward into the complex realm, more and more items, facts, knowledge, and experience from the circumscribed system must be considered, however. Hall's (1964) belief in professional nursing is grounded on the base that human beings

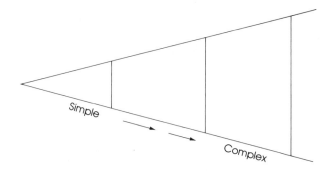

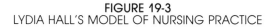

SOURCE: L. Hall, "Nursing: What is it?" The Canadian Nurse, Vol. 60, No. 2. Reprinted with permission.

FIGURE 19-3
LYDIA HALL'S MODEL OF NURSING PRACTICE

are complex, and professional nursing requires a broad range of knowledge, experience, and a process by which complex decisions can be made with and for clients. Her concept of nursing practice compares easily with Reiter's (1966) and involves three essential components as seen in Table 19-1.

It becomes evident that the system developed for providing care must be concerned with the biologic, psychologic, and sociologic facets of the individual. Figure 19-4 portrays the relationship between facets of a person. The overlapping circles illustrate the autonomy of each human aspect, as well as the inter/intrarelationship of all three.

Other lesser researched models of professional nursing practice which are based on general system theory are the following: Neuman's Health Care Systems Model (1974) and the Johnson Behavioral System Model (Grubbs, 1974; Johnson, 1968).

TABLE 19-1
COMPARISON OF LYDIA HALL'S AND FRANCES REITER'S
MODELS OF NURSING CARE

LYDIA HALL Hall, 1964)*		FRANCES REITER
"The Person"	Social Sciences Therapeutic Use of Self	"The Core"
"The Body"	Biologic and Natural Sciences Bodily Care	"The Care"
"The Disease"	Pathology and Therapeutic Sciences	"The Cure"

*Reprinted with permission from The Canadian Nurse, Vol. 60, No. 2.

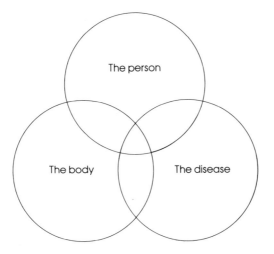

SOURCE: L. Hall, "Nursing: What is it?" The Canadian Nurse, Vol. 60, No. 2. Reprinted with permission.

FIGURE 19-4
SCHEMATIC DIAGRAM OF LYDIA HALL'S MODEL OF NURSING CARE

THE NURSING PROCESS

Definition

The nursing process is the scientific method of the nursing profession. It is the approach used to increase the effectiveness of nursing care based on the client's individual system. Grounded on scientific rather than intuitive nursing processes, it can be used continuously by a group; continuity of care is therefore implicit. As a system within itself, it is dynamic, since it moves and changes in response to the system within which it is applied. Moreover, the nursing process provides the framework upon which education of the future nurse is built.

Maintaining step with all variations of the scientific method of problem-solving processes, the nursing process is respectful of and applicable in any setting or system with any client regardless of the client's place on the health–illness continuum; the process can be interpreted within the construct of any theoretical framework of phenomenologic experience. The nursing process, plus effective actualization of the process, frames the entire profession of nursing: practice and education. It provides a strategy for individualized nursing care.

The term "nursing process" was initially coined by Hall (1955). Describing care on a scale of bad to good, four prepositions are designated in the nurse/client relationship. Moving from poor to very good, they are: nursing *at* the client, *to* the client, *for* the client, and *with* the client. The preposition *with* denotes higher processes than those prepositions preceding it. *With* implies being a part of the client's system and moving toward effective nurse/ client outcomes. The client is the leader of his or her system, and hence, also the leader in care.

Later in the fifties, Kreuter (1957) discussed the steps of the nursing process as we know them today, but did not label them as such. Coordination, planning, and evaluating nursing care were seen as promoting quality and professional practice. Johnson (1959) later included the need to assess, make decisions, and delineate actions.

Many subsequent nurse-authors have used variations on the theme in describing the nursing process. The intent remains similar. Orlando (1961) identifies three factors as the process: (1) client behavior; (2) nurse reaction; and (3) nursing actions. Knowles (1967) described nurse activity with five verbs starting with "D": discover, delve, decide, do, and discriminate. Three steps of nursing care are explicated by Orem (1971): (1) secure information from the client and make decisions regarding the need for nursing care; (2) design nursing actions and plan for delivery; and (3) control and evaluate care. Most recently, Yura and Walsh (1973) delineated the steps of the nursing process as assessment, planning, implementation, and evaluating nursing care. This author expands on these phases of the nursing process in Part I.

Summary of Components of the Nursing Process   Nursing process theories abound, but all are in essence comprised of the same elements. Let us review the phases of the nursing process as described in this book:

1. *Purpose.* This is the beginning phase—answering the questions: "Why am I doing this task?" and "What is the purpose of nursing care for the client and the client's environment?"
2. *Data Collection.* Involved in this phase are all known (surface) and surmised (underlying) facts and suppositions about the client. The health assessment, nursing history, medical history, and system analysis are included in data collection.
3. *Data Processing.* This phase provides the procedure for coordinating the pre-established responsibilities of professional nursing with the individual pieces of datum from the client. It is this point that facilitates individualization in client care.
4. *Nursing Diagnosis.* In response to the client's system, the areas of nursing responsibility, and data processing, the following question is posed: "In what areas does this client need assistance from me?" Your response develops the nursing diagnoses. Diagnoses are then ranked in priority in terms of their importance in a specific time and place.
5. *Nursing Orders/Plan of Action.* Priority diagnoses are then put into operation in terms of what must be done by the nurse with the client and the

client's system to accomplish the designated purpose of care. Specific steps are delineated for each diagnosis.

6. *Implementation.* This component involves either directly carrying out nursing orders or delegating them to other professional and/or technical nurses as the complexity of the intervention implies.
7. *Continuous Data Collection.*
8. *Continuous Evaluation.*
9. *Constant Feedback.*

Steps 7 through 9 are not sequential, as are those that precede. Evaluation of each nursing action by the nurse and client provides more data and the process flows with the additions, deletions, or alterations indicated—constantly. Feedback is received and given between all parts of the client's system; this is consistently evaluated and provides additional data. The nursing process is a dynamic process operating within and for open, dynamic systems.

The purpose of the nursing process is to use a definitive, scientific method in the delivery of quality, individualized nursing care.

SUMMARY

Chapter 19 discussed the conceptual framework of the nursing process, specifying general system theory as important and describing nursing theories that employ this approach. The nursing process has then been defined, including a discussion of its goals.

REFERENCES

American Nurses' Association's First Position on Education for Nursing. *American Journal of Nursing* 65:106-111, 1965.

Banathy, B. *Instructional systems.* Palo Alto, Calif: Fearon, 1968.

Grubbs, J. The Johnson behavioral systems model. In J. Riehl and C. Roy, *Conceptual models for nursing practice.* New York: Appleton-Century-Crofts, 1974.

Hall, L. Quality of nursing care. *Public Health News.* New Jersey: State Department of Health, June, 1955.

Hall, L. Nursing: What is it? *The Canadian Nurse* 60: 150-154, 1964.

Hersey, P., and Blanchard, K. *Management of organizational behavior: Utilizing human resources.* Englewood Cliffs, N.J.: Prentice-Hall, 1977.

Johnson, D. A philosophy of nursing. *Nursing Outlook* 7: 198-200, 1959.

Johnson, D. One conceptual model of nursing. Unpublished paper presented April 25, 1968, Vanderbilt University, Nashville, Tenn.

Knowles, L. *Decision-making in nursing: A necessity for doing.* New York: Appleton-Century-Crofts, 1967.

Kreuter, F. What is good nursing care? *Nursing Outlook* 57: 302–304, 1957.

Neuman, B. The Betty Neuman health-care systems model: A total person approach to patient problems. In J. Riehl and C. Roy, *Conceptual models for nursing practice.* New York: Appleton-Century-Crofts, 1974.

Orem, D. *Nursing: Concepts of practice.* New York: McGraw-Hill Books, Inc. 1971.

Orlando, I. *The dynamic nurse-patient relationship.* New York: G. P. Putnam's Sons, 1961.

Reiter, F. The nurse-clinician. *American Journal of Nursing* 66: 274–280, 1966.

Rogers, M. *An introduction to the theoretical basis of nursing.* Philadelphia: F. A. Davis, 1970.

Roy, Sister C. Rogers's theoretical bases of nursing. In J. Riehl and C. Roy, *Conceptual models for nursing practice.* New York: Appleton-Century-Crofts, 1974a.

Roy, Sister C. The Roy adaptation model. In J. Riehl and C. Roy, *Conceptual models for nursing practice.* New York: Appleton-Century-Crofts, 1974b.

von Bertalanffy, L. *General system theory.* New York: George Braziller Company, 1968.

Yura, H., and Walsh, M. *The nursing process: Assessing, planning, implementing, evaluating.* New York: Appleton-Century-Crofts, 1973.

SELECTED READINGS

Two selected readings follow: one studying the systems approach in professional nursing care; the other designating the components of the nursing process exemplified by a case analysis. Both are intended to amplify and reinforce the presentation by this author through other writers' perspectives.

Systems Analysis: A Logical Approach to Professional Nursing Care

Joyce Finch, R.N., M.S.

Every day nurses are called upon to make choices among possible nursing actions: Is the anxiety of a pre-operative patient within tolerable limits or does he need assistance? Is a newly diagnosed diabetic patient ready to learn about insulin administration yet? Because of nursing error the narcotic order has "run out" but the patient is in pain. What is to be done? For the care given to be truly professional, the nurse's decisions should be based on a prediction of the probable consequences of the alternative actions. Too often, however, the nurse's action is an automatic response to the situation or the result of a hunch, rather than one that is based on a rational, replicable judgment. A body of knowledge is, of course, the raw material for making sound judgments, but knowledge is of little value unless nurses know how to use it. Therefore, as nurses develop a nursing science, they should concurrently develop strategies for applying their knowledge in the care of patients.

Systems analysis is one possible resource for the development of a tool for decision-making. The faculty of the College of Nursing at Arizona State University has begun developing and testing a systems analysis approach to nursing care in connection with a major curriculum revision.

The curriculum-planning group identified two critical variables which would affect its decisions. First, the faculty's philosophical commitment required that the curriculum provide opportunities for the nursing student to learn to give patient-centered care. Second, the increase in knowledge relevant to nursing has been so rapid that to include all such knowledge in the curriculum is an impossibility. Therefore, the consensus was that the student should be provided with sufficient knowledge and skill to begin a professional career and with the competence needed to process the knowledge required for responsible decision-making.

The curriculum-planning group therefore sought an approach which would enable students to learn to focus on the patient rather than on the problem and which would enable graduates of the program to continue functioning at a high level in the future. A study of the reports by Howland and McDowell[1-3] on the use of systems engineering in hospital design and operation prompted the group to investigate the possibilities of systems analysis as an approach to the study of nursing.

Reprinted from *Nursing Forum*, Vol. 8, No. 2, with permission of Nursing Publications, Inc., 194–B Kinderkamack Road, Park Ridge, New Jersey.

In its simplest form a system is an entity "consisting of parts in interaction."[4] Systems analysis utilizes techniques that allow long-range planning and at the same time provides the means to update and maintain the current program. Techniques for evaluation of effectiveness are based upon the ongoing functioning of the program so that it can be altered to accommodate changing conditions and requirements. An example of a program that includes these techniques is SABRE, American Airlines' seat reservation system developed by the International Business Machines Corporation.[5] SABRE's long-range objective is continuous seat inventory since American Airlines must be in minute-to-minute control of reservations in order to keep seats filled at the minimum occupancy that marks the difference between profit and loss. In seconds a central computer console handles requests for reservations from interchanges along American's route and also keeps track of all related operations such as those having to do with meals, connecting reservations, and baggage. The specifications contain more than a million instructions which fill five thick volumes.

Systems analysis is based upon probability theory and concepts. Probability recognizes a random element of chance in events. Outcomes are uncertain since alternative approaches may occur. This uncertainty was expressed colloquially by President Johnson when he said, "I'll see you, God willin' and if the creeks don't rise." To predict the consequences of a decision, it is necessary to determine the relative likelihood of occurrence of each of the possible outcomes of that decision. "Mathematically, probability represents a proportion or relative frequency that specifies the degree of assurance that an event will occur."[6]

Systems analysis is particularly applicable to the study of complex problems. It involves an organization of data that is achieved by breaking a whole into its component parts in such a way that the relationships of these parts may be studied and manipulated. Example: Health care involves not only physicians, nurses, hospitals, machines, and techniques but also such diverse elements as the standard of living, the tax base, transportation, the support of mass communications, and even opinions of neighbors. Knowledge of the availability and value of health services may be outweighed by the relative difficulty of procuring these services; planning for health care, if it is to be successful, will have to include these less obvious variables. The logical relationships of such complex networks is called "organized complexity."[7]

A general systems theory is evolving "which can discuss the relationships of the empirical world."[8] This development has been stimulated by the rapid accumulation of knowledge and the resulting proliferation of specialization, which has necessitated the creation of a theoretical framework that enables one specialist to communicate with other specialists.

Systems can be closed or open. A closed system is one in which there is neither input nor output of information, materials, or energy from or to the environment. An open system is characterized by an exchange of energy in the form of information with the environment.[9] One way in which this exchange is accomplished is by feedback control mechanisms, whereby a part of the output of the system is fed back to the input in order to affect future outputs.

Example: A measurement of the response of a patient to nursing intervention is fed back into the system and thus influences the plan for continuing care. Feedback control mechanisms are present in those systems that are self-regulating, that is, goal-directed.

Open systems are governed by the principles of equifinality, which states, "The same final state may be reached with different initial conditions and in different ways."[10] Example: It is possible for a person to become an effective contributing member of his community in a number of ways. He may learn a trade or he may become a professional person. He may become a member of a charitable organization or he may be an active member of his political party. The best possible decision will be in part dependent on the person's understanding of the available approaches.

Systems tend to maintain a state of equilibrium. Cannon, who outlined a systems approach to the study of physiology, identified internal self-regulating mechanisms which operate to maintain the physiological equilibrium, or homeostasis, of the organism.[11] A consideration of only those mechanisms that regulate fluid balance will lead one to see that systems analysis is an extremely useful method of studying both multivariable causation and multiple alternatives to action.

The goal of equilibrium implies that systems, like other organisms, suffer from wear and tear of their own activities. The over-all goal of systems analysis is to intervene in this process of disorganization, or entropy.[12] Constraints, or those relationships which reduce alternatives, are useful in this intervention.[13] Example: A person who has had the choice of four routes to the office finds that the highway department has closed one route for repairs and the police department has closed a second route for an official parade, thus reducing the possible choices by one half.

Cybernetics and decision theory have contributed to systems theory. Cybernetics, the science of communication and control, assumes that a system is goal-directed and asks the question: What does it do? When a set of possibilities is identified the focus is redirected to the regulating mechanism operant in the particular instance.[14] Example: Roses have the capacity to bloom or refrain from blooming. What prevents them from blooming at certain times, and what prompts them to bloom at times? Florists apply an understanding of the relationships between light, temperature, humidity, and water so that we may have roses any day of the year.

Decision theory supplies a framework for identifying criteria to be used in "analyzing rational choices, within human organizations, based upon examination of a given situation and its possible outcomes."[15] Goodenough describes the need for decision theory when he states:

> . . . there is frequently more than one course of action that will gratify a want. Which is most effective depends on how it affects conditions pertaining to other wants that one happens to have at the same time. For this reason we must qualify our definition of a need. In any situation the need is for a course of action that will be of maximum effi-

cacy in relation to the gratification of all of one's wants. That is to say, for each want there is need for that one among the several possible means of gratifying it which will at the same time either maximally promote the gratification of other wants or minimally interfere with their continued gratification.[16]

Goodenough then describes how this process increases in complexity when the number of people is increased and the number of wants is multiplied.

General systems theory makes possible the development of models that are abstractions of the real world. The model identifies essential variables that can be manipulated for optimal problem solution and in this way provides an opportunity to simulate events that would not be feasible in an actual setting. The manned space program is an excellent example of development by simulation. Even if volunteers were foolhardy enough to offer their services, public opinion in an open society would not support the human wastage or the economic burden of trial-and-error testing of space vehicles. Models make it possible to compare the actual state with the ideal state; the consequences of the possible manipulations can then be predicted before a decision is reached. The process of selection of the best possible solution is called a "trade-off."

The simplest models are purely descriptive of the events occurring within a system. Analytical models explore alternatives that provide a logical basis for decision-making. The most sophisticated models are mathematical models developed for the purpose of predicting future outcomes.

The curriculum-planning group was intrigued by the possibilities of a systems approach to nursing care and decided to try to develop a nursing care system. In this undertaking the group has had the benefit of consultation from Dr. A. Alan B. Pritsker of the College of Engineering at Arizona State University.[17,18]

The outcome of the planning group's work was a descriptive model of professional nursing care which is based on the assumption that all nursing care is carried out through the nurse-patient relationship. The components of a nurse-patient relationship were identified as: (1) a patient who is in a state of disequilibrium that can be resolved by nursing care; (2) a nurse who is prepared to assist in the resolution of this state of disruption; and (3) the termination of the relationship when equilibrium is restored. As a group has become more knowledgeable in the use of systems it has, with Dr. Pritsker's assistance, worked gradually toward the development of an analytical model. *Figures 1 and 2* represent the current level of development of our system of professional nursing care.

The operational features of the model are as follows:

- The patient is defined as an individual or a group of individuals and is seen as entering the system with expectations of benefiting from nursing care.
- The model is conceptualized as an open system so that the nurse who seldom operates independently of other health personnel, may exchange information with other systems of health care.

- It is assumed that anyone can be trained to make observations and carry out nursing action; the professional nurse takes responsibility for assessment and decision analysis. Figure 1.
- The professional nurse makes two types of assessments. Operational assessments define the expectations of measurements related to the functional performance of the individual. Comparative assessments discriminate between measurements of an individual's current status and pre-set limits which have been established prior to the measurement.
- Strategic goals are defined as being concerned with over-all objectives of nursing care. Tactical goals are defined as being concerned with "what will help the patient feel better today."
- The patient exits from the system when the possible benefits have been derived; the nurse continues to work with the patient as long as movement toward the desired state is feasible.

When the components of the professional nursing care model (Figure 1) are visualized it becomes clear that a subsystem can be developed within each component (Figure 2). The next steps will probably be directed toward the further development and refinement of the subsystems. The ultimate objective is a mathematical model that can be used to predict outcomes accurately as well as to describe and analyze problems. Since such a model can be programmed for computers, simulated nursing problems can be worked out before the nursing student goes into an actual nurse-patient setting. The problem is to define clearly what the nurse is expected to achieve; the actual programming is then relatively simple.

The strategies dictated by the professional nursing care model constitute a basic feature of the revised curriculum. Learning experiences have been organized in two patterns. The students are given assignments concerned with general systems theory concurrent with assignments concerned with components of the nursing care system. Some of the students master the basic

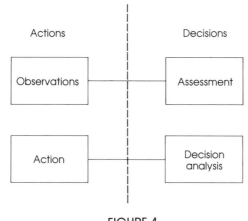

FIGURE 1
PROFESSIONAL NURSING CARE SYSTEM

concepts of systems before proceeding with the components of the nursing care model. Others work in reverse order. The student is thus allowed a degree of freedom in the selection of a learning method best suited to individual accomplishment. At succeeding levels of learning, students are given assignments in systems analysis of increasing complexity.

Final evaluation of the professional nursing care model will depend on a comprehensive evaluation of all curriculum revisions. In the meantime, current observations indicate a favorable reaction to this tool for decision-making from students and faculty alike.

The planning group has identified a number of positive values in the professional nursing care system:

- Primary focus upon the patient is maintained throughout the process.
- The plan of nursing can be altered to accommodate the changing condition and requirements of the patient, since continuous evaluation of patient responses to nursing intervention through feedback control is an integral part of the process.
- When problems in decision-making occur, the feedback control mechanism facilitates location of the point of departure from the process.
- The vocabulary of systems analysis transfers readily across the disciplinary lines. This increases the probability of accurate interpretation of the nursing care process by others.

After a year of experience with the revised curriculum, our junior students have learned to use the vocabulary of systems with confidence and are able to describe their activities meaningfully to others. They have acquired skill in looking critically at their own performance to determine where they need to focus their attention: they may need further data; their observations may have been inadequate or inaccurate; their knowledge of normal and pathological states may be faulty or inadequate; or they may have to reconsider their assessment in regard to personal bias or in relation to the ordering of the data. The ability to withhold judgement until needed data are accumulated and ordered is acquired more slowly, but learning is enhanced as students recognize their maturation in this area. Example: A student became concerned about the quality of nursing care that she had given in a single three-hour experience with an elderly lady with a handicapping chest condition. She reported, "I didn't have an opportunity to see the patient before I took care of her. I knew her diagnosis and I had studied the pathological aspects and nursing care the night before I saw her, but I didn't know anything about her as an individual. After I had taken care of her I knew she felt better, for she was no longer in respiratory distress but was relaxed and comfortable. But I still did not know what it all meant to her." In a discussion about her reaction to this situation the student was able to recognize that she was attempting to make long-range goals operational in a situation in which only short-term goals were feasible. In a subsequent discussion the student said that as she had reflected upon the nurse-patient interaction she had learned much more about the patient than she had believed possible in such a short interval.

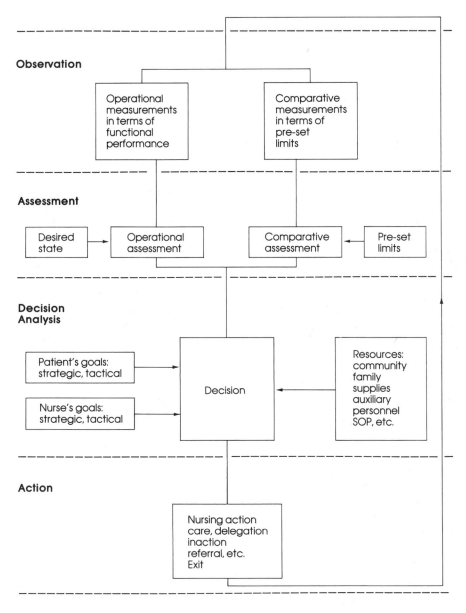

FIGURE 2
SYSTEM OF PROFESSIONAL NURSING CARE

Nurses who would have confidence in their ability to evaluate their environment would appear to have a higher probability of success in acquiring knowledge and skills requisite to rational decision-making than do those who lack this self-confidence. Example: To test the effectiveness of the curriculum with respect to the integration of public health nursing content in the other courses, the NLN Achievement Test in this area was given to the junior students, who had not yet had the course in public health nursing. One student reported, "It wasn't too bad. Of course I didn't know a lot of the answers, but I discovered that many questions were asking for either observation or assessment and I could do that."

On the negative side, the precision of observation and communication dictated by the systems approach can be extremely frustrating if the necessity for sharpening skills is identified when the means of doing so are not clear. This problem has been a recurrent one in those situations in which the content was subjective and difficult to measure. The dynamic nature of the system has also caused problems to instructors and students who have been conditioned to traditional problem-solving methods. One student expressed the feelings of many when she said, "Just once I'd like to go to bed knowing that tomorrow I can get up without something still waiting to be finished." Upon reflection, the planning group has concluded that this on-goingness is one of the elements of the nursing program that is most representative of the real world.

Although the professional nursing care system model was developed as a learning tool for students, expectations are that further development will lead to a tool for the accurate measurement of nursing care in any setting. Through the use of this tool, the nurse will be able to predict the consequences of her behavior in the nurse-patient relationship and thus to make decisions in the best interests of the patient.

The use of systems analysis also has potential for facilitating the development of a science of nursing. Basically the problem in such development is to identify what is unknown about nursing care rather than what is known. Systems seem to hold promise of the ability to identify gaps in nursing knowledge which have so far eluded professional nurses.

In all efforts to develop and use systems in nursing, we must not lose sight of the fact that systems analysis is only a tool. Wiener has cautioned against the dehumanizing characteristics of systems; it is possible for the system to become more important than the persons involved.[19] The nurse's commitment will continue to be that aspect of good nursing care that cannot be programed into any system.

REFERENCES

1. Howland, Daniel, "Approaches to the Systems Problem," *Nursing Research,* Vol. 12, No. 3, Summer 1963, pp. 172–174.

2. Howland, Daniel, "A Hospital Systems Model," *Nursing Research,* Vol. 12, No. 4, Fall 1963, pp. 232–236.

3. Howland, Daniel and Wanda McDowell, "The Measurement of Patient Care: A Conceptual Framework," *Nursing Research,* Vol. 13, No. 1, Winter 1964, pp. 4–7.

4. von Bertalanffy, Ludwig, *General System Theory,* New York: George Braziller, Inc., 1968, p. 19.

5. Burck, Gilbert, *The Computer Age and Its Potential for Management*, New York: Harper & Row, Publishers, Inc., 1965, pp. 31–34.

6. Armore, Sidney J., *Introduction to Statistical Analysis and Inference for Psychology and Education*, New York: John Wiley & Sons, Inc., 1966, pp. 187–197.

7. Rapoport, Anatol and William J. Horvath, "Thoughts on Organization Theory," *Modern Systems Research for the Behavioral Scientist*, Walter Buckley, Editor, Chicago: Aldine Publishing Co., 1968, pp. 71–75.

8. Boulding, Kenneth E., "General Systems Theory—The Skeleton of Science," *Modern Systems Research for the Behavioral Scientist*, Walter Buckley, Editor, Chicago: Aldine Publishing Co., 1968, pp. 3–10.

9. Hall, A. D. and R. E. Fagan, "Definition of System," *Modern Systems Research for the Behavioral Scientist*, Walter Buckley. Editor, Chicago: Aldine Publishing Co., 1968, pp. 81–92.

10. von Bertalanffy, *op. cit.*, p. 40.

11. Cannon, Walter B., *The Wisdom of the Body*, New York: W. W. Norton & Co., Inc., 1932.

12. Wiener, Norbert, *The Human Use of Human Beings: Cybernetics and Society*, New York: Doubleday & Company, 1950, p. 12.

13. Ashby, W. Ross, *An Introduction to Cybernetics*, New York: John Wiley & Sons, Inc., 1956, p. 127.

14. *Ibid*, pp. 1–6.

15. von Bertalanffy, Ludwig, "General System Theory—A Critical Review," *Modern Systems Research for the Behavioral Scientist*, Walter Buckley, Editor, Chicago: Aldine Publishing Co., 1968, pp. 11–30.

16. Goodenough, Ward Hunt, *Cooperation in Change*, New York: John Wiley & Sons, Inc., 1963, p. 55.

17. Pritsker, A. A. B., GERT: Graphical Evaluation and Review Techniques, Santa Monica, The Rand Corporation, 1966.

18. Pritsker, A. A. B., The Formulation of Automatic Checkout Techniques, Batelle Memorial Institute, Technical Documentary Report #ASD–TDR–62–291, 1962.

19. Wiener, *op. cit.*, pp. 187–193.

Components of
the Nursing Process

Virginia Kohlman Carrieri, M.S.

Judith Sitzman, M.S.

Nursing care is a continuous process. It must have coordination of parts without interruption or cessation. It must be set in motion and progress toward the integration of the whole individual or his highest achievable level of wellness. To achieve these goals patient care must be deliberate, systematic, and individualized through the use of the nursing process.

Many theoretical frameworks could be used to examine process as a concept. Parker defines process as "that intellectual scheme whereby relationships are put together." According to Parker, this encompasses the procedures of analysis, synthesis, and reduction to practice. Analysis involves the accumulation of, the classification of, and the distinction between differences in data. Synthesis includes establishing relationships between data, deriving trends, performing deductive and inductive analysis, and creating operational devices. Reduction to practice involves operational devices used on particular occasions in specific settings and testing for the effectiveness and validity of the operational devices.[1]

These concepts and additional resources have been used by various workers to outline the unique elements of the nursing process.[3,4,5] These elements have often been identified as: observation, inference, validation, assessment, action, and evaluation.

This model of the nursing process was deliberately utilized by the present authors while caring for patients undergoing cardiac valve replacements. The process was initiated when data regarding a patient were obtained through interaction with the patient, from other health team members, or from patient records. Relationships with these patients usually began one week prior to surgery and were maintained until discharge.

OBSERVATION

The first step of the process, observation, is defined for this investigation as a deliberate search for relevant data about a patient with concurrent assignment of meaning to these data in light of the nurse's frame of reference.

Reprinted from *Nursing Clinics of North America*, Vol. 6, No. 1, with permission from W. B. Saunders Company.

It is realized that all observations are influenced by the nurse's previous experiences; however, what makes her observations scientific is the deliberateness and special care with which she makes reliable observations. The nurse is aware that observation is constantly subject to error and can be influenced by all past theoretical and experiential knowledge.

Kaplan contrasts scientific observation with casual everyday observations: "Observation is purposive behavior, directed toward ends that lie beyond the act of observation itself: the aim is to secure materials that will play a part in other phases of inquiry, like the formation and validation of hypotheses."[2]

Observation demanded the building of a trust relationship with the patient so that he felt free to verbalize all of his concerns. This relationship facilitated the collection of a wider range of observations about the physical and psychosocial status of the patient. Only through accumulation of significant information is the nurse able to progress beyond the first step of the process toward an accurate diagnosis and plan of care.

The authors utilized both a nursing history form and a nursing diagnosis as the format for instituting the processs, recording their findings, and retrieving information about the patient. All observations were categorized and coded using the following nursing history form unique to this report.

NURSING HISTORY FORM

Character of Information
1. Personal data, i.e., age, religion, marital status, etc.
2. Socio-economic and cultural influences
3. Concept or perception of self
4. Physiologic status
5. Adaptation to illness
   a. Current illness and life pattern of illness
   b. Hospital setting or health team
6. Understanding of treatments and procedures during hospitalization
7. Specific fears, i.e., fear of death, procedures, etc.

Source of Information
A. Observation or communication with the patient
B. Review of medical record
C. Communication with health team
D. Communication with significant others

Examples of selected observations and appropriate coding regarding one cardiac surgical patient are listed herewith:

Coding	Observations
(1B)	White male, 37, Protestant, divorced 3 years ago
(1B)	3 children with wife, many unskilled jobs

(4B)   Aortic stenosis, penicillin allergy, only sx "SOB"
(6A)   "All I know is they cut you open and sew you back together again"
(5aA)   "I came here for heart surgery, but they've had their fingers in
            everything I have"
(5bA)   "They're not going to throw something in my face and make me
            sign it"
(5aA)   "I've been having too much fun for the last 4 years to lie in bed for
            surgery"
(5A)   Moving constantly in bed
(1A)   Smoking frequently
(4A)   Skin color gray-white

These are examples of the significant information obtained during one interaction with a patient which had relevance for deliberate planning of nursing care, since they are clues about the patient as an individual. These are only a few of the many observations obtained during each interview with cardiac patients during the investigation of this interpersonal process.

INFERENCE

After coding all observations, the nurse initiated the second step in the process, that of inference. Inference is defined for purposes of this report as an interpretation of patient verbalization and behavior based on the nurse's prior theoretical knowledge of the type of problem with which the patient is confronted. The nurse infers, usually without sufficient data, that a certain type of problem exists for the patient. An awareness on the nurse's part that she is using the inference process, with its reliance on intuition as well as theoretical knowledge, in making decisions about the nature of her patient's problems should be a caution to her that she may, in fact, be functioning without sufficient data, and thus lead her to seek additional information before acting on the problem as she first perceives it.

The following are exemplary observations and inferences taken from a lengthy list of patterns of observations received each day throughout one patient's hospitalization.

Observations	Inferences
Preop. Day #2	
"The only thing I hated was that tube down my nose— scared me to death"	Fear of suctioning Fear of nasogastric tube
Postop. Day #1	
"Froze all night, all I could think of was let me die warm"	Hypothermia mattress may be too high Fear of death

Observations	Inferences
Rapid, shallow breathing. Rate 32/min. Flushed skin, restless	Atelectasis, consolidation, drug reaction

Postop. Day #4
"I thought I was going to die or faint, all I could see was my open chest on that pissy floor"

"Now that I've gotten over the operation. I'll probably die of pneumonia"

Fear of death
Fear of pain
Fear of body mutilation

"My heart went all to pieces, guess I'm coming all unglued"

Postop. Day #7
"Why don't they give me pain medication before the machine?"

Pain

"Now I know what pain is, it couldn't be worse"

"All I can do is say, buddy, I'm here...sometimes I don't think they know it's you"

Hostility toward staff
Impersonalization by staff

"I came here for heart surgery but they've had their fingers in everything I have"

Mistrust and resentment of staff

Postop. Day #8
"My heart beats faster and makes more noise than it did before surgery"

Postoperative expectations of self not being met

"I'm worse than before, weak as a cat, I'd rather give them their valve back and take mine; it was better"

VALIDATION

After the nurse formulated inferences as to the possibility of existing patient problems, she entered the third step of the nursing process, validation. Validation is defined as the corroboration of the patient's definition with that of the nurse's, and, when a discrepancy between the two occurs, attaining mutual agreement.

Agreement regarding definition of the problem can be achieved by various methods. If possible, verbal exploration of the situation with the patient should confirm the nurse's definition of the problem or necessitate its reformulation. The following exchange illustrates this method.

> Patient discussing previous surgery: "The only thing I hated was that tube down my nose...scared me to death"

Based on the nurse's knowledge of the patient's previous appendectomy she inferred that he feared the nasogastric tube.

> Nurse validating: "You're scared to death of which tube? The one put down your nose to make you cough or the tube which was inserted through your nose into your stomach for drainage?"
> Patient response: "The one in my stomach that they put cold water down"

Thus, the patient confirmed the fact that in this case the nurse's definition and his own were the same. Further "hunches" explored by the authors were those based on their significance in terms of identification of patient problems.

If the problem cannot be confirmed verbally with the patient, the nurse has at her command alternate methods of identifying potential patient problems. Using all of her senses, available diagnostic tools, and/or actions on behalf of the patient, she indirectly validates her inferences.

For example, the authors observed that on the first postoperative day the patient had rapid, shallow respirations (32/min.), was restless, and had flushed skin. The following inferences were made; fever, atelectasis, consolidation, or possible drug reaction.

Nurse Validating
1. Felt skin for temperature and took temperature
2. Observed chest expansion, percussed chest, and used stethoscope to listen for quality and distribution of breath sounds
3. Observed amount and character of sputum
4. Examined chest films with M.D.
5. Checked laboratory reports for lowered arterial Po_2

Through several sources the authors were able to confirm their inference that the patient had developed right lower lobe atelectasis.

ASSESSMENT

Validation of patient problems allows the nurse to direct her attention toward assessment, the fourth component of the nursing process. The authors used assessment and the concept of nursing diagnosis interchangeably. Both of these steps were defined as relating knowledge to patient problems and determining central problems, which led to the development of alternative mitigating actions.

Peplau has summarized some of the steps involved in the process of assessment. Thought processes might include: sorting and classifying, comparing, applying concepts and relationships, and summarizing or synthesizing data.[6] Review of the literature also indicates many suggestions for categories to be used in assessing data or making a nursing diagnosis.[3,7,8]

However, the authors chose to code daily patient observations using the categories described above in the nursing history form. Inferences were made from these observations and were subsequently recorded. Based on frequency and importance, only certain validated inferences were recognized as central problems, and functioned as the assessment or nursing diagnosis. Just as the physician's diagnosis may change, the nurse's diagnosis also may vary from day to day or minute to minute. As the nurse's understanding and knowledge of the patient increases and as the patient presents new problems, the diagnosis should be revised accordingly.

A deliberative approach to diagnosis leads the nurse to decisionmaking and priority-setting in the assessment of patient needs. The process enables formulation of nursing actions with a greater probability of success because more valid and comprehensive data are received.

The authors have included below one example of a preoperative nursing assessment or diagnosis. This assessment was formed by collecting many observations and inferences, similar to those shown above, during several interactions with the patient, family, or health team. Those validated inferences that demonstrated a pattern of frequency and importance were then established as the nursing diagnosis from which a plan of care was formulated.

ACTION

Nursing action, the next step in the process, is defined as the testing of alternatives and the carrying out of those considered the most suitable. The appropriate alternative actions chosen by the authors are listed below with the nursing diagnosis to illustrate these two steps in the process.

Nursing Diagnosis
1. Decreased energy with dypsnea on exertion.
2. Possible reaction to antibiotics and other medications.
3. Apparent anxiety and need for tension release.
4. Need for knowledge of procedures as they relate to self.
5. Possible low self-esteem and low masculine self-image.
6. Possible denial of illness leading to self-destruction.
7. Fear of losing body intactness and death.
8. Unstable social environment.

Alternative Nursing Actions
1. Help patient to understand physical limitations prior to surgery in order to conserve energy; attempt to decrease environmental stressors.
2. Alert staff about possible drug reactions; observe for these reactions.

3. Assist patient to cope with illness by listening, focusing on what concerns him, and involving him in simple ward activities.
4. Investigate the patient's perception of the medical and nursing treatments in relation to himself; after investigation focus teaching on actual danger threats perceivd by patient.
5a. Collect further data to validate low male identity.
5b. Allow patient to control his environment whenever possible.
5c. Involve patient in decision-making.
6a. Collect data to validate diagnosis of denial of illness and self-destructive behavior.
6b. Assist patient to develop a more realistic perception of postoperative self by focusing on realistic outcome of surgery.
6c. Help patient to gain understanding of rationale for M.D. order to stop smoking.
7a. Recognize nurse's behavior which may interfere with patient's ability to verbalize feelings about death.
7b. Listen for clues indicating patient's desire to express feelings about death.
8a. Collect more data to validate patient's life style and pattern of illness.
8b. Seek consultation from social worker and chaplain.

Nursing actions or interventions are in part dependent upon the nurse's theory of nursing. Such actions should encompass all activities from counseling and teaching to physical care and delegated medical therapy. Another important facet with which the nurse must concern herself is the priority of intervention. Although may factors beyond the scope of this report are significant, the patient's priority of needs primarily determines the type, level, and speed of intervention. Certainly, in particular patient situations, the nurse may need to act or intervene immediately after rapidly moving through the first steps of the process.

EVALUATION

The final step of these operational processes is that of evaluation. Evaluation is defined as a continuous process through which appraisal of the effectiveness of the previous steps in meeting the patient's needs is provided. Observation of patient behavior, communication with the patient, his family, and health team members, and diagnostic measurements were used to evaluate each step in the process and the total process. Because patient and nursing goals had been clearly defined, the authors were better able to determine the degree to which these goals had been achieved.

The following patient situations are presented to illustrate the process of evaluation. Previous steps in the process have been included in an attempt to describe more clearly the flow and developing nursing process for the reader.

Patient Situation I
Postop. Day #2
  Observations:
    Flushed skin color, elevated temp., restless
    Rapid, shallow respirations, rate 32/min.
    Greater expansion of left chest than right
    Region of right lower lobe dull to percussion with diminished breath
      sounds
    Decreased sputum in last 24 hours
  Inferences:
    Possible atelectasis or drug reaction
  Validated Inference:
    Chest film and M.D. physical examination confirmed right lower
      lobe atelectasis
  Nursing Assessment/Diagnosis:
    Right Lower Lobe Atelectasis
  Nursing Actions:
    1. Frequent change of position
    2. Support incision during frequent deep breathing and coughing,
       clapping and vibrating, reemphasize need for all procedures
    3. Contact physical therapist for chest therapy
    4. Administer IPPB with bronchodilator as ordered
    5. Observe for changes in expansion, rate, and breath sounds
    6. Observe laboratory reports of blood gases for possible changes in acid-
       base balance, hypoxia
    7. Force fluids
Postop. Day #5
  Nurse Evaluation:
    Chest film confirmed cessation of atelectatic process
    Blood gases within normal limits

Patient Situation II
Postop. Days #8, 9
  Observations:
    "All I can do is say, buddy, I'm here . . . sometimes I don't think they know
      it's you."
    "They're not going to throw something in my face and make me sign it
      again."
    "That doctor is like a bull in a china shop."
  Inference:
    Impersonalization of patient by staff
  Validated Inference:
    Patient was asked his impressions of the health team, to which he replied,
      "They treat you like a guinea pig around here, sometimes I don't think
        they know it's you."

Nursing Assessment/Diagnosis:
Impersonalization by staff
Nursing Actions:
Discuss ways of personalizing care with nursing and medical staff.
1. Patient decision-making whenever possible
2. Possibility of one staff member caring for patient
3. Explain rationale for procedures before acting
4. Allow patient to express hostility
Postop. Day #13
  Nurse Evaluation:
    1. Patient's decreased frequency of negative comments about staff
    2. Also increased positive clues, such as:
       "Dr. B. didn't yank out those stitches so hard today."
       "Oh, I know that, Miss J. told me all about that pill this morning."

CONCLUSIONS

The authors formulated the following conclusions while putting this process into operation. The daily recording of all observations, inferences, diagnoses, actions, and evaluations in horizontal sequence within one notebook assisted the authors and the staff to see definite patterns of patient behavior and subsequent nursing actions for this group of patients. This method of recording and coding data also was practical, time-conserving, easy to use, and could actually be implemented in the patient setting.

It is apparent that this process requires the use of both theory and expert clinical practice in order that valid nursing actions can be derived and evaluated for effectiveness.

Continuity of care was necessarily increased as nurses gained an understanding of the process through discussions and care conferences. With increased knowledge of the process and recording designs they assisted the authors in establishing nursing histories, diagnoses, alternate actions, and evaluations. With such assistance a wider range of patient problems was identified and a unified plan of care achieved. Care plans were transferred with patients as they moved from preoperative to postoperative settings. These plans were easily communicated to other health team members and community agencies.

A trust relationship with the patient was the cornerstone of this process. The accumulation of data would have been impossible if the authors had not conveyed interest and concern, and used all their abilities to form relationships that became therapeutic catalysts.

One of the most important findings was that patients evaluated this process favorably. They expressed opinions that knowledge of procedures and potential danger threats, exposure to the intensive care unit preoperatively, and identification with one nurse throughout their hospitalization helped them to understand and anticipate events during hospitalization. Anxiety appeared to be reduced, and postoperative expectations seemed more realistic.

In conclusion, a more scientific approach to the nursing process has enabled the investigators to identify a wider range of patient problems, to apply theoretical knowledge toward the solution of identified patient needs, and to define a rationale for nursing action which has a higher probability of success. It is the authors' opinion that the use of this nursing process would help to increase understanding of individual patient problems and give insight into patterns of behavior to be used for future prediction.

REFERENCES

1. Parker, C. J., and Rubin, L. J.: Process as Content: Curriculum Design and the Application of Knowledge. Chicago, Rand McNally & Co., 1966.

2. Kaplan, Abraham: The Conduct of Inquiry: Methodology for Behavioral Science. San Francisco, Chandler Publishing Co., 1964, p. 127.

3. Lewis, L., Carozza, V., Carroll, M., Darragh, R., Patrick, M., and Schadt, E.: Defining Clinical Content Graduate Nursing Programs: Medical-Surgical Nursing. Colorado, Western Interstate Commission for Higher Education, 1967.

4. Wiedenbach, Ernestine: Clinical Nursing—A Helping Art. New York, Springer Publishing Co., 1964.

5. Orlando, Ida Jean: The Dynamic Nurse-Patient Relationship. New York, G. P. Putnam's Sons, 1961.

6. Peplau, Hildegard, E.: Process and Concept Learning. In Burd, Shirley, and Marshall, Margaret A., Eds.: Some Clinical Approaches to Psychiatric Nursing. New York, The Macmillan Co., 1963, pp. 333–336.

7. McCain, R. Faye: Nursing by assessment—not intuition. Am. J. Nursing, 65:82–84, April, 1965.

8. Little, Dolores E., and Carnevali, Doris L.: Nursing Care Planning. Philadelphia, J. B. Lippincott Co., 1969.

20

The Humanistic Approach
in Learning and
Nursing Practice

Part V has studied nursing as a helping profession, discussing the dimensions of helping according to those researchers in the area of counseling psychology. The theoretical framework of general system theory encompassing the nursing process was discussed in Chapter 19. Models of nursing care developed by various theorists focusing on the systems approach were presented. The definition of the nursing process concluded that chapter.

Chapter 20 is devoted to an added dimension, the humanistic approach to the nursing process; that, is, the humanistic approach in both practicing and learning the process. The conceptual framework for humanistic education begins the chapter discussion followed by a theoretical model which is the foundation of all the concepts presented in each chapter of this book.

THE CONCEPTUAL FRAMEWORK

It is important to remember that the nursing process involves a constant state of learning, whether in simply learning nursing techniques, or in learning about a particular client in order to provide care. The conceptual framework for this humanistic education focuses primarily on attitudinal development and then on behavioral manifestations in practice. Attitudes pervade all aspects of self: thoughts and feelings, values, experiences, desires, behaviors, and one's own body. The learner's belief systems become the core of the educational process (Combs, 1972). Attitudes are then developed and consonant behaviors follow. Rogers (1967a) has synthesized from research findings (Aspy, 1965; Barrett-Linnard, 1962; Emmerling, 1961; Schmuck, 1963, 1966) that attitudinal development as the primary focus in a learning process effectively facilitates deeper learning with self-understanding, and is a characteristic of practitioners who are regarded as effective. Recognizing the significance of research findings, it becomes necessary to explore attitudinal development.

Attitudes as Determinants of Behavior

Definition of Attitude A general characteristic of an attitude is one's tendency to evaluate an object in a certain way (Katz and Stotland, 1959). This definition was elucidated earlier by Campbell (1947) when he described a social attitude as a syndrome of response consistency towards social objects. Perceptual sets (see Chapter 7) formulated in past experience is another dimension added by Asch (1948, 1952). Yet all of these definitions include an essential similarity: an attitude is a posture toward an object or person within an individual's mind, leading to behavior.

Attitudinal Structure Social psychologists break down attitudes into three highly correlated aspects: affective, cognitive, and behavioral (Katz and Stotland, 1959). Lott (1973) viewed the *affective* facet as relating to the dichotomous feelings of good/bad, like/dislike, approach/avoidance, etc. He stated that the affective aspect of attitudes was seen by many theorists as providing the motivational energy for behavior.

The *cognitive* dimension is useful in determining the information and beliefs about an object or person (Katz and Stotland, 1959) and was seen by Osgood (1962) and Osgood, Suci, and Tannenbaum (1957) as having evaluative dimensions. This implies there is no neutrality in cognition and thereby couples the cognitive and affective aspects.

The third aspect of attitudinal structure is termed *behavioral* or action and is seen as the predisposed response to a certain stimulus (Lott, 1973). The strength of this aspect directly relates to elicited responses (Lott, 1973). It can be concluded at this point that attitudes have a positive relationship with behavior.

Hersey and Blanchard (1977) simplify attitudinal structure by saying that behavior is a function of motives and goals. Motives are defined as needs, wants, desires, and unconscious and/or conscious beliefs within an individual; goals are seen as external factors influencing the individual and, among others, include incentives, responsibilities, anticipated results, or behavioral outcomes. Both combine to yield behavior (Hersey and Blanchard, 1977).

Since it becomes evident that attitudes are responsible for behavior as well as behavioral intent, positive attitudinal development toward nursing care becomes paramount; this positive attitude is integrated with knowledge and experience. If clear understanding and positive attitudes are not developed, the negative ramifications will extend throughout one's nursing career: it is the seed from which all grows. Moreover, since negative experience requires extra effort to first neutralize and then relearn (Carkhuff, 1969c) it becomes paramount that initial contact with the nursing process be positive and firmly based in individual belief systems. This will provide the opportunity to truly learn and know, to integrate the foundations of nursing practice with personal meaning and individual experience.

The Existential Base

Attitudes have been described as being composed of an individual's beliefs, values, response sets, and perceptions about an object, person or process. These, plus motives, lead to behavior. For a nurse's behavior to be based on positive attitudes paralleled with an awareness of what must be accomplished in helping, education must focus on both dimensions. The awareness of requirements for helping is usually developed in educational systems and practice experience in nursing. The high correlation of attitudes to behavior mandates that attitudes be equally studied. Attitudinal development involves primary focus on internal processes of the learner: it involves *knowing* rather than *knowing about;* it includes understanding self.

The conceptual model used by the author for facilitating knowing in a learner is existentially based. One knows only because one experiences and is so aware—uniquely. This concept is crystallized in the words of Axline (1964, p. 20) in which she states, "Even though we do not have the wisdom to enumerate the reasons for the behavior of another person, we can grant that every individual does have his private world of meaning, conceived out of the integrity and dignity of his personality."

Grounded on the position that every human being is a unique entity, it becomes possible to visualize the differences among people's thoughts, interpretations, and beliefs. Pain/pleasure, harmony/dissonance, and beauty/ugliness then become real when one explores one's own feelings and thoughts regarding an object, person, or process. Weisman (1965) has said that all persons regard themselves as a unique, significant entity. Thoughts and feelings are valid and cannot be excused as prejudice or preference—thoughts and feelings are reality, valuable only to the individual (Weisman, 1965).

Existentialism is the philosophy that provides the foundation for a humanistic approach to learning and using the nursing process. Existentialism describes an attitude and an approach to human beings. It is concerned with human longing and man's search for importance within self. Beck (1963) views the existential philosophy as that which emphasizes the view of reality that is most meaningful to a person—the person's own existence and being. Camus (1946, 1955, 1956, 1972) has written extensively on the aspect of being, pointing out three corollaries (1955). The first is that we can understand another human being only as we see what that human is moving towards, what that person is becoming; we can understand ourselves only as we project our potentialities into action.

The second aspect of *being*, according to Camus (1955), is that it is not an inherent given. In other words, being does not unfold automatically as the flower from a seed, but it can be forfeited or sloughed off. Self-consciousness is an inseparable element from the human being; humans are the particular beings who must become aware of themselves if they are to become themselves.

The third distinctive aspect described by Camus (1955) is that humans are the beings who know that at some future moment they will not be; in effect, the person is in relation with non-being—death. If one is to grasp what it means to exist, one must confront the fact that at any moment one may cease to exist and that death will inescapably arrive at some moment in the future. With this awareness of non-being, however, existence takes on vitality and immediacy, and the individual experiences a heightened consciousness of self, the world, and others at the same time.

Harper (1959) states that in existential therapy, emphasis is placed on the importance of the individual's goals and values with attention directed towards understanding an individual's personal world and carousel of values. Existentialists analyze the meaning structure of each person's unique world of values by consciously attempting to strip themselves of preconceived notions about the nature and values of man-at-large.

Existentialism Applied to Nursing It has been shown that attitudes relate positively to behavior; therefore, *one's beliefs about the nursing process will affect practice.* Referring back to the question of how to develop positive attitudinal development in nurses, and integrating the described conceptual framework, the following conclusions can be synthesized. A nurse must be aware of personal experience in relation to the nursing process, recognize this as valid and true, and respond to clients in concert with the individual reality of both oneself and the client. The objective is to have motives and goals in harmony with elicited behavior.

The conceptual framework has discussed the underlying philosophy of humanistic education: individuality and self-knowledge as the basis in learning. This has been portrayed by La Monica and Parisi (1975) in the PELLEM Pentagram (Figure 20-1).

PELLEM Pentagram

The PELLEM Pentagram (named for its originators Elaine L. La Monica and Eunice M. Parisi) is a model of self, comprised of five interrelated yet separate, composite parts. These are:

1. Thoughts, Feelings
2. Philosophy, Values
3. Desires
4. Behaviors
5. Experiences

It is symbolized by a five-pointed star as shown in Figure 20-1. Each point represents one aspect of self. These aspects merge in the center to form the total self. Represented by a circular line running through each point is the body.

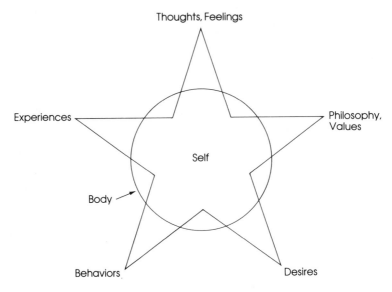

Thoughts, Feelings

Experiences

Philosophy, Values

Self

Body

Behaviors

Desires

SOURCE: La Monica and Parisi (1975).

FIGURE 20-1
PELLEM Pentagram

It is symbolized in this way because of the interrelating effect of the body on how and what one experiences, feels, thinks, and behaves.

The points of the model represent what is thought by theorists to be operating within a person's total experience. An individual's body is the vehicle for self-expression and, therefore, crosses all facets of the pentagram; it is one's language. Self, signified by the center of the model, is the blending of all.

Absent from the model is the influence of psychic powers and mystical phenomena that may play a part. To date, their influence is undetermined and indeed looked upon by many "concrete scientists" as superstitions or at best unknowns. These energies are neither denied nor claimed as fact.

The self is studied holistically. It is the interplay of all parts that produces the unique phenomenon of the individual. Likewise, it is all the components acting in unison that provide the reasons for experience at any given moment. To deny the importance of any one of these parts is to deny an important aspect of our being.

This model provides a simple way to view the complexities of a person. It stems from a personal and professional struggle to know, understand, and be self-directive. In analyzing why people are perceived in certain positions with observable feelings, the areas of the PELLEM Pentagram should be explored. When these are studied, problem areas and actions seem to fall into place. A feeling of more fully knowing oneself can lead to self-acceptance concurrent with self-worth even though the life process usually prohibits ultimate truth. Ultimate truth exists only if the knowing process occurs in an atmosphere of complete safety and trust.

Use of the model in learning the nursing process becomes important because the process is the professional guideline for *all* nursing practice. The nurse who is aware of the complex nature of self is also likely to be aware of the complexities of the client, thus leading to care based on the whole person.

Actualizing the humanistic approach becomes the next step. Humanism refers to anything that involves thought and human ideals. Therefore, humanism refers to the process of learning as well as the affective part of learning in particular. Equally important in dealing with the whole person are the cognitive and psychomotor aspects of learning. In this book, the theory of the nursing process is provided as well as guidelines for utilizing the humanistic approach in learning the psychomotor skills necessary to implement the process; concurrently, this book provides guidelines for exploring and developing affective attitudes. A dynamic, personal learning experience is necessary in learning and utilizing the nursing process; it is accomplished by human relations education.

The Human Relations Educational Mode in Attitudinal Development

Looking at the history of the human relations model, Matarazzo (1965) reviewed counseling and psychotherapeutic processes and concluded that the group helping process was a self-taught art with few guiding principles. There were controversies between practitioners who concentrated upon the individual helpee within the group, those who fixed upon interpersonal relationships within the group, and others who gave chief attention to the interaction between the group and the individual, with no definite conclusions being reached. Out of the traditional model of group psychotherapy, there developed a number of experiential types. For example: growth groups (Gazda, Asbury, Balzer, Childers, Desselle, Walters, 1973; Lubin and Lubin, 1967), encounter and marathon groups (Bach, 1966; Moustakas, 1972; Murphy, 1969; Stoller, 1967), the self-directed groups (Berzon and Soloman, 1966; Rogers, 1967b), sensitivity and "T" groups (Benne, 1969; Bradford, Gibb, and Benne, 1964; Schein and Bennis, 1965), and humanistic-experiential ones (Berne, 1964; Perls, 1969; Schutz, 1967).

The human relations training model, which grew out of the T-group model, was developed at Bethel by the organization called the National Training Laboratories. The model has been documented as being effective (Appley and Winder, 1973).

There are several underlying assumptions about the nature of the learning process distinguishing T-groups and human relations training from other models of learning. All of these assumptions are directly applicable to the nursing process. According to Seashore (1970, pp. 15–16),* these assumptions are:

- *Learning Responsibility.* Each participant is responsible for his own learning. What a person learns depends upon his own style, readiness, and the relationships he develops with other members of the group.
- *Staff Role.* The staff person's role is to facilitate the examination and understanding of the experiences in the group. He helps participants to focus on the way the group is working, the style of an individual's participation, or the issues that are facing the group.
- *Experience and Conceptualization.* Most learning is a combination of experience and conceptualization. A major T-group aim is to provide a setting in which individuals are encouraged to examine their experiences together in enough detail so that valid generalizations can be drawn.
- *Authentic Relationships and Learning.* A person is most free to learn when he establishes authentic relationships with other people and thereby increases his sense of self-esteem and decreases his defensiveness. In authentic relationships persons can be open, honest, and direct with one another so that they are communicating what they are actually feeling rather than masking their feelings.
- *Skill Acquisition and Values.* The development of new skills in working with people is maximized as a person examines the basic values underlying his behavior, as he acquires appropriate concepts and theory, and as he is able to practice new behavior and obtain feedback on the degree to which his behavior produces the intended impact.

The goals and outcomes of human relations training are classified according to potential learning involving individuals, groups, and organizations (Seashore, 1970). The metagoals of the laboratory method involve inquiry, collaboration, rational conflict resolution, and the freedom to exercise choice. These processes are shared by the staff and the participants (Appley and Winder, 1973). These researchers further stated that in a relatively safe world, members can test and learn trust, risk-taking, openness, and interdependence. Studies by Gibb (1971), Harrison and Lubin (1965), and Miles (1965) have all found the T-group method an effective one for increasing interpersonal communication.

Carkhuff, Collingwood, and Renz (1969) investigated the effects of didactic training upon trainee levels of discrimination and communication. Their results indicated that exclusively didactic training yielded significant

---

*Reprinted with permission from NTL Institute.

improvement in discrimination but very little generalization of learning in communication skills.

Carkhuff and Truax (1965) evaluated the effects of an integrated didactic and experiential approach to training. They found that these two combined were basic to the training program, in addition to having a trainer who was a role model in offering high levels of empathy, respect, concreteness, and genuineness.

Carkhuff (1969e), Carkhuff and Banks (1970), and Carkhuff and Bierman (1970) discovered that to effect differences in communication, training must employ a behavioristic, interpersonal approach preceding practice in communication.

Several studies confirmed the need and success of providing experiential, interpersonal, and intrapersonal group training for helping professionals (Berenson, Carkhuff, and Myrus, 1966; Foulds, 1969; Martin and Carkhuff, 1968; Truax, Silbur, and Wargo, 1966; Vitalo, 1971).

With conclusions based on research and experience, Carkhuff (1969d, p. 130)* offered several propositions that led him to prefer the group training mode:

- *Proposition I.* "The core of functioning or dysfunctioning (health or psychopathology) is interpersonal."
- *Proposition II.* "The core of the helping process (learning or relearning) is interpersonal."
- *Proposition III.* "Group processes are the preferred mode of working with difficulties in interpersonal functioning." Group processes can obviously insure the greatest amount of learning for the greatest number of people at one time.
- *Proposition IV.* "Systematic group training in interpersonal functioning is the preferred mode of working with difficulties in interpersonal functioning."

Carkhuff (1969d) made use of all sources of learning: experiential, didactic, and role-modeling. He stressed that the key in all group helping processes is the level of functioning of the leader (Carkhuff, 1969a, 1969b). The use of high functioning leaders results in an atmosphere whereby trainees/helpees can move toward higher levels of functioning, as well as providing multiple potential helpers/trainers for individual group members (Carkhuff, 1969d).

The advantages of human-relations-modeled group processes that include all sources of learning under the direction of a high functioning leader are numerous. They apply in both training and helping.

Each helpee has the following opportunities, according to Carkhuff (1969d, p. 181):*

*Reprinted by permission. Copyright 1969 by Holt, Rinehart and Winston, Inc.

1. to act out his characteristic behaviors;
2. to observe the characteristic behaviors of others;
3. to communicate directly with another person other than the helper;
4. to dispense with unsuccessful defenses and express himself freely in the context of a facilitative group atmosphere;
5. to share in the helper's clarification and interpretation of the behavior of another;
6. to try out new behaviors directly with others;
7. to have the experience of helping as well as being helped;
8. to be valued by more than one person;
9. to focus upon the generalities of experience within the group;
10. to obtain a definition of social reality.

Advantages of group over individual processes for the trainer/helper are also significant.

According to Carkhuff (1969d, p. 181),* the helper has an opportunity to:

1. observe directly the behaviors of the individual helpees;
2. facilitate communication between individual helpees;
3. create a facilitative group atmosphere within which each group member may come to serve as a helper;
4. focus directly upon the generalities in the group experience;
5. utilize his resources in such a way as to get a maximum return in human benefits for a minimum of investment of time and energy on the part of the helper.

It is important to note the limitations of group processes for the helper/ trainer and helpee/trainee. They may be more difficult for the helper to control, since there are more individuals and interactions to which the helper must attend. An effective leader can minimize these conditions, however, and handle group crises just as the leader would handle a crisis in individual treatment. If necessary, individual treatment can be offered concurrent with group processes (Carkhuff, 1969d).

Several conclusions can be reached regarding the preference of the human relations model in training and treatment. This model is goal and action directed and provides a work oriented structure through which experiential and therapeutic processes can take place. It emphasizes practice in the behavior one wishes to effect and leaves the trainee/helpee with tangible and usable skills. Longer retention of these skills is promoted, since they are learned as a result of direct teaching, shaping, and modeling. Group members can be systematically selected and there is a built-in means for assessing the effectiveness of the program because the very nature of systematic training involves steps that lead to measurable outcomes (Carkhuff, 1969d). States

*Reprinted by permission. Copyright 1969 by Holt, Rinehart and Winston, Inc.

Carkhuff (1969d, p. 184):* "In summary, what can be accomplished individually can be accomplished in groups—and more! What can be accomplished in groups can be accomplished in systematic training—and more!"

APPLICATION OF HUMANISTIC LEARNING TO NURSING PRACTICE

Throughout this book it has been stressed that learning continually occurs. Therefore, the elements of humanistic learning are easily applied to nursing practice.

Humanistic learning emphasizes the individuality of the student. The student, of course, can be the actual student nurse. Or, in the case of giving client care, the care-giver may be the student, learning about the client as data are collected, processed, compiled into a care plan, and evaluated. Indeed, all members of the health care system learn as care is given. Humanistic education emphasizes long-term changes in behavior through attitudinal development. Therefore, both care-givers and care-receivers experience learning throughout the nursing process as behaviors are studied and changed to coincide with good health. Members of the health care system learn from each other and with each other.

By integrating content with knowledge and experience and, of course, feelings, the care-giver and care-receiver can work together to achieve an individualized, quality care plan which will help the client towards the all-important (and oft-repeated) goal: the client's fullest health potential.

In addition, the humanistic approach emphasizes change. Therefore, in nursing practice the nurse becomes aware of change in personal perceptions, change in both client and health team attitudes, change in the client's conditions, and a change in personal experience. Each of these aspects builds on the nurse's experiential foundation; the nurse can only grow.

Humanism emphasizes the interrelationship of persons, the environment, and the inner self. In giving care, therefore, all concerning the client—and all concerning the nurse—is taken into consideration. The result is humanistic care of the whole person; the nursing process achieves its ultimate goal.

SUMMARY

The humanistic approach utilized throughout this book and conceptualized in this chapter is a combination of many facets of learning theory. Content material, outside experiences related to actual practice, and direct nursing care are elements of the humanistic approach to learning and applying the

*Reprinted by permission. Copyright 1969 by Holt, Rinehart and Winston, Inc.

nursing process as presented in this book. The continuous bond between elements of humanistic learning is that the learning is intended to focus on the individuality of the student. In other words, the designs are built so that the student can take a new body of knowledge; use background, expectations, and experience; and work through an exercise related to the content needing to be learned. Sharing with fellow students enables one to be aware of a broader range of perceptions, all adding to self-learning. Through this personalization of content, one brings outside experiences into one's life, adding significance. This significance is necessary if learning is to bring long-term change in behavior, since this type of change will greatly help in insuring that students continue to strive toward carrying the high ideals learned in academic environments to service institutions. Humanistic psychologists have documented that people learn more fully when the learning involves themselves (Combs and Syngg, 1959; Jourard, 1971; Rogers, 1965). Ultimately then, through humanistic learning of the nursing process, a behavior pattern is established in which the nurse later applies a humanistic approach to exploring client care, giving client care, and, indeed, learning about the individual client.

REFERENCES

Appley, D., and Winder, A. *T-Groups and therapy groups in a changing society.* San Francisco: Jossey-Bass, 1973.

Asch, S. The doctrine of suggestion, prestige, and imitations in social psychology. *Psychological Review* 55:250–276, 1948.

Asch, S. *Social psychology.* Englewood Cliffs, N.J.: Prentice-Hall, 1952.

Aspy, D. A study of three facilitative conditions and their relationship to the achievement of third grade students. Unpublished doctoral dissertation, University of Kentucky, 1965.

Axline, V. *Dibs: In search of self.* New York: Ballantine Books, 1964.

Bach, G. The marathon group: I. Intensive practice of intimate interaction. *Psychological Reports* 18:995–1002, 1966.

Barrett-Lennard, G. Dimensions of therapist response as causal factors in therapeutic change. *Psychological Monographs* 76: No. 562, 1962.

Beck, C. *Philosophical foundations of guidance.* Englewood Cliffs, N.J.: Prentice-Hall, 1963.

Benne, K. *The self, the group or the task: Differences among growth groups.* Paper presented at: The growth groups: Encounter, marathon, sensitivity and 'T." Ninth Annual Conference, Personality Theory and Counseling Practice, University of Florida, Gainesville, January, 1969.

Berenson, B., Carkhuff, R., and Myrus, P. The interpersonal functioning and training of college students. *Journal of Counseling Psychology* 13:441–446, 1966.

Berne, E. *Games people play: The psychology of human relationships.* New York: Grove Press, 1964.

Berzon, B., and Soloman, L. Research frontiers: The self-directed therapeutic group. *Journal of Counseling Psychology* 13:491–497, 1966.

Bradford, P., Gibb, J., and Benne, K. (eds.). *T-Group theory and laboratory method: An innovation in re-education.* New York: John Wiley and Sons, 1964.

Campbell, D. The generality of social attitudes. Unpublished doctoral dissertation, University of California, Berkeley, 1947.

Camus, A. *The stranger.* New York: Alfred A. Knopf, 1946.

Camus, A. *The myth of Sisyphus.* New York: Random House, 1955.

Camus, A. *The rebel.* New York: Alfred A. Knopf, 1956.

Camus, A. *The plague.* New York: Vintage Books, 1972.

Carkhuff, R. *Critical perspectives on group processes.* Presented at: The growth groups: Encounter, marathon, sensitivity and "T." Ninth Annual Conference, Personality Theory and Counseling Practice, University of Florida, Gainesville, January, 1969a.

Carkhuff, R. Critical variables in effective counselor training. *Journal of Counseling Psychology* 16:238–245, 1969b.

Carkhuff, R. *Helping and human relations: A primer for lay and professional helpers,* Vol. II. New York: Holt, Rinehart and Winston, 1969d.

Carkhuff, R. *Helping and human relations: A primer for lay and professional Helpers,* Vol. II. New York: Holt, Rinehart and Winston, 1969d.

Carkhuff, R. The prediction of the effects of didactic training in discrimination. *Journal of Clinical Psychology* 25:460–461, 1969e.

Carkhuff, R., and Banks, G. Training as a preferred mode of facilitating relations between races and generations. *Journal of Counseling Psychology* 17:413–418, 1970.

Carkhuff, R., and Bierman, R. Training as a preferred mode of treatment of parents of emotionally disturbed children. *Journal of Counseling Psychology* 17:157–161, 1970.

Carkhuff, R., and Truax, C. Training in counseling and psychotherapy: An evaluation of an integrated didactic and experiential approach. *Journal of Consulting Psychology* 29:333–336, 1965.

Carkhuff, R., Collingwood, T., and Renz, L. The effects of didactic training upon trainee levels of discrimination and communication. *Journal of Clinical Psychology* 25:460–461, 1969.

Combs, A. *Educational accountability: Beyond behavioral objectives.* Washington, D.C.: Association for Supervision and Curriculum Development, 1972.

Combs, A., and Syngg, D. *Individual behavior.* New York: Harper and Row, 1959.

Emmerling, F. A study of the relationships between personality characteristics of classroom teachers and pupil perceptions. Unpublished doctoral dissertation, Auburn University, Auburn, Alabama, 1961.

Foulds, M. Self-actualization and the communication of facilitative conditions during counseling. *Journal of Counseling Psychology* 16:132–136, 1969.

Gazda, G., Asbury, F., Balzer, F., Childers, W., Desselle, R., and Walters, R. *Human relations development: A manual for educators.* Boston: Allyn and Bacon, 1973.

Gibb, J. The effects of human relations training. In A. Bergin and S. Garfield (eds.). *Handbook of psychotherapy and behavior change.* New York: John Wiley and Sons, 1971.

Harper, R. *Psychoanalysis and psychotherapy.* Englewood Cliffs, N.J.: Prentice-Hall, 1959.

Harrison, R., and Lubin, B. Personal style, group composition and learning. *Journal of Applied Behavioral Science* 3:286–301, 1965.

Hersey, P., and Blanchard, K. *Management of organizational behavior.* Englewood Cliffs, N.J.: Prentice-Hall, 1977.

Jourard, S. *The transparent self.* New York: Van Nostrand Reinhold Co., 1971.

Katz, D., and Stotland, E. A preliminary statement to a theory of attitude structure and change. In S. Koch (ed.), *Psychology: A study of a science,* Vol. 3. New York: McGraw-Hill Books, Inc., 1959.

La Monica, E., and Parisi, E. The PELLEM Pentagram. Unpublished material, University of Massachusetts, 1975.

Lott, A. Social psychology. In B. Wolman (ed.), *Handbook of General Psychology.* Englewood Cliffs, N.J.: Prentice-Hall, 1973.

Lubin, B., and Lubin, A. *Group psychotherapy: A bibliography of the literature from 1956 to 1964.* East Lansing, Michigan: Michigan State University Press, 1967.

Martin, J., and Carkhuff, R. Changes in personality and interpersonal functioning in counselors in training. *Journal of Clinical Psychology* 24:109–110, 1968.

Matarazzo, J. Psychotherapeutic processes. *Annual Review of Psychology* 16:181–219, 1965.

Miles, M. Changes during and following laboratory training: A clinical experimental study. *Journal of Applied Behavioral Science* 1:215–242, 1965.

Moustakas, C. *The authentic teacher: Sensitivity and awareness in the classroom.* Cambridge, Mass.: Howard A. Doyle, 1972.

Murphy, M. *The growth center phenomenon.* Presented at: The growth groups: Encounter, marathon, sensitivity and "T." Ninth Annual Conference, Personality Theory and Counseling Practice, University of Florida, Gainesville, January, 1969.

Osgood, C. Studies on the generality of affective meaning systems. *American Psychologist* 17:10–28, 1962.

Osgood, C., Suci, G., and Tannenbaum, P. *The measurement of meaning.* Urbana: University of Illinois Press, 1957.

Perls, F. *Gestalt therapy verbatim.* Lafayette, Calif.: Real People Press, 1969.

Rogers, C. *On becoming a person.* Boston: Houghton Mifflin Co., 1965.

Rogers, C. The interpersonal relationship in the facilitation of learning. In R. Leeper (ed.). *Humanizing education: The person in the process.* Washington, D.C.: Association for Supervision and Curriculum Development, 1967a.

Rogers, C. A plan for self-directed change in an educational system. *Educational Leadership* 24:717–731, 1967b.

Schein, E., and Bennis, W. (eds.). *Personal and organizational change through group methods: The laboratory approach.* New York: John Wiley and Sons, 1965.

Schmuck, R. Some relationships of peer liking patterns in the classroom to pupil attitudes and achievement. *The School Review* 71:337–359, 1963.

Schmuck, R. Some aspects of classroom social climate. *Psychology in the Schools* 3:59–65, 1966.

Schutz, W. *Joy: Expanding human awareness.* New York: Grove Press, 1967.

Seashore, C. What is sensitivity training? In R. Golembiewski and A. Blumberg (eds.). *Sensitivity training and the laboratory approach: Readings about concepts and applications.* Itasca, Ill.: F. E. Peacock, 1970.

Stoller, F. The long weekend. *Psychology Today* 1:28–33, 1967.

Truax, C., Silbur, L., and Wargo, D. Training and change in psychotherapeutic skills. Mimeographed manuscript, Arkansas Rehabilitation and Research Center, University of Arkansas, 1966.

Vitalo, R. Teaching improved interpersonal functioning as a preferred mode of treatment. *Journal of Clinical Psychology* 27:166–171, 1971.

Weisman, A. *The existential core of psychoanalysis.* Boston: Little, Brown and Company, 1965.

SELECTED READINGS

Two articles written by pioneers in the area of humanistic education are included for further reading. Both discuss humanistic learning philosophy as it was originally developed. Humanism as a philosophy has its roots in educational systems. The essence of these articles, among others, has been synthesized and applied in nursing practice. Practice implies education and the circularity of this process becomes evident. Each article is intended to provide a clearer understanding of the historical development of humanism in our nursing profession.

The Human Side of Learning

Arthur W. Combs

Anyone who doesn't know that education is in deep trouble must have been hiding somewhere for the last fifteen years. Somehow we have lost touch with the times, so we find young people opting out, copping out, and dropping out of the system. The processes of education have become concerned with nonhuman questions, and the system is dehumanizing to the people in it. Earl Kelley once said, "We've got this marvelous school system with beautiful buildings and a magnificent curriculum and these great teachers and these marvelous administrators, and then, damn it all, the parents send us the wrong kids."

For a number of generations now, we have been dealing with learning from a false premise. Most of us are familiar with Pavlov's famous experiment conditioning a dog to respond to a bell. The principles he established then are the ones we still use to deal with the problems of learning in our schools today. But Pavlov's system depended on: 1) separating his dogs from all other dogs, which made the learning process an isolated event; 2) tying his dogs down so that they could only do precisely what he had in mind, a technique not very feasible for most elementary teachers; 3) completely removing the dogs from all other possible sources of stimuli, a hard thing to do in a classroom.

This point of view has taught us to deal with the problem of learning as a question of stimulus and response, to be understood in terms of input and output. Currently it finds its latest expression in behavioral objectives, performance based criteria for learning that systematically demand that you: Establish your objectives in behavioral terms; set up the machinery to accomplish them; and then test whether or not you have achieved them. Such an approach seems straightforward, businesslike, and logical; and that's what is wrong with it. I quote from Earl Kelley again, who once said, "Logic is often only a systematic way of arriving at the wrong answers!"

I'm not opposed to behavioral objectives. Nobody can be against accountability. The difficulty with the concept is that its fundamental premise is only partly right. The fact is that behavioral objectives are useful devices for dealing with the simplest, most primitive aspects of education, the things we already do quite well. Unfortunately, they do not serve us so well when they are applied to other kinds of objectives, such as intelligent behavior requiring a creative approach to a problem. Behavioral objectives do not deal with the problem of holistic goals. They do not help us in dealing with the things that make us truly human—the questions of human beliefs, attitudes, feelings,

Reprinted with permission from *The National Elementary Principal* (January 1973). Copyright 1973 by *The National Elementary Principal*.

understandings, and concerns—the things we call "affective." Nor do they deal with the problems of self-actualization, citizenship, responsibility, caring, and many other such humanistic goals of educators.

Using this approach, we are evaluating schools and circumstances on the basis of what we know how to test. As a result, we are finding that our educational objectives are being established by default because the things we know how to test are the simplest, smallest units of cognitive procedures, which don't really matter much anyway.

We are spending millions and millions of dollars on this very small aspect of dealing with the educational problem, while the problems of self-concept, human attitudes, feelings, beliefs, meanings, and intelligence are going unexplored.

Although I do not oppose behavioral objectives, I do believe that those who are forcing accountability techniques on us need also to be held accountable for what they are doing to American education.

Performance based criteria is the method of big business, a technique of management, and we are now in the process of applying these industrial techniques to education everywhere. We ought to know better. When industry developed the assembly line and other systematic techniques to increase efficiency, what happened? The workers felt dehumanized by the system and formed unions to fight it. And that is precisely what is happening with our young people today. They feel increasingly dehumanized by the system, so they are fighting it at every possible level. Applying industrial techniques to human problems just won't work. A systems approach, it should be understood, is only a method of making sure you accomplish your objectives. Applied to the wrong objectives, systems approaches only guarantee that your errors will be colossal.

The trouble with education today is not its lack of efficiency, but its lack of humanity. Learning is not a mechanical process, but a *human* process. The whole approach to learning through behavioral objectives concentrates our attention on the simplest, most primitive aspects of the educational endeavor, while it almost entirely overlooks the human values. I believe we can get along better with a person who can't read than with a bigot. We are doing very little to prevent the production of bigots but a very great deal to prevent the production of poor readers.

Learning is a human problem always consisting of two parts. First, we have to provide people with some new information or some new experience, and we know how to do that very well. We are experts at it. With the aid of our new electronic gadgets, we can do it faster and more furiously than ever before in history. Second, the student must discover the meaning of the information provided him. The dropout is not a dropout because we didn't give him information. We told him, but he never discovered what that information meant.

I would like to give an alternate definition to the S-R theory most of us cut our teeth on: Information will affect a person's behavior only in the degree to which he has discovered its personal meaning for him. For example, I read in this morning's paper that there has been an increase in the number of cases of pulmonic stenosis in the state of Florida in the past two years. I don't know what pulmonic stenosis is, so this information has no meaning for me. Later in the day I hear a friend talking about pulmonic stenosis, so I look it up and find that it's a disorder that produces a closing up of the pulmonary artery. It's a dangerous disorder, and it produces blue babies. Now I know what it is, but it still doesn't affect my behavior very much. Later in the day I received a letter from a mother of one of my students who says, "Dear Teacher, we have taken Sally to the clinic, where we learned that she has got pulmonic stenosis, and she's going to have to be operated on when she reaches adolescence. In the meantime, we would appreciate it if you would keep an eye out for her."

This information has more meaning to me now because it's happening to one of my students, and my behavior reflects that meaning. I protect the girl, and I talk to other people on the faculty: "Did you hear about Sally? Isn't it a shame? She's got pulmonic stenosis. Poor child, she's going to have to be operated on."

Let's go one step further. Suppose I have just learned that my daughter has pulmonic stenosis. Now this information affects my behavior tremendously, in every aspect of my daily life.

This explains why so much of what we do in school has no effect on students. Sometimes we even discourage them from finding the personal meaning of a piece of information. We say, "Eddie, I'm not interested in what you think about that, what does the book say?" which is the same as telling him that school is a place where you learn about things that don't matter.

What do we need to do, then, if we're going to humanize the business of learning? We have to see the whole problem of learning differently. We have to give up our preoccupation with objectivity. In our research at the University of Florida, we find that objectivity correlates negatively with effectiveness in the helping professions we have so far explored.

Freud once said that no one ever does anything unless he would rather. In other words, no one ever does anything unless he thinks it is important. So the first thing we must do to humanize learning is to believe it is important.

Let me tell another story by way of illustration. In the suburbs of Atlanta there was a young woman teaching first grade who had beautiful long blonde hair which she wore in a pony tail down to the middle of her back. For the first three days of the school year she wore her hair that way. Then, on Thursday she decided to do it up in a bun on top of her head. One of the little boys in her class looked into the room and didn't recognize his teacher. He was lost. The bell rang, school started, and he didn't know where he belonged. He was out in the hall crying. The supervisor asked him, "What's the trouble?" and he said, "I can't find my teacher." She said, "Well, what's your teacher's name? What room are you in?" He didn't know. So she said, "Well, come on, let's see if we can find her." They started down the hall together, the supervisor and the little boy, hand-in-hand, opening one door after another without much luck until they came to the room where this young woman was teaching. As they stood there in the doorway, the teacher turned and saw them and she said, "Why, Joey, it's good to see you. We've been wondering where you were. Come on in. We've missed you." And the little boy pulled away from the supervisor and threw himself into the teacher's arms. She gave him a hug, patted him on the fanny, and he ran to his seat. She knew what was important. She thought little boys were important.

Suppose the teacher hadn't thought little boys were important. Suppose, for instance, she thought supervisors were important. Then she would have said, "Why good morning, Miss Smith. We're so glad you've come to see us, aren't we boys and girls?" And the little boy would have been ignored. Or the teacher might have thought the lesson was important, in which case she would have said, "Joey, for heaven's sake, where have you been? You're already two pages behind. Come in here and get to work." Or she might have thought that discipline was important, and said, "Joey, you know very well when you're late you must go to the office and get a permit. Now run and get it." But she didn't. She thought little boys were important. And so it is with each of us. We have to believe humanizing learning is important.

To humanize learning we must also recognize that people don't behave according to the facts of a situation, they behave in terms of their beliefs. In the last presidential election, those who thought that the Democrats would save us and the Republicans would ruin us voted for the Democrats. And those who thought the Republicans would save us and the Democrats would ruin us voted for the Republicans. Each of us behaved not in terms of "the facts," but in terms of our beliefs. A fact is only what we believe is so. Sensitivity to the beliefs of the people we work with is basic to effective behavior. In our research on the helping professions, we found the outstanding characteristic of effective helpers was that the good ones are always concerned with how things look from the point of view of the people they are working with.

Let me give another illustration of what I mean by being aware of the other person's point of view. A supervisor and a teacher were talking about a little boy: "I don't know what to do with him," the teacher said. "I know that he can do it; I tell him, 'It's easy, Frank, you can do it; but he won't even try.' " The supervisor said, "Don't ever tell a child something is easy. Look at it from the child's point of view. If you tell him it's easy and he can't do it, he can only conclude that he must be stupid, and if he can do it, you have robbed it of all its thrill! Tell him it's hard, that you know it's hard, but you're pretty sure he can do it. Then if he can't do it, he hasn't lost face, and if he can do it, what a glory that is for him."

So much of what we do in teaching is not concerned with people. It is concerned with rules, regulations, order, and neatness. I visited a school some years ago, and as I sat in the principal's office one of the bus drivers came in with a little boy in one hand and a broken arm from one of the seats of the bus in the other hand. How did this principal behave? He became very angry. It was as if the little boy had broken the principal's arm. And, in a sense, the boy had, I suppose.

In contrast to that, I am reminded of a visit I made to a school in Michigan. As I walked down the hall with the principal, a teacher and a group of children came out of one of the rooms of this very old building. We walked into the room and saw that it was in complete havoc. The principal said, "It's a mess isn't it? And it can stay that way. The teacher has raised the reading level of her classes by two grades every year she's had them. If that's the way she wants to teach, it's all right with me!"

We walked along to the gymnasium and looked in. He said as we looked at the floor, "That's the third finish we've had on that floor this year. We use it in the evenings for family roller skating!" There is a man whose values are clear. He is more concerned with people than things.

There are hundreds of ways we dehumanize people in our schools, and we need to make a systematic attempt to get rid of them.

In *Crisis in the Classroom*, Charles Silberman says that he believes one of the major problems in American education is "mindlessness." We do so many things without having the slightest idea of why we're doing them. One dehumanizing element is the grading system. Grades motivate very few people, nor are they good as an evaluative device. Everyone knows that no two teachers evaluate people in exactly the same terms. Yet we piously regard grades as though they all mean the same thing, under the same circumstances, to all people at all times.

I remember my son coming home from college and asking, "Dad, how can you, as an educator, put up with the grading system? Grading on the curve makes it to my advantage to destroy my friends. Dad, that's a hell of a way to teach young people to live." I'd never thought of it that way before.

Another thing we need to understand is the serious limitation of competition as a motivational system. Psychologists know three things about motivation:

1. The only people who are motivated by competition are those who think they can win. And that's not very many. Everyone else sits back and watches them beat their brains out.
2. People who do not feel they have a chance of winning and are forced to compete are not motivated. They are discouraged and disillusioned by the process, and we cannot afford a discouraged and disillusioned populace.
3. When competition becomes too important, morality breaks down, and any means becomes justified to achieve the ends—the basketball team begins to use its elbows and students begin to cheat on exams.

Grade level and grouping is another mindless obstacle to humanizing. All the research we have on grouping tells us that no one method of grouping is superior to any other. And yet we go right on, in the same old ways, insisting that we must have grade levels. As a result, we might have an eleven-year-old child in the sixth grade reading at the third-grade level. Every day of his life we feed him a diet of failure because we can't find a way to give a success experience to such a child.

If we want to humanize the processes of learning, we must make a systematic search for the things that destroy effective learning and remove them from the scene. If we're going to humanize the processes of learning, we must take the student in as a partner. Education wouldn't be irrelevant if students had a voice in decision making. One of my friends once said that the problem of American education today is that "all of us are busy providing students with answers to problems they don't have yet." And that's true. We decide what people need to know and then we teach it to them whether they need it or not. As a result some students discover that school is a place where you study things that don't matter and so they drop out. It's intelligent to drop out. If it isn't getting you anywhere, if it doesn't have any meaning, if it doesn't do something for you, then it's intelligent to drop out. But we seldom think of it that way. Most of us regard the dropout as though there is something wrong with him.

Part of making education relevant to the student is allowing him to develop responsibility for his own learning. But responsibility can only be learned from having responsibility, never from having it withheld. The teacher who says, "You be good kids while I'm out of the room" is an example of what I'm talking about. When she comes back the room is bedlam. "I'll never leave you alone again," she says. By this pronouncement she has robbed the children of any opportunity to learn how to behave responsibly on their own.

Not long ago, I arrived at a school just after the election for student body president, and the teachers were upset because the student who was elected president had run on a platform of no school on Friday, free lunches, free admissions to the football games, and a whole string of other impossible things. The teachers thought it was "a travesty on democracy" and suggested that the student body have another election. I said, "If you do that, how are these kids ever going to discover the terrible price you have to pay for electing a jackass to office?"

We know that what a person believes about himself is crucial to his growth and development. We also know that a person learns this self-concept from the way he is treated by significant people in his life. The student takes his self-concept with him wherever he goes. He takes it to Latin class, to arithmetic class, to gym class, and he takes it home with him. Wherever he goes, his self-concept goes, too. Everything that happens to him has an effect on his self-concept.

Are we influencing that self-concept in positive or negative ways? We need to ask ourselves these kinds of questions. How can a person feel liked unless somebody likes him? How can a person feel wanted unless somebody wants him? How can a person feel acceptable unless somebody accepts him? How can a person feel he's a person with dignity and integrity unless somebody treats him so? And how can a person feel that he is capable unless he has some success? In the answers to those questions, we'll find the answers to the human side of learning.

Humanistic Education

Alfred S. Alschuler

In the Symposium, Alcibiades praised Socrates by saying, "He is exactly like the busts of (the god) Silenus which are set up in the statuaries' shops, holding pipes and flutes in their mouths; they open in the middle and have images of gods inside them. When I opened him (Socrates) and looked within at his serious purpose, I saw divine and golden images of such fascinating beauty that I was ready to do in a moment whatever Socrates commanded." Silenus was a minor Greek deity, a follower of Dionysus, disconcertedly homely, and nearly human. Usually he was seen drunk, sitting precariously on the back of an ass, yet he was renowned for the unsurpassed wisdom and knowledge of past and future that emerged, as with Socrates, in any dialogue. Silenus was a popular god, for he symbolized the universal desire to be discovered and valued for one's inner virtues. All of us want to be a Silenus and to have our Alcibiades. "His words are ridiculous when you first hear them," continues Alcibiades, "but he who opens the bust and sees what is within will find that they are the only words which have a meaning in them, and also the most divine, abounding in fair images of virtue and extending to the whole duty of a good and honorable man." As Humanistic Educators, we are Alcibiades for our students, opening them up, discovering their inner virtues and drawing forth (literally, "educating") the "good and honorable man."

Only a small number of events in a lifetime radically change the way a person lives—a deeply religious experience, getting married or divorced, having a child, the death of parents, involvement in a serious accident. These dramatic, singular events transform a person's outlook, relation to others and view of himself. By comparison, daily learning experiences in school are undramatic, regularized and designed to promote steady, small increments in external knowledge rather than rapid changes in motives, values and relationships. Obviously we do not want to create regular apocalyptic events that drastically change students' personal lives. However, the ultimate teaching goal of Humanistic Education is to develop effective strategies and humane technology for educating inner strengths as profoundly as these rare life-changing events.

UNIQUELY HUMAN LEARNING

Inchoate work in Humanistic Education exists. Scattered across the United States a handful of individuals working in isolated independence have

Reprinted with permission from *Educational Technology Magazine*. Copyright 1970 by *Educational Technology Magazine*.

created programmatic approaches to the discovery and enhancement of inner strengths. These Humanistic Education courses respond directly to previously unanswered student questions about setting goals, clarifying values, forming identity, increasing their sense of personal efficacy and having more satisfying relationships with others. The array of humanistic education courses include training in: achievement motivation, awareness and excitement, creative thinking, interpersonal sensitivity, affiliation motivation, joy, self reliance, self esteem, self assessment, self renewal, self actualization, self understanding, strength training, development of moral reasoning, value clarification, body awareness, meditative processes and other aspects of ideal adult functioning.* The variety of virtuous sounding titles testifies to the extent of developmental efforts underway, and also reflects the absence of a definitive description of ideal end states. In spite of this diversity, most of these courses share four general goals, in addition to their unique and specific emphases.

First, most courses attempt to develop a person's *imagination* by using procedures that encourage a constructive dialogue with one's fantasy life. In Synectics training, a creativity course, students are asked to "make the strange familiar" by fantasizing themselves inside a strange object, or to "make the familiar strange" by fantasizing about a common object. In other creativity courses, remote associations are encouraged in order to attain a new, useful and creative perspective on some problem. In other courses, students are taken on guided tours of day dreams and night dreams and on fantasy trips into their own body. In achievement motivation courses, students are encouraged to fantasize about doing things exceptionally well and are taught how to differentiate between achievement imagery and plain old task imagery. Later in the course, these achievement images are tied to reality through careful planning and projects. These procedures often bring previously ignored aspects of one's personality into awareness. Usually this is a joyful, enhancing experience in contrast to psychoanalytic dream analysis and free association, which are oriented to uncovering unconscious conflicts. The implication is that most adults don't make constructive use of their fantasy life and have forgotten how to enjoy fantasy in a childlike but healthy way.

Second, most courses try to develop better *communication skills* by using non-verbal exercises, such as silent theater improvisations, free expression dance movements, meditation, the exaggeration of spontaneous body movements and a wide variety of games. In sensitivity training and encounter groups, non-verbal exercises are used to increase channels of communication. Some personal feelings can be expressed more effectively in motions than in words. Other times, dance and theater improvisations are used because they increase one's expressive vocabulary and are simply joyful experiences. As

---

*Descriptions of a number of these courses along with a comprehensive bibliography are contained in *New Directions in Psychological Education,* A. S. Alschuler, *Educational Opportunities Forum,* whole issue, January, 1970, State Education Department, Albany, New York. The three most well developed sets of curriculum materials exist for: (1) *Teaching Achievement Motivation,* by A. Alschuler, D. Tabor, J. McIntyre, Education Ventures, Inc., Middletown, Connecticut, 1970; (2) "Urban Affairs and Communications," T. Borton and N. Newberg, specialists in Humanistic Education, Philadelphia Board of Education Building, Philadelphia, Pa.; (3) "Value Clarification," see *Values and Teaching,* L. Raths, M. Harmon, S. Simon, Columbus, Ohio: Charles Merrill Books, 1966.

with constructive fantasizing, proponents of these methods believe that this type of expression, communication and learning is underdeveloped in most people.

A third goal common to these courses is to develop and explore individuals' *emotional responses* to the world. In most courses, how people feel is considered more important than what they think about things. Without these emotional experiences, ranging from laughter and exhilaration to tears and fear, the teacher is likely to consider the course a failure. For example, if an adolescent is scaling a cliff in an Outward Bound course and does not feel any fear, he will not increase his self confidence through his accomplishment. In Achievement Motivation courses, strong group feelings are developed to help support the individual in whatever he chooses to do well. In all of these courses, there is a shared belief that affect increases meaningful learning and that the capacity for the full range of affective responses is a crucial human potentiality often underdeveloped in adults. As a result, a wide range of techniques to enhance affect have been created.*

A fourth goal emphasizes the importance of *living fully and intensely* "here and now." The emphasis takes many forms. In Gestalt awareness training, the goal is philosophically explicit. In most courses, it is subtle and implicit. Usually courses are held in retreat settings which cut people off from past obligations and future commitments for brief periods of time. The isolated resort settings dramatize the "here and now" opportunities. In general there is little emphasis on future "homework" or past personal history as an explanation for behavior. A vivid example is Synanon, a total environment program for drug addicts, which promotes "self actualization," and in the process curses addiction. Synanon requires the addict to kick drugs immediately upon entering the program. Other "bad" behavior which stands in the way of self actualization is pointed out as it occurs. Historical explanations for bad behavior are considered excuses and are not tolerated. In other Humanistic Education programs, the games, exercises, group process, etc., are model opportunities to explore, discover and try out new behavior here and now. The assumption is that if a person can't change "here and now," where the conditions for growth are optimal, he is not likely to continue growing outside and after the course.

The existing procedures for developing new thinking, action and feelings in the "here and now" constitute humane methods for educating inner strengths. These methods make it possible to create, without trauma, the sequence of uniquely human learning that occurs during and after rare, dramatic, life-changing events.

In most of these naturally occurring events there is a strong focus of attention on what is happening "here and now." Whether it is a mother's labor during birth, the taking of marriage vows, the shock of realizing your arm is broken, or the ecstasy of a religious vision, the intensity of the experience crowds out familiar reactions. One characteristic that sets these experiences apart is the simultaneous intensity of radically new thoughts, actions and

*Human Relations Education: A Guidebook to Learning Activities, prepared by the Human Relations Project of Western New York, reprinted by the University of the State of New York, the State Education Department, Curriculum Development Center, Albany, New York, 1969.

feelings. Usually these experiences break established relationships, as when a parent dies. Often they disrupt habitual patterns of living, or dissolve longtime beliefs. Whether the experience is revelatory or traumatic in nature, it breaks basic continuities in a person's life. After the peak of the experience has passed, there is a period of some confusion and puzzlement, during which the person attempts to make sense out of what happened and to establish meaningful new continuities. This attempt takes many forms, from conversation with friends to meditation and prayer. Even if the experience is never fully understood, in time the consequences become clearer—how relationships are altered, what goals and values are different, and what new behaviors occur. After a while these changes seem more familiar and practiced. For example, new roles become less confusing. As the newness of being a parent wears off, the role becomes an integral part of a person's life, with its own rich set of relationships, behaviors and meanings. Similarly, in time, the traumatic loss of a loved one results in new relationships, behaviors and meanings that we internalize in our way of living.

This sequence of learning can be conceptualized as a six-step process and used as a guideline in planning Humanistic Education courses and sequencing existing humanistic procedures.

1. Focus attention on what is happening here and now by creating moderate novelty that is slightly different from what is expected.
2. Provide an intense, integrated experience of the desired new thoughts, actions and feelings.
3. Help the person make sense out of his experience by attempting to conceptualize what happened.
4. Relate the experience to the person's values, goals, behavior and relationships with others.
5. Stabilize the new thought, action and feelings through practice.
6. Internalize the changes.

This teaching strategy is not simply a heuristic device. A considerable amount of support for the validity of these guidelines exists in the theoretical and empirical research literature on personality change.*

This strategy indicates a number of ways that Humanistic Education differs from more traditional academic training. The most effective way to proceed through this learning sequence is to set aside a large block of time, often as long as a week or more, in a special location for a concentrated workshop. The untypical setting helps create moderate novelty, reduces distractions and helps focus attention on the new experiences. The concentrated time period is needed to allow the participants to follow new thoughts, to try out new behavior and to stick with their feelings to a natural conclusion.

---

*The most relevant summaries of this literature can be found in D. C. McClelland, "Toward a Theory of Motive Acquisition," *American Psychologist*, May, 1965; D. C. McClelland and D. G. Winter, *Motivating Economic Achievement*, Free Press, 1969; Campbell, J., Dunnette, M., "Effectiveness of T-Group Experience in Managerial Training and Development," *Psychological Bulletin*, August, 1968, pp. 73–104.

Emotions, in contrast to *thoughts,* tend to be non-reversible and difficult to stop quickly at the end of a 45-minute class period. This inhibits the expression of feelings, just as longer time periods encourage the expression of feelings. In this sense, Humanistic Education is experience based and inductive, in contrast to academic learning—which tends to be more abstract, logical and deductive.

A less obvious difference is the integration and simultaneous development of thoughts, feelings and actions. Learning achievement motivation, for example, involves developing a specific cognitive pattern of planning, a special type of excitement and a set of related action strategies. Most normal learning situations differ by rewarding expertise as a "thinker" in academic courses, or as a doer in physical courses like vocational education or athletics. This makes it especially difficult for teachers to be concerned in practice with educating the "whole child." However, there is some justification for the way schooling fragments human functioning into component parts. It does prepare students for adult lives in which separate role performances are played out in many directions. Just as students move from class to class during the day, adults move from role to role. We work in one place, have our intimate, loving relationship in another place, and usually travel to still other places for recreation. In each role adults are known for a narrow set of behaviors, just as students are known by their teachers as a math student, or typing student and rarely as a complex, many-sided individual. Experience-based learning integrates human functioning in the service of balanced maturation.

The art and technology of Humanistic Education, in large part, lies in the creation of productive learning experiences. Only the outlines of this technology are clear at this time. Teachers must be insightful diagnosticians of children's experience, so that moderately novel situations can be created. These situations bridge the gap between where the child is and where he can be. Thus, teachers must know a wide range of Humanistic Education procedures and be knowledgeable about the goals of human development. This expertise allows them to help students conceptualize, relate and apply their new experiential knowledge. Few learning experiences require extensive hardware and materials. Most procedures involve the person in relation to his own body, feelings and imagination or in relation to his environment and other people. A comprehensive source book of humanistic methods would be useful, but ultimately each teacher must adapt and sequence these methods to create the course of learning, i.e., the curriculum. In this sense, curriculum innovation is constant, and Humanistic Educators need to become adept at improvising sequences of learning that lead to internalization.

Compared to typical school goals, Humanistic Education courses aim for long-term internalization, not short-term gains in mastery. More precisely, these courses attempt to increase "operant" behavior as well as respondent behavior. Operant behavior is voluntary, seemingly spontaneous and certainly not required by the situation. What a person does with his leisure time is an indication of his operant behavior. Respondent behavior requires external cues and incentives before it will occur, just as an examination question brings forth respondent knowledge that otherwise probably would not have been demonstrated. In practice, most school learning calls for respondent behavior: multiple choice and true-false questions, reading assigned chapters, solving a given set of mathematics problems correctly, or writing an essay to a prescribed theme. To be most meaningful to a student, Humanistic Education must result in operant, internalized behavior, since after the course is over there will not be anyone to follow him around defining the problems, presenting the alternatives, guiding the response and evaluating the results. Paradoxically, the most important thing to do in helping a person develop long-term operant behavior is to stop doing anything. Support must be gradually transferred from external sources to the person's own inner resources. The problem is to leave on time—not too soon, because guidance is needed in the early phases, and not too late because that retards essential self reliance. At the present time, staging perfectly timed exits is an art in need of becoming a technology.

HUMANIZING SCHOOLS

Educating the "good and honorable man" is a ubiquitous aim of schooling. The problem is not the legitimacy of humanistic goals for public education, but how to translate these goals fully into practice. Specifically, it is unethical to develop students' ability to relate more warmly and directly their achievement motivation, their capacity for creative thinking through Humanistic Education courses, and then send them back into normal classrooms where these processes are not functional. For example, many Humanistic Education courses teach people how to develop collaborative and trusting relationships. Only in schools are there so few structured opportunities for practicing team-work and cooperation. From the humanistic point of view, the way people learn is just as important as what they learn. Ideally, there should be at least as much variety in the teaching-learning process within a single school as exists outside and after school, where students are variously required, ordered, coached, coaxed, persuaded, led, followed, threatened, promised, lectured, questioned, joined, challenged and left alone. Compared to this handsome array of naturally occurring learning processes, the typical range within a school is embarrassingly narrow. As Humanistic Education courses are introduced in schools, corresponding new processes should be available in regular courses in order for students to *practice what they have learned.*

How students learn is determined in large part by the rules of the implicit learning game and the teacher's leadership style. Both rules and leadership styles can be modified easily, although these methods of changing the processes of learning generally are not used. One of the first errors made by teachers who decide to increase the number of alternative learning processes is to decrease the number of rules and amount of teacher leadership, because this seems to decrease authoritarianism while increasing the possibility of many types of student initiative and learning styles. The key to a systematic variation in learning processes, however, is not how many rules and directions, but *what kind.* For example, such highly rule-governed activities as baseball and square dancing are non-authoritarian, and stimulate specific human processes. A variety of desired learning processes can be aroused by changing the rules which govern the nature of the scoring system, the type of obstacles to success and how decisions about strategy and tactics are made.* Implementing a variety of "learning games" requires of teachers great flexibility and repertoire of personal styles; they must have actualized many of the "divine and golden images" within themselves.

Just as it is unethical to develop inner strengths in students and put them into classrooms with a narrow range of legitimate learning styles, so too is it unethical to expect this flexibility within teachers or among a school faculty in a school that does not encourage, support and reward this variety. Ultimately, the administrative style, rules and rewards in a whole school must implement a pluralistic philosophy of education. The task of humanizing schools is, of necessity, multi-leveled and holistic.

The technology of planned change in schools is just now emerging. As recently as 1965 there was only one book devoted exclusively to the problem. Since then, the Office of Education and the National Training Laboratories have sponsored a large-scale investigation of how to increase innovation in teaching, learning and human relations at all levels in school systems—The Cooperative Project for Educational Development (COPED). The results of COPED suggest a four-phased strategy for maximizing the likelihood of effectively introducing Humanistic Education in a school.†

1. *Selection*

The top administrator and other key decision makers should be committed in principle to innovation in advance of specific training programs. Representatives from all groups within the school should be eligible for the special training programs.

2. *Diagnosis*

Organizational strengths and weaknesses need to be assessed. This can be done most effectively through interviews with potential participants prior to the major change efforts. Information is obtained on such factors as the reward system, rules, communication patterns, current school issues and individual goals. Often it helps if these data are shared with the school system in a "diagnostic workshop." The purpose of this collaborative meeting is to further clarify the problem and place priorities on the goals of change.

3. *Introductory Training*

A training program is designed to meet the defined needs. This workshop introduces the members of the school to relevant aspects of Humanistic Education. The workshop follows the six-step sequence described earlier.

*For a complete explication of this position see "The Effects of Classroom Structure on Motivation and Performance," A. S. Alschuler, *Educational Technology*, August, 1969, and "Motivation in the Classroom," Chapter 3 in *Teaching Achievement Motivation*, A. Alschuler, D. Tabor, J. McIntyre, Education Ventures, Inc., Middletown, Connecticut, 1970.

†Based on a private conversation with Dr. Dale G. Lake, Director of COPED and editor of the *COPED, Final Report*, April, 1970, ERIC Files, U.S. Office of Education, Division of Research.

During the final phase, the school is encouraged to select an ongoing "change management team" with representatives from all groups in the school.

4. *Follow Through*

After the initial training the aim is to build into the school system a permanent team of self-sufficient change management experts and well-trained Humanistic Educators. The "change management team" coordinates this development, and conscientiously supports the introduction of Humanistic Education. These changes can be accomplished through internal task forces, additional specialized training or a variety of organizational development services from outside consultants. To start the "follow through," the team is encouraged to implement a high visibility project likely to succeed.

This strategy for change differs markedly from traditional approaches through graduate school teacher education and curriculum reform. It more closely resembles the creation of a Research and Development group within a corporation. This comparison highlights the fact that businesses often spend as much as 10–15% of their budget on R & D activities whereas the typical corresponding allocation by schools is less than 1%. The absence of this strong coordinating group in schools vitiates the effectiveness of "new curricula" and restricts the influence of well-trained new teachers. The creation of an effective change management team coordinates and internalizes curriculum innovation within the school.

Although the existence of this coordinating group does facilitate changes in the character of schooling, it does not guarantee perfect guidance towards ultimate human goals. For instance, some teachers make humanistic methods ends in themselves. The use of game simulations and role playing, ipso facto, is considered good. Creativity training courses are endorsed whether or not the problems to be solved are meaningful. Courses in Theater Improvisation are introduced to develop non-verbal behavior independent of significant personal relationships and goals. As a result, these courses and methods often fail precisely in what they are trying to accomplish. Strengthening imagination simply becomes bizarre fantasizing; a narrow focus on feelings leads to misunderstanding; exclusive attention to non-verbal communication stimulates anti-intellectual distrust of rational, goal-directed behavior.

Major advances in Humanistic Education are not likely to come simply from the proliferation of methods, training, teacher-curriculum-developers or the creation of self renewing schools, although each of these tasks are worthy. We need guiding visions of the "good and honorable man" and utopian models for the places where we live. Human abilities are strengthened, integrated, balanced and given meaning only in the pursuit of these goals. The essentially heuristic value of these unattainable ideals is conveyed in the word "Utopia," a pun made by Thomas More on "Eutopia" (good place) and "Outopia" (no place). In the last century, over 200 utopian communities were started—and none has survived. The longest-lived utopian communities are those which face the question of life and death daily (kibbutzem, Synanon) or which surround a single charismatic leader (Ashrams with their gurus) or those which share an ultimate faith (Amish, Oneida). In the United States, most of us no longer face daily life-death issues. We are surrounded by anti-heroes, who command our sympathy by their stand against those public figures who would be our gurus. Ultimate faith is being replaced by immediate action concerns against visible injustice and for personal pleasure. This is reflected in our schools, where pluralistic demands for innovation often mask the loss of an ultimate sense of mission.

The consequences of this value crisis are to leave key ethical questions unanswered for all types of education: What kind of teaching and subject matter is in the best interests of students? Who is to decide? How? How do you know when a teacher is competent? How do you know when teaching is effective, ineffective or negative? Choices about what new curricula to develop, how to train teachers, what kinds of learning outcomes to assess and how best to humanize schooling depend on answers to these ethical questions. Obviously, there is no single set of definitive conclusions; but, instead, there is the opportunity for all educators to engage in a uniquely human search for values. The continuing attempt to discover "divine and golden images" and to draw forth the "good and honorable man" is the mission of Humanistic Education.

EPILOGUE
THE GOLDEN HELPING RULE

Whenever you feel unable to respond to a client;
Whenever you do not know what to say;
Whenever you want to help but do not know
    what would be helpful . . . .

Place yourself in the client's world;
Be in that time and space;
Ask yourself the questions asked you;
Feel what you think the client feels . . . .

Then say what you would like to hear;
Do what you would like to have done.

Elaine Lynne La Monica

HUMANISTIC EXERCISES

PART V
NURSING: A HELPING PROFESSION*

EXERCISE 1
Getting Acquainted and Ice-Breaking
EXERCISE 2
Getting Acquainted and Ice-Breaking
EXERCISE 3
Thoughts and Feelings
EXERCISE 4
Thoughts and Feelings
EXERCISE 5
Philosophy and Values
EXERCISE 6
Philosophy and Values
EXERCISE 7
Desires and Goals
EXERCISE 8
Behaviors
EXERCISE 9
Behaviors
EXERCISE 10
Experiences
EXERCISE 11
Experiences
EXERCISE 12
Body Expression
EXERCISE 13
Body Expression
EXERCISE 14
Self: My Nursing Shield

*Jointly created and designed by Eunice M. Parisi and Elaine L. La Monica.

EXERCISE 1
Getting Acquainted and Ice-Breaking

PURPOSES
1. To introduce the participants to each other.
2. To begin formation of the group.
3. To establish an atmosphere conducive to humanistic learning.

FACILITY
Large room.

MATERIALS
None.

TIME REQUIRED
One hour.

GROUP SIZE
Unlimited groups of two.

DESIGN
1. Pair group members, including self.
2. Request that each pair share information about themselves with their partner—thoughts, experiences, backgrounds, goals and hobbies, etc. (20 minutes).
3. Form large group.
4. Ask each member of the pair to introduce each other to the rest of the class.
5. Provide an overview of the course to the entire class.

VARIATIONS
1. Have members wear name tags on which they have only drawn a picture. Instruct them to mill around and find a partner. Then proceed with design.
2. Use adjectives in the above variation instead of a picture.

EXERCISE 2
Getting Acquainted and Ice-Breaking

PURPOSES
1. To facilitate development of positive group member relationships.
2. To create an atmosphere of openness and sharing.
3. To encourage self-expression.

FACILITY
Large room to accommodate class size and extra space for working.
(tables or carpeted floor)

MATERIALS

Construction paper	Scissors
Magazines	Paste
Crayons	Assorted media

TIME REQUIRED
One hour.

GROUP SIZE
Unlimited groups of six.

DESIGN
1. Using the materials provided, ask each individual to develop a collage that represents a self portrait (20 minutes).
2. In groups of six, have everyone share their collages, telling what each item means, how their feelings are represented in the design, their beliefs, etc. (20 minutes).
3. Discuss the experience in the total group.

VARIATIONS
1. This exercise can be done with any media available or just crayons and paper.
2. A second collage can be done on a self portrait as a nurse, comparing the two in a group discussion.

EXERCISE 3
Thoughts and Feelings

PURPOSES
1. To identify feelings aroused in the course of one's work.
2. To form a composite of feelings which gives an indication of the emotional climate and attitudes one faces in the nursing profession.

FACILITY
A room large enough for groups of five to talk without disturbing each other.

MATERIALS
Crayons—assorted colors for each participant
Paper—36" x 24"

TIME REQUIRED
45 minutes.

GROUP SIZE
Unlimited groups of five—preferably at least ten total participants.

DESIGN

CONCEPT LIST

helping	life	client
death	doctor	hospital
baccalaureate degree	nursing history	NLN
professionalism	dedication	ANA
nurse	associate degree	education
uniform	community	discharge
Florence Nightingale	sacrifice	client

1. Each participant has assorted colored crayons and papers. Participants are told that the purpose of the exercise is to identify the feelings that are constantly flowing within them at work.
2. Twelve (or more) concepts are going to be given slowly, with a pause between each word. The participant is to identify the major feeling the person has when thinking of that word. Then the person is to choose a color and draw with it.
3. Upon completion, the participants are given some time to reflect upon their product, its major characteristics, meaning, and use of colors.
4. Request that individuals share their collages in five-person groups.

5. Have each person speak out to the large group the one or two words which best represent their emotional state while they are at work in a clinical agency.
6. Discuss the experience.

VARIATIONS

1. Mill around, holding collage in view. Find one or two others whose collages strike you in a particular way. Discuss your collages together.
2. Mill around, holding collages in view. Find the one or two persons whose collages are most dissimilar to yours. Share the differences and their meaning.

EXERCISE 4
Thoughts and Feelings

PURPOSE   To identify the thoughts and feelings generated by particular nursing situations.

FACILITY   A room large enough for groups of five to converse without disturbing others or being disturbed.

MATERIALS   Paper, pencils, or pens.

TIME REQUIRED   45 minutes +.

GROUP SIZE   Unlimited groups of five.

STORIES   1. It is 8 p.m. in the Emergency Room. The telephone call a few minutes ago said the ambulance is on its way. There has been an automobile accident: One dead and two injured. The ambulance arrives. I meet it at the door. I feel _____

_____

_____ .

I think _____

_____

_____ .

I do _____

_____

_____ .

2. I have been working in Room 310 for three hours with no break. The light in 311 goes on. I walk in _____

_____ .

3. Ms. R., age 25, is scheduled to leave at 11 a.m. today. She has recovered from a panhysterectomy. It is my task to discharge her. I enter the room _____

_____ .

4. It is noon. All clients are having lunch. I am waiting to go to the cafeteria. The loud speaker comes on— "Code Blue, cardiac intensive care." I feel _____

_____

_____ .

I think _____

_____

_____ .

I do _____
_____
_____ .

DESIGN

1. The participants are informed of the goal of the exercise and are instructed as to the nature of the experience. They are told to complete a story using the first person—I—approach. Focus should be on what they think, feel, and would do in response to the situation. This assists in realizing the differences and interrelatedness of the three experiences.
2. Read one or two situations to the participants, allowing them ten minutes to finish a story.
3. Divide into groups of five to share the stories with all the drama they desire.
4. After sharing, have them discuss in small groups the similarities and differences in thoughts and feelings among persons and how the feelings could affect their behavior during each situation.
5. The process can be repeated with each story if desired.
6. Discuss the experience.

VARIATIONS

1. The facilitator writes a nursing-focused story, leaving out all adjectives and descriptive words. These are to be filled in by the participants and discussed.
2. Within small groups, a couple of volunteers each write situations from their own experiences similar to the examples given. The other participants finish the stories as they would respond personally. These are then shared and compared with the writer's experience.
3. Give the participants all four situations, of which they are to choose one to finish. In the sharing, ask them to explain why they chose that particular one.

DISCUSSION

Thoughts and feelings may have an impact on how you behave, as well as your relationship to self, other staff members, and clients.

EXERCISE 5
Philosophy and Values

PURPOSES

1. To identify what nursing means to each participant.
2. To identify any generalization among nurses as to what values underlie the profession.

FACILITY

Rooms large enough for groups of five to converse undisturbed.

MATERIALS

None.

TIME REQUIRED

One hour.

GROUP SIZE

Unlimited groups of five. A minimum of ten is preferable for the entire group.

DESIGN

1. Each participant is to lie on the floor and relax, breathing deeply.
2. The facilitator asks the participants to think back to when they first felt like nurses.
   a. When was it?
   b. What did it feel like?
   c. What did it mean to feel like a nurse?
   Time should be provided to have participants be able to appreciate the experience fully.
3. After individually responding to the above questions, groups of five or the total group should form to devise a consensual list as to what the underlying values are.
4. Participants should compare their own lists to the consensual one and think about some of the following questions.
   a. How similar or different is it?
   b. Does this say anything about me? If so, what does it say?
   c. When is the last time I felt like a nurse?
   d. Do I feel like a nurse all the time? When do I and when don't I?
   e. Do we as a group have a value system or philosophy of nursing? Does it match what is written in nursing history and literature?

Ask whether or not the feelings of being a nurse have changed since the first time they thought of themselves as nurses. Have the participants trace the development of these feelings.

DISCUSSION   What happens if we as nurses do not experience what we value? What kind of an effect is there on us? How much room is there for diverse value systems? What are the parameters? Discuss the importance of philosophy and values as a framework and pathway in nursing. It is our philosophy and values that dictate **how we work and why,** if we work, why we work, and how comfortable and satisfied we are in our journey.

EXERCISE 6
Philosophy and Values

PURPOSES
1. To identify the values underlying self as a nurse.
2. To compare values and philosophies with other nurses.

FACILITY
A room large enough for groups of eight to converse without disturbance.

MATERIALS
Paper, pencils.

TIME REQUIRED
45 minutes.

GROUP SIZE
Unlimited groups of eight.

SENTENCE COMPLETIONS

1. I am a nurse because _____ .

2. As a nurse I should be _____ .

3. As a nurse I should not _____ .

4. The most important thing for me to remember as a nurse is _____ .

5. I am different from other nurses in that_____ .

6. The one thing all nurses have in common is _____ .

7. The thing I like most about nursing is _____ .

8. Some nurses make me angry because _____ _____ .

DESIGN
1. Give the instruction for participants to complete the above eight sentences. Read them to the group, allowing time for participants to respond thoughtfully.
2. Once completed, the participants should form groups of eight to discuss their responses and identify the similarities and differences between them. After discussion the group is then asked if they can make any generalized statements about nurses and themselves as nurses.
3. Discuss the experience.

VARIATIONS Choose one or two people whom you would expect to have answers very different from yours. Discuss responses, where they came from, and why you expected them to be different.

DISCUSSION Explore the effect of values on the everyday operation of nursing. Stress the importance of values as a personal framework within which a person functions and a generalized direction or path for the profession.
How do great similarities or great discrepancies in values among nurses affect the individual nurse or the "nursing profession"?

EXERCISE 7
Desires and Goals:
What I Want In Nursing

PURPOSES
1. To discuss the facets of nursing practice that prevent it from being personally fulfilling.
2. To begin to explore the areas of nursing practice that one may wish to change.

FACILITY
Large, comfortable room.

MATERIALS
Paper, pen or pencil.

TIME REQUIRED
One hour.

GROUP SIZE
Groups of six, maximum number of total group— eighteen.

SENTENCE COMPLETIONS

1. If there is one thing I would change about myself as a nurse, it would be _____ .

2. If there is one thing I would change about my profession, it would be _____ .

3. In five years I would like to be _____ .

4. Nursing is more than _____ ,

it is _____ .

5. An aspect of nursing that is missing for me is _____ .

6. In nursing school, the experience is/was _____ .

7. Now, nursing is _____ and I feel _____ about this.

DESIGN
1. Have participants complete the statements individually.
2. In groups of six, ask members to share their completions one by one. Advise them to react to each other's statements and note significant or dissimilar/similar thoughts. Look at how the thoughts evolved and why they are important.
3. Discuss small group activities.
4. Ask the small groups to come together and form a total group. Have each small group report their significant and similar feelings.
5. Discuss the similarities and differences among the group.
6. Request that individuals think about what they have learned from others in the experience.

VARIATIONS
Ask members of the group to add any sentence completions which seem appropriate.

DISCUSSION
To isolate problem areas, one has to discriminate perceived reality from the ideal. This exercise begins to uncover the discrepancy.

EXERCISE 8
Behaviors

PURPOSES

1. To find out how others perceive your behavior.
2. To learn possible alternative ways of behaving.

FACILITY

Room with ample size to sit in dyads without being cramped.

MATERIALS

None.

TIME REQUIRED

30 minutes.

GROUP SIZE

Unlimited dyads.

DESIGN

1. Explain the purpose of this exercise and the importance of feedback from someone who knows you.
2. The participants are asked to form dyads with the person who best knows them.
3. The first person describes to the other how he or she thinks he or she is generally viewed by others. Next the first person is asked to focus on his or her behavior in situations he or she has a problem handling; then in situations which he or she feels he or she handles well.
4. The partner confirms or denies these self-perceptions. The partner may share the effects of the other's behavior on self. Alternative suggestions for ways of behaving can then be developed by the first person and checked with the partner.
5. The roles are now reversed and the design repeated.
6. Discuss the experience.

VARIATIONS

1. Members may meet in larger groups to get a number of perceptions. This is a bit riskier but may give a more reliable picture to the person.
2. In dyads, each participant takes a few moments to think not only of self but of the partner. Then the person describes the situations that he or she feels the partner has the most trouble with and the situations that the partner handles well. The partner compares these perceptions with his or her own. These are shared and the discussion reversed.

DISCUSSION   Feedback can be a helping process. Without feedback from others on the effect of one's behavior, one's self-perception may not be accurate. One must work toward an accurate view of how one is affecting others to be successful in reaching one's own ends. In support of these statements people may be encouraged to discuss times when they have been misunderstood.

EXERCISE 9
Behaviors

PURPOSES
1. To receive feedback from others in the profession.
2. To learn some behavioral alternatives to situations.

FACILITY
A room large enough to allow for the milling around of participants. As little furniture as possible is ideal.

MATERIALS
Roles for various participants—if desired. Costumes may be devised.

TIME REQUIRED
1½ hours.

GROUP SIZE
Approximately twenty.

ROLE-PLAY SITUATIONS
1. A head nurse's or team conference meeting concerning a client or a particular problem.
   a. Ms. Rudcliff in Room 313 will not take her medicine and is very uncooperative.
   b. The team is in "bad" shape. No one helps each other; there is no direct hostility; it's just that no one seems to care. This attitude has had an effect on the client. The atmosphere is gloomy. Something has to be done.
2. The same person should star in all three following scenes to determine the behavioral differences between situations if they should occur:
   a. Two nurses talking about a client in the client's room.
   b. Two nurses talking about a client while standing in the hall.
   c. Two nurses talking about a client in the parking lot after work.
3. A nurse feeding four clients dinner.
   Client A—impatient, irritable.
   Client B—seems lonely, wants to talk.
   Client C—extremely concerned about her condition.
   Client D—apathetic, does not seem to care about anything, including dinner.
4. A student nurse with the instructor and a client. The student is being evaluated by the instructor.

DESIGN

1. A participant who wishes to receive feedback is selected to star in a role-play situation. The participant is asked to choose one of the four situations, either the one the person feels most identified with or the one the person feels most distant from. Two stars may be required.
2. The supporting cast (all group members) is given a minute to think about the roles they wish to play. They may portray any attitude or role they desire.
3. The supporting cast's job is to observe the behavior of the star(s) and provide feedback as to its effect both to the other role players and themselves in their role. If appropriate, more effective ways of behaving can be suggested.
4. The sequence is repeated with new actors or actresses or subsequent stories.
5. Discuss the experience.

VARIATIONS

1. Each participant dons a sign bearing key words that describe the person as a practicing nurse. Examples may be: operating room, ICU, staff nurse, supervisor, or student. These signs are to include the position and area of nursing they are identified with. The participants mill around and group with others bearing the same or similar sign. This group makes up a short role play typifying a situation in which they are likely to be involved. The audience observes, giving feedback to each role player on the effect of the person's behavior on other role players and on the person.
2. Suggestions to more effective ways of behaving may be offered. Feedback may be provided for all role players instead of just the star.

DISCUSSION

Emphasize the importance of knowing how you affect others on the job. Intent may not always match behavior. Stress also the value of developing a trusting support system where honest reactions are a norm.

EXERCISE 10
Experiences

To begin to get in touch with the experiences one has had that have affected the choice of nursing as a profession.

FACILITY Large room, preferably with a carpet. If room is not carpeted, participants can be asked to bring their own blankets.

MATERIALS None.

TIME REQUIRED 45 minutes to one hour.

GROUP SIZE Groups of three; maximum number in groups depends on size of the room.

DESIGN
1. Each participant is asked to lie down on the floor and take several slow, deep breaths.
2. Speaking quietly and slowly, tell participants to gradually turn off everything in their personal worlds and concentrate only on the air they are breathing, their moving bodies, and the floor on which they rest.
3. After a few minutes of quiet, ask the participants to look back into their history and ponder the following questions. State each in a slow, subdued voice, to maintain the mood of oneness with the time, place, and thoughtfulness. Allow time between questions.
4. Questions:
   a. Who was the most impressive nurse you remember in your life?
   b. How old were you when you first met this nurse?
   c. What was the nurse like physically?
   d. What was the nurse like as a person?
   e. What was there about the nurse that impressed you?
   f. Why was the nurse so important in your life?
5. After allowing about fifteen minutes of reminiscence, ask the members to get up and form triads. Instruct them to share their thoughts with the other two members of their groups. You may place these questions on a blackboard or piece of newsprint for easier recall.

6. Following sharing in triads, ask each group of three to identify any particularly significant or similarly shared experiences.
7. Move into large group to share and discuss significant or similar factors.
8. Discuss the experience.

DISCUSSION   It is important to become aware of the sets and expectations that nurses have had in their past experience to enable them to formulate their real goals and rationale in the present framework. The identification and modeling process is influential in our sociologic development.

EXERCISE 11
Experiences

PURPOSE   To look at past experiences that most affected one's
                 practice in nursing.

FACILITY   Large, comfortable room where people can sit in small
                 groups.

MATERIALS   Drawing paper or newsprint.
                 Crayons or felt-tipped pens.

TIME REQUIRED   One hour.

GROUP SIZE   Unlimited groups of six.

DESIGN   1. Having six participants sit in a circle, instruct them to
                    draw a picture of the most critical experience they
                    have had in their nursing practice.
                 2. When members are finished, have them share their
                    picture with others in their group. In sharing, have
                    them explain the incident and how they pictured it,
                    discuss why it was critical, and look at how it affects
                    them presently. Other members of the group may
                    react to the incidents.
                 3. Discuss the experience in small groups.

DISCUSSION   Looking at important points in one's career is useful in
                 raising consciousness on who a nurse is in the here-and-
                 now. Discovering incidents that are critical in one's
                 experience may tend to formulate reasons for present
                 behavior.

EXERCISE 12
Body Expression

PURPOSE   To explore changes in body language when one plays a professional role.

FACILITY   Large room.

MATERIALS   None.

TIME REQUIRED   One hour.

GROUP SIZE   Unlimited groups of twelve.

DESIGN
1. In the middle of a large circle have participants individually or in pairs act out one of the following scenes:
   a. Strolling on the beach with someone of the opposite sex.
   b. Chatting in the hall with a friend.
   c. Introducing one good friend to another good friend.
   Then have them act out one of the next scenes:
   d. A nurse in a client's room when the client is of the opposite sex.
   e. A nurse speaking with the head nurse.
   f. A nurse on a break in the lounge.
2. Ask the observers to give feedback to the role players. They should be concerned with the following:
   a. How did the role player use his/her body in the scenes? Were there any differences between the two scenes? What were they?
   b. What changes occurred in the physical being of the role player between scenes? In which did the person appear more comfortable?
3. Ask the role player to discuss feelings in the two scenes and respond to the feedback.
4. Discuss the experience.

DISCUSSION   When one gets into a role, one may change. The kind of change may be important to be aware of.

EXERCISE 13
Body Expression

PURPOSE

To develop an image of one's physical self-concept and how one relates through it in nursing practice.

FACILITY

Large comfortable room.

MATERIALS

Drawing paper or newsprint.
Crayons.

TIME REQUIRED

45 minutes to one hour.

GROUP SIZE

Unlimited groups of six.

DESIGN

1. Using paper and crayons, have individuals draw and color a uniform that they feel would best suit their body.
2. In groups of six, have them describe their uniform, the reason for the colors, and their bodies in it. Have them think about and share thoughts related to the following questions:
   a. How does it differ from the uniform I wear?
   b. Why is it me?
   c. What does my body feel like in it?
   d. Why does it most suit me?
   e. Why does it least suit me?
3. Discuss the experience.

VARIATIONS

1. Have people draw as described and then draw another picture of what they actually wear while practicing. Compare and share the pictures and what they feel like in each.
2. Ask members to draw the ideal nurse's uniform. Ask what it represents in terms of physical self-image. Share these sketches in small groups.

DISCUSSION

It is important to look at the feelings, values, and emphasis that one places on a uniform. Clothing is an extension of one's self-concept. Learning and awareness may be derived from exploring the similarities and/or differences between nursing and personal values.

EXERCISE 14
Self: My Nursing Shield

PURPOSES

1. To look at the thoughts, feelings, and experiences that developed one's desire to become a nurse.
2. To become aware of one's personal values or philosophy of nursing.
3. To explore one's desires and beliefs in ideal nursing practice.
4. To probe into the ways one actually practices while in a nursing position.

FACILITY

Large room, preferably with small tables.

MATERIALS

Construction paper.
Felt-tipped pens or crayons.

TIME REQUIRED

One hour.

GROUP SIZE

Groups of four, maximum twenty-four.

DESIGN

1. In groups of four, have participants draw a large shield on paper and divide it into six parts as shown.

NAME

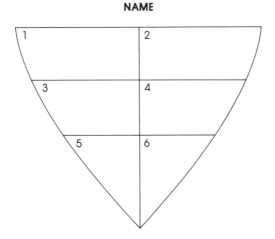

2. Have them place their names at the top of the shield. Explain that this is their personal nursing shield and symbolizes various aspects of themselves as nurses.

3. Request that the areas in the shield be numbered from one to six.
4. Ask participants to draw in the designated area pictures or symbols that answer the following six questions:
   a. What or who was significant to me in developing a desire to become a nurse?
   b. Describe the "best" nurse I knew.
   c. What do I believe the essence of nursing to be?
   d. What signifies my personal practice in nursing?
   e. How do I experience my body at work?
   f. In five years, if all were ideal, how would I be as a nurse?
5. After completing the shield, ask the groups of four to discuss their shields with each other. Suggest that they explore the symbols, reasons, thoughts, and feelings that went into each picture.
6. Discuss the experience.

VARIATIONS

The questions to be answered and pictured in the shield can be changed according to the needs of the group.

DISCUSSION

It is necessary for a person to explore globally the various feelings and experiences that formulated what the person is professionally today. From this point, the person can begin to conceptualize the ideal versus reality.

APPENDIX
Key to Abbreviations

AC	before meals
ANA	American Nurses' Association
B.I.D.	twice per day
B/P	blood pressure
BRP	bathroom privileges
BS	blood sugar
BUN	blood urea nitrogen
CBC	complete blood count
CCU	coronary care unit
c̄	with
c/o	complains of
ECG	electrocardiogram
FBS	fasting blood sugar
h	hour
HS	hour of sleep
ICU	intensive care unit
I & O	intake and output
IV	intravenous
lb	pound
L & W	living and well
mg	milligram
MI	myocardial infarction
min	minute
MS	morphine sulfate
NLN	National League of Nurses
O²	oxygen
OOB	out of bed
PC	after meals
PO	given orally

PRN	according to necessity
pt	patient
PVC	premature ventricular contraction
Q	every
QD	every day
Q 2h	every two hours
Q h	every hour
QHS	every night
QID	four times per day
S/A	sugar and acetone
SC	subcutaneously
S. Car.	South Carolina
STT	particular waves on an ECG
TBL	tablespoon
TPR	temperature, pulse, and respiration
U-100	units of insulin—100
VDRL	venereal disease research laboratory—test for syphilis

INDEX